Small Ruminants

Editors

MICHELLE ANNE KUTZLER
CINDY WOLF

VETERINARY CLINICS
OF NORTH AMERICA:
FOOD ANIMAL PRACTICE

www.vetfood.theclinics.com

Consulting Editor
ROBERT A. SMITH

March 2021 • Volume 37 • Number 1

ELSEVIER

1600 John F. Kennedy Boulevard • Suite 1800 • Philadelphia, Pennsylvania, 19103-2899

http://www.vetfood.theclinics.com

VETERINARY CLINICS OF NORTH AMERICA: FOOD ANIMAL PRACTICE Volume 37, Number 1
March 2021 ISSN 0749-0720, ISBN-13: 978-0-323-77546-5

Editor: Katerina Heidhausen
Developmental Editor: Nicole Congleton

Veterinary Clinics of North America: Food Animal Practice (ISSN 0749-0720) is published in March, July, and November by Elsevier Inc., 360 Park Avenue South, New York, NY 10010-1710. Subscription prices are $262.00 per year (domestic individuals), $628.00 per year (domestic institutions), $100.00 per year (domestic students/residents), $283.00 per year (Canadian individuals), $672.00 per year (Canadian institutions), $335.00 per year (international individuals), $672.00 per year (international institutions), $100.00 per year (Canadian students), and $165.00 (international students). To receive student/resident rate, orders must be accompanied by name of affiliated institution, date of term, and the signature of program/residency coordinator on institution letterhead. *Clinics* subscription prices. All prices are subject to change without notice. **POSTMASTER:** Send address changes to *Veterinary Clinics of North America: Food Animal Practice*, Elsevier Health Sciences Division, Subscription Customer Service, 3251 Riverport Lane, Maryland Heights, MO 63043. Customer Service (orders, claims, online, change of address): Elsevier Health Sciences Division, Subscription **Customer Service, 3251 Riverport Lane, Maryland Heights, MO 63043. Tel: 1-800-654-2452 (U.S. and Canada); 314-447-8871 (ouside U.S. and Canada). Fax: 314-447-8029. E-mail: journalscustomerservice-usa@elsevier.com (for print support); journalsonlinesupport-usa@elsevier.com (for online support).**

Reprints. For copies of 100 or more, of articles in this publication, please contact the Commercial Reprints Department, Elsevier Inc., 360 Park Avenue South, New York, NY 10010-1710. Tel.: 212-633-3874; Fax: 212-633-3820; E-mail: reprints@elsevier.com.

Veterinary Clinics of North America: Food Animal Practice is covered in *Current Contents/Agriculture, Biology and Environmental Sciences, MEDLINE/PubMed (Index Medicus), and Excerpta Medica.*

Contributors

CONSULTING EDITOR

ROBERT A. SMITH, DVM, MS
Diplomate, American Board of Veterinary Practitioners; Veterinary Research and
Consulting Services, LLC, Greeley, Colorado, USA; Veterinary Research and Consulting
Services, LLC, Stillwater, Oklahoma, USA

EDITORS

MICHELLE ANNE KUTZLER, MBA, DVM, PhD
Diplomate, American College of Theriogenologists; Associate Professor, Animal and
Rangeland Sciences, Oregon State University, Corvallis, Oregon, USA

CINDY WOLF, DVM
Associate Clinical Professor ad Honorem, Veterinary Population Medicine, College of
Veterinary Medicine, University of Minnesota, Saint Paul, Minnesota, USA

AUTHORS

DANELLE A. BICKETT-WEDDLE, DVM, MPH, PhD
Diplomate, American College of Veterinary Preventive Medicine; Associate Director,
Center for Food Security and Public Health, Iowa State University, Ames, Iowa, USA

N. ISAAC BOTT, DVM
Mountain West Animal Hospital Inc, Springville, Utah, USA

RENÉE D. DEWELL, DVM, MS
Lead Public Health Veterinarian, Center for Food Security and Public Health, Iowa State
University, Ames, Iowa, USA

TASMAN FLORA, BS
Department of Animal and Rangeland Sciences, Oregon State University, Corvallis,
Oregon, USA

HAYDER MOHAMMED HASSAN HABEEB, PhD
Department of Animal Production, College of Agriculture, Al-Qasim Green University,
Hella, Iraq

MEERA HELLER, DVM, PhD
Diplomate, American College of Veterinary Internal Medicine (Large Animal Internal
Medicine); Associate Professor, Department of Medicine and Epidemiology, University of
California, Davis School of Veterinary Medicine, Davis, California, USA

MELISSA N. HEMPSTEAD, PhD
Department of Veterinary Diagnostic and Production Animal Medicine, College of
Veterinary Medicine, Iowa State University, Ames, Iowa, USA

MICHELLE ING, DVM
Granite Bay Alpacas, Granite Bay, California, USA

JENNIFER JOHNS, DVM, PhD
Diplomate, American College of Veterinary Pathologists (Clinical Pathology); Assistant Professor, Department of Biomedical Sciences, Oregon State University Carlson College of Veterinary Medicine, Corvallis, Oregon, USA

MICHELLE ANNE KUTZLER, MBA, DVM, PhD
Diplomate, American College of Theriogenologists; Associate Professor, Animal and Rangeland Science, Oregon State University, Corvallis, Oregon, USA

TAYLOR M. LINDQUIST, BS
Department of Veterinary Diagnostic and Production Animal Medicine, College of Veterinary Medicine, Iowa State University, Ames, Iowa, USA

CHARLES E. McINTOSH, BS
Student Intern, Center for Food Security and Public Health, Iowa State University, Ames, Iowa, USA

ERICA McKENZIE, BSc, BVMS, PhD
Department of Clinical Sciences, Carlson College of Veterinary Medicine, Oregon State University, Corvallis, Oregon, USA

PAULA MENZIES, DVM, MPVM
Diplomate, European College of Small Ruminant Health Management; Professor Emerita, Department of Population Medicine, Ontario Veterinary College, University of Guelph, Guelph, Ontario Canada

PAUL PLUMMER, DVM, PhD
Diplomate, American College of Veterinary Internal Medicine (Large Animal Internal Medicine); Diplomate, European College of Small Ruminant Health Management; Professor, Department of Veterinary Diagnostic and Production Animal Medicine, College of Veterinary Medicine, Iowa State University, Ames, Iowa, USA

JENNIFER SCHLEINING, DVM, MS
Diplomate, American College of Veterinary Surgery - Large Animal; Clinical Associate Professor, College of Veterinary Medicine and Biomedical Sciences, Texas A&M University, College Station, Texas, USA

CLARE M. SCULLY, MA, DVM, MS
Diplomate, American College of Theriogenologists; Assistant Professor of Food Animal Health Maintenance, Department of Veterinary Clinical Sciences, Louisiana State University School of Veterinary Medicine, Baton Rouge, Louisiana, USA

JAN K. SHEARER, DVM, MS
Department of Veterinary Diagnostic and Production Animal Medicine, College of Veterinary Medicine, Iowa State University, Ames, Iowa, USA

CLIFFORD F. SHIPLEY, DVM
Diplomate, American College of Theriogenologists; Professor Emeritus, Department of Veterinary Clinical Medicine, College of Veterinary Medicine, University of Illinois, Urbana, Illinois, USA

MARY SMALLMAN, MS
Instructor, Department of Animal and Rangeland Sciences, Oregon State University, Corvallis, Oregon, USA

JOE S. SMITH, DVM, MPS, PhD
Diplomate, American College of Veterinary Internal Medicine (Large Animal Internal Medicine); Diplomate, American College of Veterinary Clinical Pharmacology; Assistant Professor, College of Veterinary Medicine, University of Tennessee, Knoxville, Tennessee, USA

JAMIE L. STEWART, DVM, PhD
Diplomate, American College of Theriogenologists; Assistant Professor in Production Management Medicine, Department of Large Animal Clinical Sciences, Virginia-Maryland College of Veterinary Medicine, Virginia Polytechnic Institute and State University, Blacksburg, Virginia, USA

SUSANNE M. STIEGER-VANEGAS, Dr med vet, PhD
Department of Clinical Sciences, Carlson College of Veterinary Medicine, Oregon State University, Corvallis, Oregon, USA

CINDY WOLF, DVM
Associate Clinical Professor ad Honorem, Veterinary Population Medicine, College of Veterinary Medicine, University of Minnesota, Saint Paul, Minnesota, USA

Contents

Ultrasonography can often achieve a diagnosis in small ruminants, with ease of use and virtually no contraindications. Radiography also provides a relatively comprehensive overview, but reduced penetration of the abdomen in larger animals and summation of abdominal organs can limit its diagnostic value. Computed tomography is a newer imaging modality that provides summation-free imaging but can have limited availability and financial restrictions.

sheep and goat milk production, to concentrate work and labor cost, and to plan for the lambing and kidding time. Breeders can also use estrus synchronization to stimulate ewes and does to exhibit estrus and ovulate outside of the breeding season, although both the ovulation rate and pregnancy rate may be decreased. To increase the ovulation rate outside of the breeding season, a variety of estrus synchronization methods have been used.

 Video content accompanies this article at http://www.vetfood. theclinics.com.

Hysteroscopy in alpacas and llamas allows for the identification of abnormalities on the surface or within the endometrium that cannot be identified with other methods. Hysteroscopy also allows for site-directed endometrial cytology, culture, and biopsy to achieve a definitive diagnosis. Even when no cause for infertility can be found, previously infertile females tend to become pregnant and maintain their pregnancies to term following the hysteroscopic procedure. This therapeutic effect may be a response to pre-hysteroscopy estrogen treatment, dilation of the uterine horns during hysteroscopy, and/or posttreatment uterine lavages. Complications following hysteroscopy have not been reported in camelids.

 Video content accompanies this article at http://www.vetequine. theclinics.com/.

Staphylococcus aureus is the most important cause of clinical mastitis in goats, and non-aureus staphylococci is the most common isolate from subclinical mastitis. Environmental streptococci are a severe problem. Somatic cell counts and California mastitis test are a screening test for mastitis and an indicator of poor udder health, but values should be interpreted differently than with dairy cattle. Somatic cell scores likely are a more useful way of viewing data. High bacterial counts in milk are common; mastitis may be involved as a cause. Proper udder preparation, milking procedure, and post-milking management are key factors in mastitis control.

 Video content accompanies this article at http://www.vetfood. theclinics.com.

Neonatal maladjustment syndrome is characterized by depressed consciousness, neurologic signs, and reduced or nonexistent suckle reflex. Resuscitation compression (squeezing) has been used in newborn foals and calves to reduce the behavioral symptoms of neonatal maladjustment syndrome. In this review, the authors describe how resuscitation compression can be used in newborn sheep. This technique can improve abnormal neonatal lamb behavior and encourage suckling in resistant lambs.

Anemia is a clinically important syndrome in small ruminants. Anemia can be divided into regenerative and nonregenerative forms. Differentials for regenerative anemia include hemorrhage owing to gastrointestinal or external parasitism or hemostatic disorders, and hemolysis owing to infectious, osmotic, toxic, and nutritional causes. Differentials for nonregenerative anemia include inflammatory and chronic diseases, renal failure, pancytopenia, copper deficiency, and heavy metal toxicosis. Iron deficiency anemia can be caused by chronic gastrointestinal and external hemorrhage or nutritional deficiency and may be mildly regenerative or nonregenerative. Appropriate diagnostic tests are described along with treatments, including blood transfusion, parasite control, and prevention.

Small ruminant lentiviruses (SLRVs) have been recognized throughout the world for decades. SLRVs are a heterogenous group of viruses that can infect sheep, goats, and wild ruminants. Evidence supports cross-species infection. These viruses cause lifelong infections where they target specific organs, which can result in production losses due to diminished milk production, consequential increases in neonatal death and diminished growth, and premature culling of prime age animals. No vaccine or treatments have proved effective. Control programs rely on an understanding of viral transmission and application of highly sensitive, specific, and frequent testing regimens.

Sheep operations will be subject to movement controls during a US foot and mouth disease outbreak and should be prepared to manage animal and product movement disruptions. The voluntary Secure Sheep and Wool Supply (SSWS) Plan for Continuity of Business provides tools for the sheep industry to develop contingency plans, write enhanced, operation-specific biosecurity plans, and learn about disease surveillance opportunities and challenges. The SSWS Plan is science-based and risk-based, funded by the American Sheep Industry Association, and developed collaboratively with industry, government officials, and veterinarians at Iowa State University. For more information, visit www.securesheepwool.org.

Video content accompanies this article at http://www.vetfood. theclinics.com.

There are hundreds of small reindeer operations scattered across the continental United States. These facilities house small groups of reindeer, typically between 2 and 30 animals. Small ruminant practitioners often are called on to help diagnose and treat a variety of conditions in these reindeer herds. This article discusses the restraint, anesthesia, reproductive management, common diseases, and problems that a veterinarian may encounter when providing care for Rangifer species.

VETERINARY CLINICS OF NORTH AMERICA: FOOD ANIMAL PRACTICE

FORTHCOMING ISSUES

July 2021
Ruminant Ophthalmology
Annette O'Connor, *Editor*

November 2021
Honey Bee Veterinary Medicine
Jeffrey R. Applegate, Jr. and Britteny Kyle,
Editors

RECENT ISSUES

November 2020
Toxicology
Steve Ensley and Timothy J. Evans, *Editors*

July 2020
Bovine Respiratory Disease
Amelia Woolums and Douglas L. Step,
Editors

SERIES OF RELATED INTEREST

Veterinary Clinics of North America: Equine Practice

THE CLINICS ARE NOW AVAILABLE ONLINE!
Access your subscription at:
www.theclinics.com

Preface

Small Ruminant Practice

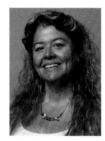 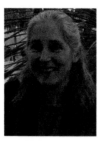

Michelle Anne Kutzler, MBA, DVM, PhD   Cindy Wolf, DVM

Editors

This issue of *Veterinary Clinics of North America: Food Animal Practice* is dedicated to small ruminant practice. Small ruminant practice remains a field rich in discovery through veterinary and biomedical research as well as through clinical practice. It has been over 15 years since the last issue of *Veterinary Clinics of North America: Food Animal Practice* focused on this subject area. Since then, there has been remarkable progress on the understanding of many physiologic and pathologic processes, leading to new and alternative therapies for many conditions.

This issue of *Veterinary Clinics of North America: Food Animal Practice* brings together a group of talented practicing veterinarians and academicians that have extensive clinical and research small ruminant experience. Each article is designed to contain relevant scientific information on the topic, while remaining practical and helpful. Our wide range of topics connects a diversity of small ruminant practice areas from hematology, urology, theriogenology, and imaging to pain management and animal welfare. It also includes an article on veterinary care for reindeer, a novel method to reduce lamb mortality, and much more.

We are grateful to the authors for their contributions. We are certain that readers will appreciate these diagnostic and treatment recommendations. Patients and clients alike will benefit from the presentation of new expertise. We hope that the Small

Vet Clin Food Anim 37 (2021) xiii–xiv
https://doi.org/10.1016/j.cvfa.2020.12.006
0749-0720/21/© 2020 Published by Elsevier Inc.

vetfood.theclinics.com

Ruminant Practice issue of *Veterinary Clinics of North America: Food Animal Practice* will serve as a useful resource for years to come.

Michelle Anne Kutzler, MBA, DVM, PhD
Animal and Rangeland Sciences
Oregon State University
112 Withycombe Hall
Corvallis, OR 97331, USA

Cindy Wolf, DVM
Veterinary Population Medicine
College of Veterinary Medicine
University of Minnesota
PO Box 422
Rushford, MN 55971, USA

E-mail addresses:
michelle.kutzler@oregonstate.edu (M.A. Kutzler)
wolfx006@umn.edu (C. Wolf)

Pain Management in Small Ruminants and Camelids

Analgesic Agents

Joe S. Smith, DVM, MPS, PhD[a],*, Jennifer Schleining, DVM, MS[b],
Paul Plummer, DVM, PhD[c]

KEYWORDS

- Alpaca • Analgesia • Goat • Llama • Pain • Sheep • Small ruminant

KEY POINTS

- Pain management of sheep, goats, llamas, and alpacas has historically been overlooked. Herein, we provide an evidence-based overview of the important aspect of pain control in these species.
- Economical options for pain management are available and efficacious.
- Multiple drug classes, such as nonsteroidal anti-inflammatories, opioids, local anesthetics, and GABA analogues can be applied in small ruminant practice.

INTRODUCTION

Similar to other animal species, small ruminants and camelids experience pain following noxious stimuli. The noxious stimuli may come in the form of a management procedure (eg, tail docking or castration) or may be the direct or indirect result of a naturally occurring physiologic abnormality (eg, urethral obstruction or surgery for orthopedic or obstetric condition). The most important aspect of pain management is the prompt identification of the painful activity, and the swift implementation of plans to manage the pain observed. In cases in which the pain results from a management procedure, it is preferable for the veterinary practitioner to anticipate the pain. This way the practitioner can develop and implement preemptive pain management strategies before conducting the procedure in accordance with appropriate animal welfare principles. The goal of this article was to review the current understanding of pain management in sheep, goats, and camelids. We first review the methods used

[a] College of Veterinary Medicine, University of Tennessee, 2407 River Drive, Knoxville, TN 37996-4500, USA; [b] College of Veterinary Medicine and Biomedical Sciences, Texas A&M University, 500 Raymond Stotzer Parkway, College Station, TX 77845, USA; [c] College of Veterinary Medicine, Iowa State University, 1809 South Riverside Drive, Ames, IA 50011, USA
* Corresponding author.
E-mail address: joesmith@utk.edu

Vet Clin Food Anim 37 (2021) 1–16
https://doi.org/10.1016/j.cvfa.2020.12.001
0749-0720/21/© 2020 Elsevier Inc. All rights reserved.
vetfood.theclinics.com

to evaluate pain in these species and outline management goals for pain control. A discussion of the predominant pharmacologic interventions follows.

REGULATORY CONCERNS

Currently in the United States and Canada, there are no drug formulations labeled for use in sheep, goats, llamas, or alpacas for the management or control of pain. As such, the use of all drugs for analgesia would be considered extra-label drug use and fall under the principles of the Animal Medical Drug Use Clarification Act (AMDUCA). When treating pain in food animals, practitioners should use the Food Animal Residue Avoidance Databank (FARAD; United States; www.farad.org) or the Canadian Global Food Animal Residue Avoidance Databank (Canada; www.cgfarad.usask.ca) for appropriate meat and milk withdrawal recommendations. Frequent submissions are encouraged, as the recommendations of FARAD are frequently updated with the results from emerging research.

GOALS OF ANALGESIC MANAGEMENT

For sheep, goats, llamas, and alpacas, pain management should be both clinically effective and economically feasible for the owner while adhering to the principles of appropriate meat and milk withdrawal recommendations. Because of the differences in physiology across ruminant species, cautious extrapolation should be used when comparing studies from large ruminants (eg, cattle) with small ruminants (eg, sheep, goats, llamas, alpacas). The best practices for pain management in these smaller species should rely on scientific evidence whenever possible. Pain management goals should be focused on preemptive analgesia when possible (ie, preoperative administration of anti-inflammatories and/or other pharmacologic agents), interventions that provide continuous analgesia, and strategies that minimize negative side effects. A current challenge in interpreting pharmacologic data is the lack of published therapeutic concentrations for most of the available medications for use in small ruminants and camelids. Many of the therapeutic concentration ranges are extrapolated from companion animals or humans and may not truly reflect the concentration of drug required for analgesia in small ruminant species.

RECOGNITION OF PAIN IN SMALL RUMINANT SPECIES

One of the challenges in pain management is the recognition of pain in certain small ruminants, especially sheep and camelids, that tend to be stoic and do not readily show overt signs of discomfort. As prey species, small ruminants often do not exhibit pronounced painful behavior, especially in the early stages of experiencing pain. Subtle deviations from normal in behavior, appetite, urination, or defecation can be used to determine if a patient is experiencing pain. The Guidelines for Recognition and Assessment of Animal Pain is published online by the Royal (Dick) School of Veterinary Studies, Edinburgh, Scotland, and can serve as a resource for pain recognition strategies in livestock.[1]

THERAPEUTIC OPTIONS

There are generally 3 primary classes of pharmacologic agents routinely used to control pain in small ruminants and camelids (**Table 1**). These classes are essentially the same as those used in other food-producing and fiber-producing species and have been reviewed previously.[2] One other significant difference between the broad classes of pharmacologic agents is that some of these agents are considered

Table 1
Analgesic dosing strategies for sheep, goats, and camelids

Drug	Mechanism of Action	Dose	Route	Frequency	Comments	Reference
Analgesic dose table for sheep						
Opioids						
Morphine	μ agonist	0.05–0.1 mg/kg	PO	q 4–6 h	Not recommended	George et al,[23] 2003
Fentanyl	μ agonist; κ antagonist	2.5 μg/kg/h	TD	Patch applied q 72–96 h	Careful preparation of patch application site	Burke et al,[24] 2017
			IV		Not recommended due to rapid clearance	Ahern et al,[25] 2010
Tramadol	Weak μ agonist; inhibitor of serotonin reuptake		PO		Not recommended	
Buprenorphine	Partial μ and κ agonist, δ antagonist	0.01 mg/kg	IV	q 6 h	Not superior to fentanyl patches for postoperative orthopedic pain; effective based on behavioral score post orthopedic procedure	Ahern et al,[26] 2009
Butorphanol	μ antagonist to partial agonist; κ agonist	0.2 mg/kg	IM	q 6 h		
Nalbuphine	Partial μ and κ agonist, δ antagonist	1 mg/kg	SC	Once	Peak analgesia at 30 min and started to decline at 120 min	O'Hair et al,[12] 1988
NSAIDs						
Phenylbutazone	Nonselective COX inhibitor		IV, SC, PO		Not recommended	

(continued on next page)

Table 1
(continued)

Drug	Mechanism of Action	Dose	Route	Frequency	Comments	Reference
Meloxicam	Slight to moderate COX-2 inhibitor	0.5 mg/kg	IV	q 12 h		Shukla et al,[27] 2007
		2.0 mg/kg	PO	Loading dose		Plummer & Schleining,[2] 2013
		1.0 mg/kg	PO	q 24 h following loading dose		Plummer & Schleining,[2] 2013
Flunixin Meglumine	Nonselective COX inhibitor	1.1 mg/kg	IV	q 12–24 h		Cheng et al,[28] 1998 and Welsh et al,[29] 1994
Carprofen	Slight to moderate COX inhibitor	4 mg/kg	IV	once, preoperatively		Otto et al,[30] 2004
Lidocaine	Local anesthetic: sodium channel inhibitor	40 mg	IA			Shafford et al,[31] 2004
		1 mL/50 kg	EP			Ivany and Muir,[32] 2004[a]
			IV	CRI		Raske et al,[33] 2010
Bupivacaine	Local anesthetic: sodium channel inhibitor	10 mg	IA			Shafford et al,[31] 2004
		1–2 mg/kg	SC			Hellyer et al, Lumb and Jones,[34] 2007
Ketamine	NMDA receptor antagonist	10 µg/kg/min	IV	CRI		Raske et al,[33] 2010
Analgesic dose table for goats						
Opioids						
Morphine	µ agonist	0.05–0.1 mg/kg	IV or SC	q 4–6 h		George et al,[23] 2003
			PO		Not recommended	
		0.1 mg/kg	EP			Hendrickson et al,[35] 1996

Drug	Mechanism	Dose	Route	Interval	Comments	Reference
Fentanyl	μ agonist; κ antagonist		TD		Not supported by EBM	Carroll et al,[36] 1999
			IV	Not recommended due to rapid clearance		Carroll et al,[36] 1999
Butorphanol	μ antagonist to partial agonist; κ agonist	0.1 mg/kg	IV	4–6 h	Altered behavior in less painful animals	Carroll et al,[37] 2001
		0.1 mg/kg	IM	4–6 h	Altered behavior in less painful animals	Carroll et al[37], 2001
Tramadol	Weak μ agonist; inhibitor of serotonin reuptake	2–4 mg/kg	IV	q 6 h		De Sousa et al[38], 2007
		2 mg/kg	PO		Not recommended	De Souza et al[38], 2007
NSAIDS						
Phenylbutazone	Nonselective COX inhibitor		IV, SC, PO		Not recommended	
Meloxicam	Slightly/moderately selective COX-2 inhibitor	0.5 mg/kg	IV	q 8 h		Shukla et al[27], 2007
		0.5 mg/kg	PO	q 24 h		Ingvast-Larsson et al[39], 2010
		0.5 mg/kg	IM	q 24 h		Ingvast-Larsson et al[39], 2010
Flunixin Meglumine	Nonselective COX inhibitor	1.1 mg/kg; 2.2 mg/kg	IV	q 12 h (1.1 mg/kg)		Smith et al[5], 2020; Reppert et al[40], 2019
		1.1 mg/kg	SC	q 12 h		Smith et al[5], 2020
		3.3 mg/kg	TD	once	Low bioavailability	Reppert et al[40], 2019

(continued on next page)

Table 1
(continued)

Drug	Mechanism of Action	Dose	Route	Frequency	Comments	Reference
Firocoxib	Highly Selective COX-2 Inhibitor	0.5 mg/kg	IV, PO	Once	High volume of distribution could lead to residue risk; currently no clinical studies	Stuart et al., 2019 (9)
Lidocaine	Local anesthetic: sodium channel blocker	1 mL/50 kg	EP			Ivany and Muir[32], 2004[a]
		1 mL/15 kg	EP			Van Metre[41], 2010[a]
		1–2 mg/kg	SC			Hellyer et al[34], Lumb and Jones 2007
		2.5 mg/kg	IV	Loading dose	Administer slowly	Doherty et al[42], 2007
		0.1 mg/kg/min	IV	CRI following loading dose		Doherty et al[42], 2007
Analgesic dose table for llamas and alpacas						
Opioids						
Morphine	μ agonist		PO		Not recommended	
		0.1 mg/kg	IV, IM	q 4 h		Abrahamsen[43], 2009[a]
Fentanyl (Llama)	μ agonist; κ antagonist	4–7.5-mg patches per adult llama	TD	Place new patch q 48 h		Grubb et al[44], 2005
Fentanyl (Alpaca)	μ agonist; κ antagonist	2 μg/kg/h	TD	Place new patch q 48–72 h		Lovasz et al[45], 2017
Butorphanol	μ antagonist to partial agonist; κ agonist	0.05–0.1 mg/kg	IV, IM	q 4–6 h		Abrahamsen et al,[43] 2009[a]. Carrol et al,[46] 2001

Drug	Mechanism	Dose	Route	Frequency	Notes	Reference
Tramadol (Llama)	Weak μ agonist; Inhibitor of serotonin reuptake	2.0 mg/kg	IV, IM	q 2–3 h		Cox et al,[47] 2011
Tramadol (Alpaca)	Weak μ agonist; Inhibitor of serotonin reuptake	3.4–4.4 mg/kg	IV	oral	Side effects; oral administration not recommended	Edmondson et al,[48] 2012
NSAIDs						
Phenylbutazone	Nonselective COX inhibitor		IV, SC, PO		Not recommended	
Meloxicam	Slightly/Moderately Selective COX-2 inhibitor	1.0 mg/kg	PO	q 3 d		Kreuder et al,[49] 2012
Flunixin Meglumine	Nonselective COX inhibitor	0.5 mg/kg	IV	once		Kreuder et al,[49] 2012
		1.1 mg/kg	IV	q 8 h		Plummer & Schleining,[2] 2013[a]
Flunixin Meglumine (Alpaca)	Nonselective COX inhibitor	3.3 mg/kg	TD	Not recommended	Transdermal formulation not recommended due to low bioavailability	Reppert et al,[40] 2019
CRI-trifusion						
Butorphanol	μ antagonist to partial agonist; κ agonist	0.05–0.1 mg/kg	IV or IM	Loading dose		Abrahamsen et al,[43] 2009[a]
		0.022 mg/kg/h	IV	CRI		Abrahamsen et al,[43] 2009[a]
Lidocaine	Local anesthetic: sodium channel blocker	1.0 mg/kg	IV	Loading dose	Administer slowly	Abrahamsen et al,[43] 2009[a]
		3.0 mg/kg/h	IV	CRI		Abrahamsen et al,[43] 2009[a]
Ketamine	NMDA receptor antagonist	0.6 mg/kg/h	IV	CRI	No loading dose needed	Abrahamsen et al,[43] 2009[a]

(continued on next page)

Table 1
(continued)

Drug	Mechanism of Action	Dose	Route	Frequency	Comments	Reference
Morphine	μ agonist	0.025 mg/kg/h	IV	CRI	No loading dose needed	Abrahamsen et al,[43] 2009[a]
Lidocaine	Local anesthetic: sodium channel blocker	1.0 mg/kg	IV	Loading dose	Administer slowly	Abrahamsen et al,[43] 2009[a]
		3.0 mg/kg/h	IV	CRI		Abrahamsen et al,[43] 2009[a]
Ketamine	NMDA receptor antagonist	0.6 mg/kg/h	IV	CRI	No loading dose needed	Abrahamsen et al,[43] 2009[a]
Lidocaine	Local anesthetic: sodium channel blocker	1 mL/50 lbs	EP		Using 2% lidocaine	Plummer & Schleining,[2] 2013[a]
Xylazine		0.1 mg/kg	EP			Plummer & Schleining,[2] 2013[a]

Abbreviations: COX, cyclooxygenase; CRI, continuous rate infusion; IM, intramuscular; IV, intravenous; NMDA, N-methyl-D-aspartate; NSAID, nonsteroidal anti-inflammatory drug; PO, per os; q, every; SC, subcutaneous; IA, intra-articular; EP, epidural; EBM, evidence-based medicine; TD, transdermal.
[a] Indicates published doses that are based on clinical experience.

"controlled drugs" that require Drug Enforcement Administration (DEA) registration and additional regulatory paperwork and drug security issues. This is especially true of the opioid class of compounds. Mobile veterinary practices should consult with their local veterinary medical association, the state board of pharmacy, and the DEA regional office regarding the appropriate storage and transportation of these compounds, as these regulations are frequently updated and can vary from state or province.

Nonsteroidal Anti-inflammatory Drugs

This class of compounds provides analgesia indirectly by decreasing the inflammatory response to tissue injury. Damage to tissue results in the production of inflammatory mediators (eg, kinins, prostaglandins) that activate primary afferent neurons and result in pain. By blocking the cyclooxygenase (COX) pathway, nonsteroidal anti-inflammatory drugs (NSAIDs) prevent the formation of prostaglandins and other signals.[3] As such, the analgesic potency of NSAIDs can be increased by preemptive administration before surgery or potentially painful management procedures. NSAIDs have several benefits when compared with other classes, such as opioids and α_2 adrenergic agonists. First, NSAIDs do not result in sedation of the patient, a side effect of the other 2 classes of drugs. Second, NSAIDs provide a longer duration of analgesia and a slower plasma half-life. NSAIDs are generally considered most effective against pain of low to moderate intensity and originating from the somatic or integumentary systems. The general side effects of this class of drugs includes gastrointestinal ulceration and nephropathy (especially in patients that are hypovolemic or dehydrated). Although NSAIDs may be helpful in the management of chronic pain, the clinician should consider these side effects in developing treatment plans and should monitor for complications when long-term therapy is necessary. In cases in which patients present with severe dehydration, fluid therapy to restore perfusion and glomerular filtration rate may be warranted before the initiation of NSAID therapy due to its propensity to cause renal insult.

Flunixin Meglumine

Flunixin is generally administered as a parenteral formulation to small ruminants and camelids. It is a nonselective COX inhibitor. Although oral formulations exist for horses, their pharmacokinetics and bioavailability in the rumen environment have not been determined. Furthermore, a study evaluating the pharmacokinetics of an orally administered granule form of flunixin meglumine in goats documented low bioavailability (58%).[4] Therefore, oral use of flunixin cannot currently be advocated. Traditionally, commercially available formulations of flunixin as a single drug (ie, not mixed with an antimicrobial) were labeled for use by the intravenous route in cattle. Intramuscular injection of these products can result in severe tissue damage, as well as prolonging the drug withdrawal time, and has the potential to result in an anaerobic environment that predisposes to clostridial myositis. Because of these potential complications, the Food and Drug Administration (FDA) has warned that they view the use of flunixin by a route of administration other than that labeled on the product as a violation of AMDUCA in cattle. Interestingly, a recent study that administered flunixin via the subcutaneous route in dairy goats did not identify any obvious tissue damage after single or multiple dosing.[5] Of the commonly used NSAIDs, flunixin is believed to have the most potent effects on relieving visceral pain. Although flunixin has a longer half-life than the opioid and α_2 adrenergic agonist, it does still generally need to be administered every 12 to 24 hours.

Meloxicam

In recent years, meloxicam has increased in popularity as an NSAID for small ruminant use. Meloxicam is a selective COX2 inhibitor that decreases the untoward side effects seen after administration of nonselective COX drugs. The product is available in the United States as a small animal injectable product, but in this preparation is cost prohibitive for use in large animals. Currently, the human generic oral formulation (7.5-mg or 15-mg tablets) of meloxicam is most widely used and validated in small ruminants and camelids. Comparative pharmacokinetics suggest that the oral formulation is highly bioavailable in sheep, goats, and camelids. Current cost for the generic tablets allows treating large animals very reasonably at less than $0.20 per 50 kg of body weight when dosed at 1 mg/kg. Although the tablets can be easily crushed and top dressed onto grain for cattle, small ruminants tend to be more selective in their eating habits such that the crushed tablets need to be mixed in molasses on grain or with water and drenched. Meloxicam also has the advantage of having a longer plasma half-life than that of flunixin or phenylbutazone and can be administered orally every 24 to 48 hours while maintaining plasma levels believed to provide sufficient analgesia.

Phenylbutazone

Phenylbutazone is a potent nonselective COX inhibitor NSAID that is typically believed to provide good musculoskeletal pain control. It is available as both an oral and injectable product in the United States, with the oral product historically being most commonly used in small ruminants and camelids.[2] The injectable product shares the side effects of tissue necrosis with flunixin and should be administered only intravenously. Intramuscular administration of phenylbutazone will result in a significant local muscle necrosis,[6] meat carcass defects, and may predispose to clostridial myositis. Because of reports of an idiosyncratic serum-sickness–type hypersensitivity reaction in humans consuming milk contaminated with phenylbutazone, the use of this drug is prohibited in all female dairy cattle older than 20 months. Although not specified by the FDA, the use of this drug in commercial dairy goats or dairy sheep should be avoided. In addition, with the advantages of newer NSAIDs (eg, meloxicam), phenylbutazone has fallen out of favor as an analgesic drug for small ruminants.

Carprofen and Firocoxib

Carprofen and firocoxib are selective COX-2 inhibitors. Carprofen has been used in small animal and equine practice for the treatment of orthopedic pain, particularly osteoarthritis. More recently, carprofen has been used for controlling pain in lambs after mulesing, as well as part of a postoperative analgesia in goats undergoing claw amputation.[7,8] A recent study of firocoxib has identified a prolonged half-life and good absorption in goats.[9] However, use of firocoxib is challenging at this time because of the lack of tissue residue studies to guide determination of milk and meat withdrawal times.

Aspirin

Although aspirin (acetylsalicylic acid) has been on the market for a considerable time, it is not widely used in small ruminants or camelids. Well-designed studies of aspirin in cattle have failed to demonstrate significant benefits to its use. Despite a high bioavailability in sheep, goats, and camels,[10] no studies exist to support its use for analgesia in these species.

Opioids

The opioid class of compounds is a broad group of drugs that bind to opioid receptors in the nervous system. These drugs are subclassified by their action as agonist, agonist-antagonist, or antagonist of one of several opioid receptors. Common opioid receptors include mu (μ), delta (δ), and kappa (κ). Mu receptor actions typically result in analgesia and sedation, whereas kappa receptor activation can lead to central analgesia. Like the α_2-adrenergic agonist, stimulation of the opioid receptors results in stimulation of the G-coupled protein pathways and the ultimate hyperpolarization of postsynaptic neurons. These compounds are generally believed to provide potent visceral analgesia.

Most opioids are considered controlled substances and are regulated by the DEA (United States). They require special licenses and additional records to possess, order and prescribe and need to be stored in an approved manner (eg, double-locked box with an inventory record).

As a general class of drugs, opioids have the potential to induce some degree of sedation, respiratory depression, decreased gastrointestinal motility, and decreased appetite. In some cases, they can induce a hyperexcitable state that will mask their sedative properties.[11] They do have potent analgesic activity that can vary with some degree in potency between the specific compounds.

Morphine

Morphine is the prototypical opioid agonist. It is generally administered as an injectable product by the intravenous, intramuscular, or epidural routes. It has a relatively short plasma half-life and must be re-administered frequently. In the United States, morphine is a scheduled drug and requires proper DEA licensing and recordkeeping. In comparison with some of the other opioid products, morphine is generally less expensive, but its analgesic potency is also less than many of the other opioids. The analgesic potency of morphine is similar to that of the α_2-adrenergic agonist.

Butorphanol

Butorphanol is a synthetic opioid with both agonist and antagonist properties. In comparison with morphine, butorphanol is 3 to 5 times more potent in its analgesic effects.[11] Butorphanol also has a less negative effect on the respiratory system in comparison to morphine, but costs considerably more at the present time. In recent years, increased use of a combination of butorphanol, xylazine, and ketamine for restraint in small ruminants and camelids has demonstrated potent analgesic effects. Butorphanol is a scheduled narcotic and requires DEA licensure and appropriate recordkeeping.

Nalbuphine

Nalbuphine is a lesser known opioid agonist/antagonist that was originally a schedule CII drug, but was removed from DEA schedule in most (but not all) states. This would allow for the use of nalbuphine without DEA licensure in the states where it is not a scheduled substance. Comparable to butorphanol in its analgesic efficacy, nalbuphine is typically much cheaper than butorphanol. It is supplied as an injectable product and can be substituted for butorphanol in many applications. There have been few published studies demonstrating its use in small ruminants or camelids for analgesia. In sheep, subcutaneous administration of nalbuphine (1 mg/kg) resulted in analgesia within 15 to 30 minutes.[12] Clinical experience of the authors suggests nalbuphine performs equally well to butorphanol in these species.

Fentanyl

Fentanyl is a potent opioid analgesic that is available as both an injectable and transdermal formulation. Because of cost, as well as the human abuse potential, the injectable formulation is rarely used in small ruminants or camelids. However, the transdermal formulation can provide for moderately long potent analgesia. The transdermal patch can be applied to a hairless area of the skin in a portion of the body where the animal is not likely to consume the patch. The patch can provide stable plasma concentrations for 2 to 3 days.[13]

Alpha₂-Adrenergic Agonists

Alpha₂-adrenergic agonists are routinely used on small ruminants and camelids for both their sedative and analgesic properties. Examples of these drugs include xylazine, detomidine, and medetomidine. The analgesic potency of these compounds is generally considered to be similar to that of the opioids, given that they use the same effector mechanisms and are located on many of the same neurons of the brain as the mu-opioid receptor.[14] On binding to the α_2-adrenergic receptor in neurons of the brain, α_2-adrenergic agonists induce signaling of the membrane-associated G-coupled proteins that results in activation of potassium channels in the postsynaptic neuron. This process allows an influx of potassium into the cell, resulting in hyperpolarization making them unresponsive to stimulation.[14]

Ruminants and camelids are generally more sensitive to α_2-adrenergic agonists than other species like horses and small animals. Hence, appropriate dosing is of importance when dosing. For this reason, large animal preparations of xylazine (ie, 100 mg/mL xylazine) may not be appropriate for use in animals with a small body size. Many practitioners use a lower concentration formulation of xylazine (20 mg/mL) and may even dilute it further with sterile water as needed to a 1 to 2 mg/mL concentration when appropriate for the size of the animal being dosed. Similar dilution of other α_2-adrenergic agonists may be necessary. These drugs are eliminated from the plasma rapidly and have short elimination half-lives. For this reason, use of these drugs in an intramuscular or epidural manner may prolong the period of analgesia over that of intravenous dosing, albeit slower in onset than intravenous.[15]

Although there are limited data on the duration of analgesia, what data are available suggest that intramuscular dosing of xylazine provides approximately 60 minutes of analgesic efficacy with onset of action and the magnitude of effect being dose dependent.[16] Xylazine does cause cardiovascular depression with a dose-dependent decrease in heart rate and cardiac output.[15] In pregnant animals, xylazine will also decrease fetal heart rate and can induce uterine contractility. Xylazine has also been associated with decreased lung compliance, tachypnea, pulmonary edema, and hypoxia.[15] A transient hyperglycemia is often observed following use of xylazine in ruminants. This hyperglycemia will result in increased urine output and can induce a short-term diuresis. Although this side effect generally has minimal impact on the patient, it should be considered if the drug is being used to provide analgesia for a small ruminant that is experiencing an ongoing urethral obstruction.

The analgesic effect and side effects of detomidine and medetomidine are similar to those described for xylazine.[15] Because of their short duration of potent analgesia, detomidine and medetomidine are most helpful in the management of acute and surgical pain in small ruminants and camelids. In some cases of chronic severe pain, a loading dose followed by continuous rate infusions (CRIs) of these drugs is helpful; however, analgesia is typically accompanied with a dose-dependent sedation. Given that the analgesic and sedative properties are both dose-dependent, high-dose analgesia typically results in profound sedation. The use of the epidural route in administering these drugs may lessen the sedation compared with other routes.

One benefit to the use of α_2-adrenergic agonist class is that their effects (including their side effects) can be rapidly reversed with the use of α_2-adrenergic antagonists (eg, tolazoline and yohimbine). It is of paramount importance to realize that when these antagonists are used, the analgesic properties of the drug are also reversed, potentially leaving the patient painful if alternate means of analgesia are not instituted. For this reason, multimodal analgesia protocols are encouraged when feasible and appropriate.

Ketamine

In addition to its dissociative anesthetic effects, ketamine has potent analgesic effects at subanesthetic doses. Evidence suggests that the analgesia is more effective for somatic pain than for visceral pain.[17] Although it has a short plasma half-life, CRIs and epidural use of ketamine can be used in concert with other drugs to provide long-term analgesia when necessary. Ketamine does not depress the respiratory system and actually stimulates the cardiovascular system. It is a scheduled drug and consequently requires DEA licensure and appropriate paperwork.

Lidocaine

Lidocaine is a local anesthetic that blocks the depolarization of neurons and hence prevents the propagation of action potentials. It also has the potential to act as a systemic analgesic when administered as a continuous rate infusion.[11] Consequently, lidocaine is used in 2 specific modalities for pain control in small ruminants and camelids. Lidocaine is routinely used clinically to perform local nerve blocks and as a local anesthetic during management procedures required for production of these species. Second, lidocaine can be used as part of a multimodal analgesic protocol with either CRI or epidural administration. One downside to lidocaine injection for local anesthesia is that, in humans, it burns intensely at the site of injection due to the acidic pH of the commercial product. The burning sensation can be ameliorated by mixing 8.4% sodium bicarbonate with the lidocaine in a 1:10 dilution (ie, 1 mL of 8.4% sodium bicarb into 10 mL of lidocaine). Unfortunately, the lidocaine will not stay in solution long-term if the pH is neutralized, hence only the volume of lidocaine needed for a given procedure should be neutralized for immediate use. Addition of sodium bicarbonate to lidocaine has the added advantages of speeding the onset of action, prolonging and enhancing anesthesia and analgesia, while decreasing pain associated with administration of the block.[18–21]

GABA Analogues

Gabapentin is a GABA analogue that was initially developed to treat epilepsy in humans. Gabapentin is also effective as an analgesic for chronic or neuropathic pain and is used for this function in human medicine. Gabapentin binds to calcium voltage gated channels and inhibits neuroexcitation. Initial studies done in beef calves have demonstrated synergism between gabapentin and NSAIDs (meloxicam) in relieving pain-associated lameness.[22] The authors have used gabapentin several times for treating chronic lameness in sheep, goats, and llamas with apparent success; however, no formal clinical trials have been done at this time.

Through this review we have described multiple analgesic agents described for the use in sheep, goats, llamas, and alpacas. Pain management in small ruminants is affordable, with the cost of oral meloxicam less than $0.20 per 50 kg of body weight every 1 to 3 days depending on the target species. The goal of this article has been to provide an evidence-based, comprehensive, exploration of pain management drugs for sheep, goats, and camelids. Individualized pain management strategies can be necessary because of the differences among cases, species, and applications.

CLINICS CARE POINTS

- Anticipation of potentially painful procedures is critical for the mitigation of pain in small ruminants.
- NSAIDs are a potent, inexpensive, and easy to administer form of analgesia for sheep, goats, llamas, and alpacas.
- Care should be taken to obtain appropriate residue avoidance guidance for pain management in small ruminants, as almost all analgesic agents would be considered extra-label drug use.

REFERENCES

1. Kent JE, Molony V. Guidelines for the recognition and assessment of animal pain. Edinburgh (Scotland): Royal (Dick) School of Veterinary Studies; 2012. Available at: http://www.link.vet.ed.ac.uk/animalpain/Default.htm.
2. Plummer PJ, Schleining JA. Assessment and management of pain in small ruminants and camelids. Vet Clin North Am Food Anim Pract 2013;29(1):185–208.
3. Thurmon J, Tranquilli W, Benson GJ. Perioperative pain and distress. In: Thurmon J, Tranquilli W, Benson GJ, editors. Lumb and jone's veterinary anesthesia. 3rd edition. Philadelphia, PA: Williams and Wilkins; 1996.
4. Konigsson K, Torneke K, Engeland IV, et al. Pharmacokinetics and pharmacodynamic effects of flunixin after intravenous, intramuscular and oral administration to dairy goats. Acta Vet Scand 2003;44(3–4):153–9.
5. Smith JS, Marmulak TL, Angelos JA, et al. Pharmacokinetic parameters and estimated milk withdrawal intervals for domestic goats (Capra aegagrus hircus) after administration of single and multiple intravenous and subcutaneous doses of flunixin meglumine. Front Vet Sci 2020;7:213.
6. Ferre PJ, Laroute V, Braun JP, et al. Simultaneous and minimally invasive assessment of muscle tolerance and bioavailability of different volumes of an intramuscular formulation in the same animals. J Anim Sci 2006;84(5):1295–301.
7. Fekry U, Rizk A, Mosbah E, et al. Assessment of a multimodal analgesia protocol in goats undergoing claw amputation. Mansoura Vet Med J 2019;20(4):37–46.
8. Paull DR, Lee C, Colditz IG, et al. The effect of a topical anaesthetic formulation, systemic flunixin and carprofen, singly or in combination, on cortisol and behavioural responses of Merino lambs to mulesing. Aust Vet J 2007;85(3):98–106.
9. Stuart AK, KuKanich B, Caixeta LS, et al. Pharmacokinetics and bioavailability of oral firocoxib in adult, mixed-breed goats. J Vet Pharmacol Ther 2019;42(6):640–6.
10. Ali BH. Comparative pharmacokinetics of salicylate in camels, sheep and goats. Eur J Drug Metab Pharmacokinet 2003;28(2):125–8.
11. Galatos AD. Anesthesia and analgesia in sheep and goats. Vet Clin North Am Food Anim Pract 2011;27(1):47–59.
12. O'Hair KC, Dodd KT, Phillips YY, et al. Cardiopulmonary effects of nalbuphine hydrochloride and butorphanol tartrate in sheep. Lab Anim Sci 1988;38(1):58–61.

13. Ahern BJ, Soma LR, Rudy JA, et al. Pharmacokinetics of fentanyl administered transdermally and intravenously in sheep. Am J Vet Res 2010;71(10):1127–32.

14. Thurmon J, Tranquilli W, Benson GJ. Preanesthetics and anesthetic adjuncts.. In: Thurmon J, Tranquilli W, Benson GJ, editors. Lumb and jones' veterinary anesthesia. 3rd edition. Philadelphia, PA: Williams and Wilkins; 1996.

15. Kastner SB. A2-agonists in sheep: a review. Vet Anaesth Analg 2006;33(2):79–96.

16. Grant C, Upton RN, Kuchel TR. Efficacy of intra-muscular analgesics for acute pain in sheep. Aust Vet J 1996;73(4):129–32.

17. Lin HC. Dissociative anesthetics. In: Thurmon J, Tranquilli W, Benson GJ, editors. Lumb and jone's veterinary anesthesia. 3rd edition. Philadelphia, PA: Williams and Wilkens; 1996.

18. Curatolo M, Petersen-Felix S, Arendt-Nielsen L, et al. Adding sodium bicarbonate to lidocaine enhances the depth of epidural blockade. Anesth Analg 1998;86(2): 341–7.

19. Sinnott CJ, Garfield JM, Thalhammer JG, et al. Addition of sodium bicarbonate to lidocaine decreases the duration of peripheral nerve block in the rat. Anesthesiology 2000;93(4):1045–52.

20. Everest PH, Goossens H, Sibbons P, et al. Pathological changes in the rabbit ileal loop model caused by Campylobacter jejuni from human colitis. J Med Microbiol 1993;38(5):316–21.

21. McKay W, Morris R, Mushlin P. Sodium bicarbonate attenuates pain on skin infiltration with lidocaine, with or without epinephrine. Anesth Analg 1987;66(6): 572–4.

22. Coetzee JF, Mosher RA, Kohake LE, et al. Pharmacokinetics of oral gabapentin alone or co-administered with meloxicam in ruminant beef calves. Vet J 2011; 190(1):98–102.

23. George L. Pain control in food animals. In: Steffey E, editor. Recent advances in anesthetic management of large domestic animals. Ithaca (NY): International Veterinary Information Services; 2003.

24. Burke MJ, Soma LR, Boston RC, et al. Evaluation of the analgesic and pharmacokinetic properties of transdermally administered fentanyl in goats. J Vet Emerg Crit Care (San Antonio) 2017;27(5):539–47.

25. Ahern BJ, Soma LR, Rudy JA, et al. Pharmacokinetics of fentanyl administered transdermally and intravenously in sheep. Am J Vet Res 2010;71(10):1127–32.

26. Ahern BJ, Soma LR, Boston RC, et al. Comparison of the analgesic properties of transdermally administered fentanyl and intramuscularly administered buprenorphine during and following experimental orthopedic surgery in sheep. Am J Vet Res 2009;70(3):418–22.

27. Shukla M, Singh G, Sindhura B, et al. Comparative plasma pharmacokinetics of meloxicam in sheep and goats following intravenous administration. Comp Biochem Physiol C Toxicol Pharmacol 2007;145(4):528–32.

28. Cheng Z, McKeller Q, Nolan A. Pharmacokinetic studies of flunixin meglumine and phenylbutazone in plasma, exudate and transudate in sheep. J Vet Pharmacol Ther 1998;21(4):315–21.

29. Welsh EM, Nolan AM. Effects of non-steroidal anti-inflammatory drugs on the hyperalgesia to noxious mechanical stimulation induced by the application of a tourniquet to a forelimb of sheep. Res Vet Sci 1994;57(3):285–91.

30. Otto K, Adams HA. Experimental studies on the central analgesic effect of the non-steroidal anti-inflammatory drug carprofen in a sheep model – preliminary results. Anasthesiol Intensivmed Notfallmed Schmerzther 2005;40(1):25–31 [in German].

31. Shafford HL, Hellyer PW, Turner AS. Intra-articular lidocaine plus bupivacaine in sheep undergoing stifle arthrotomy. Vet Anaesth Analg 2004;31(1):20–6.
32. Ivany J, Muir W. Farm animal anesthesia. In: Fubini S, Ducharme N, editors. Farm animal surgery. St Louis (MO): Saunders; 2004. p. 102–3.
33. Raske TG, Pelkey S, Wagner AE, et al. Effect of intravenous ketamine and lidocaine on isoflurane requirement in sheep undergoing orthopedic surgery. Lab Anim (NY) 2010;39(3):76–9.
34. Hellyer P, Robertson S, Fails A. Lumb & Jones' veterinary anesthesia and analgesia. Ames (IA): Blackwell Publishing; 2007.
35. Hendrickson DA, Kruse-Elliott KT, Broadstone RV. A comparison of epidural saline, morphine, and bupivacaine for pain relief after abdominal surgery in goats. Vet Surg 1996;25(1):83–7.
36. Carroll GL, Hooper RN, Boothe DM, et al. Pharmacokinetics of fentanyl after intravenous and transdermal administration in goats. Am J Vet Res 1999;60(8):986–91.
37. Carroll GL, Boothe DM, Hartsfield SM, et al. Behavioral changes and pharmacokinetics of butorphanol in goats following intravenous and intramuscular administration. Vet Anaesth Analg 2001;28(2):102–3.
38. de Sousa AB, Santos AC, Schramm SG, et al. Pharmacokinetics of tramadol and o-desmethyltramadol in goats after intravenous and oral administration. J Vet Pharmacol Ther 2008;31(1):45–51.
39. Ingvast-Larsson C, Hogberg M, Mengistu U, et al. Pharmacokinetics of meloxicam in adult goats and its analgesic effect in disbudded kids. J Vet Pharmacol Ther 2011;34(1):64–9.
40. Reppert EJ, Kleinhenz MD, Montgomery SR, et al. Pharmacokinetics and pharmacodynamics of intravenous and transdermal flunixin meglumine in meat goats. J Vet Pharmacol Ther 2019.
41. Van Metre D, editor Small Ruminant Tips. 128th Annual Meeting of the Iowa Veterinary Medical Association; 2010. Ames, IA.
42. Doherty T, Redua MA, Queiroz-Castro P, et al. Effect of intravenous lidocaine and ketamine on the minimum alveolar concentration of isoflurane in goats. Vet Anaesth Analg 2007;34(2):125–31.
43. Abrahamsen EJ. Chemical restraint, anesthesia, and analgesia for camelids. Vet Clin North Am Food Anim Pract 2009;25(2):455–94.
44. Grubb TL, Gold JR, Schlipf JW, et al. Assessment of serum concentrations and sedative effects of fentanyl after transdermal administration at three dosages in healthy llamas. Am J Vet Res 2005;66(5):907–9.
45. Lovasz M, Aarnes TK, Hubbell JA, et al. Pharmacokinetics of intravenous and transdermal fentanyl in alpacas. J Vet Pharmacol Ther 2017;40(6):663–9.
46. Carroll GL, Boothe DM, Hartsfield SM, et al. Pharmacokinetics and pharmacodynamics of butorphanol in llamas after intravenous and intramuscular administration. J Am Vet Med Assoc 2001;219(9):1263–7.
47. Cox S, Martin-Jimenez T, van Amstel S, et al. Pharmacokinetics of intravenous and intramuscular tramadol in llamas. J Vet Pharmacol Ther 2011;34(3):259–64.
48. Edmondson MA, Duran SH, Boothe DM, et al. Pharmacokinetics of tramadol and its major metabolites in alpacas following intravenous and oral administration. J Vet Pharmacol Ther 2012;35(4):389–96.
49. Kreuder AJ, Coetzee JF, Wulf LW, et al. Bioavailability and pharmacokinetics of oral meloxicam in llamas. BMC Vet Res 2012;8(1):85.

Pain Management in Small Ruminants and Camelids

Applications and Strategies

Joe S. Smith, DVM, MPS, PhD[a],*, Jennifer Schleining, DVM, MS[b],
Paul Plummer, DVM, PhD[c]

KEYWORDS

- Alpaca • Analgesia • Epidural catheter • Goat • Llama • Pain
- Regional limb perfusion • Sheep

KEY POINTS

- Pain management of sheep, goats, llamas, and alpacas has historically been overlooked. Herein, we provide an evidence-based overview of the strategies of pain control in these species.
- Economical options for pain management are available and efficacious. These can be monotherapies as well as multimodal therapies.
- Regional analgesic techniques, such as epidural administration, and regional perfusions are reported for other species and can be used to augment pain management in small ruminants and camelids.
- Multiple husbandry and production practices, as well as postoperative case management can be improved with attention to pain management.

INTRODUCTION

Sheep, goats, and camelids experience pain following noxious stimuli that can come from a range of conditions ranging from trauma and disease to production management procedures. The methods to provide analgesia are as varied as the causes of pain themselves, ranging from oral administration to focused regional anesthesia, such as epidural administration. The goal of this article was to review the current understanding of pain management in sheep, goats, and camelids. Whereas the first article in this series focused on the agents used for pain management, this article reviews the strategies for implementation of pain management and routes of

[a] College of Veterinary Medicine, University of Tennessee, 2407 River Drive, Knoxville, TN 37996-4500, USA; [b] College of Veterinary Medicine & Biomedical Sciences, Texas A&M University, 500 Raymond Stotzer Parkway, College Station, TX 77845, USA; [c] College of Veterinary Medicine, Iowa State University, 1809 South Riverside Drive, Ames, IA 50011, USA
* Corresponding author.
E-mail address: joesmith@utk.edu

vetfood.theclinics.com

administration, including oral, intramuscular, intravenous, local versus regional, epidural, transdermal, and intra-articular.

ORAL STRATEGIES

Oral medication has the benefit of ease of administration, as most owners can administer an oral bolus, and most oral medications are relatively cost-effective. However, a disadvantage is that the rumen (or C1 in camelids) can inactivate certain medications, rendering them useless. This is an area in which the literature should be consulted for pharmacologic studies for small ruminant species.

Morphine

Oral administration of morphine is not recommended because of inactivation by the rumen. In a study conducted in sheep, only one-third of the animals achieved good analgesia following oral administration.[1] Given the high variability, it does not make a good option for consistent pain control.

Gabapentin

The use of gabapentin in small ruminants has not been described in the literature. Anecdotally, it appears to offer analgesia to ruminants experiencing neuropathic pain, and the pharmacokinetics have been described in beef and dairy cattle.[2,3] Oral gabapentin at a dosage of 5 mg/kg once daily has been used to manage recurrent neck and shoulder pain in a camel, which was unresponsive to previous administration of phenylbutazone and ketoprofen.[4] This case may support extrapolation to llamas and alpacas.

Nonsteroidal Anti-inflammatory Drugs

Meloxicam

The use of meloxicam as an analgesic is becoming more common. Its advantages include that it preferentially binds to the cyclooxygenase-2 isoenzyme, thereby decreasing the risk for harmful side effects common to nonpreferential nonsteroidal anti-inflammatory drugs (NSAIDs) and ease of administration. However, this has not been confirmed in small ruminants. Generic meloxicam is available in tablet form in 7.5-mg and 15-mg tablets and is extremely cost-effective. In llamas, oral dosing at 1.0 mg/kg maintains serum levels above 0.2 μg/mL for up to 72 hours with 76% bioavailability. This would suggest that oral dosing every 3 days would be appropriate for llamas.[5]

A study looking at the comparative pharmacokinetics of meloxicam between sheep and goats determined that meloxicam is metabolized at very different rates between the 2 species, with goats metabolizing the drug faster than sheep.[6] The elimination half-life in sheep was determined to be 10.9 hours, whereas in goats it was only 6.3 hours, but both species exhibited a similar small volume of distribution. The article extrapolated an effective concentration target of 0.73 μg/mL from prior equine results and concluded that meloxicam should be administered by the intravenous route every 12 hours in sheep and every 8 hours in goats to maintain levels considered to be analgesic. Following oral administration to goats, meloxicam was found to have high bioavailability (79%) and a half-life of nearly 11 hours. Based on these data, once-daily oral dosing at 0.5 mg/kg was recommended. In kids undergoing disbudding with cautery, there was a significant increase in comfort level in the first 24 hours following disbudding after receiving intramuscular injections of meloxicam (0.5 mg/kg) at the time of disbudding compared with the placebo group.[7] The oral bioavailability of meloxicam in sheep is 72%. Therefore, in sheep a reasonable loading dose of meloxicam is 2 mg/kg followed by oral daily administration at 1 mg/kg.[8] For extended dosing (beyond 5–7 days), the authors have used to 0.5 to 1 mg/kg every 48 hours with clinical success.

Carprofen, firocoxib

These selective NSAIDs have high oral bioavailability and are good candidates for oral administration. Oral administration of carprofen has been shown to have absorption to therapeutic concentrations within 2 hours in lambs that persist for at least 24 hours.[9]

Phenylbutazone

The use of phenylbutazone in food producing species is not recommended for reasons including human food safety as well as inducing blood dyscrasias. Because of these concerns, residues in meat and milk have zero tolerance, meaning that residue detection is likely to come with a severe penalty.

INJECTABLE STRATEGIES
Intramuscular

Butorphanol

Butorphanol as an intramuscular injection provides a more sustained, yet lower peak concentration of analgesia when compared with an intravenous bolus. However, when used concurrently with another form of analgesia (such as an NSAID), pain relief can be more efficacious than when butorphanol is used alone. In addition, the lower peak concentration reduces the risk of untoward side effects (ie, sedation).[10]

Flunixin meglumine

Although studies are available in sheep citing the use and efficacy of flunixin intramuscularly,[11,12] this would constitute an extra-label drug use as the label indicates the drug should be given intravenously. In addition, extensive muscle necrosis secondary to drug acidity and an extended withdrawal time would support use of this product in the route as labeled.

Tramadol

A pharmacokinetic study in llamas revealed that tramadol when given either intravenously (IV) or intramuscularly (IM) at 2.0 mg/kg produced therapeutic concentrations consistent with analgesia in humans.[13] However, the half-life when administered IV was only 2.1 hours and IM was only 2.5 hours. There is no known clinical data available regarding the use of tramadol in small ruminants.

Intravenous

Morphine

Although ineffective after oral administration, morphine is effective when administered parenterally. The dose range, however, varies greatly and superior analgesia may not be evident until a 10 mg/kg dose is achieved.[1]

Fentanyl

IV administered fentanyl is rapidly acting; however, it has a very short duration of activity (~20 minutes) and should be used as a constant rate infusion to maintain analgesic levels. In a recent pharmacokinetic study in sheep, the half-life of IV administered fentanyl was only 3 hours.[14] In goats, the half-life after an IV bolus of 2.5 µg/kg was only 1.2 hours.[15] Because of its repeat dosing requirement, cost, and serious diversion concerns, there is minimal clinical value of IV fentanyl at the current time.

Butorphanol

Butorphanol use is common in camelid practice as both a sedative and an analgesic. Butorphanol can be used as an IV bolus or as an IM injection. When used together with an NSAID, analgesia may be more pronounced than when used alone.[10]

Flunixin meglumine

Flunixin meglumine is labeled for the treatment of pyrexia associated with respiratory disease and mastitis as well as treatment of endotoxemia-induced inflammation in cattle. However, its use extends to small ruminants given the efficacy in cattle. A pharmacokinetic study in sheep showed a single IV dose of flunixin administered at 1.1 mg/kg had good distribution into areas of inflammation but had slow penetration and elimination from these areas.[16] In addition, IV flunixin administered at 1.0 mg/kg attenuated hyperalgesia in sheep following noxious stimulus in an in vivo pain model study.[17]

Continuous Rate Infusions

Continuous infusions for fentanyl, lidocaine, ketamine, morphine, and butorphanol have been previously reviewed.[18]

REGIONAL PAIN MANAGEMENT STRATEGIES
Epidural Administration

The epidural space can be accessed at the lumbosacral space (cranial or "high" epidural) or at the sacrococcygeal or first coccygeal space (caudal or "low" epidural) quite easily in most small ruminants, although sheep with docked tail can provide challenges to access. The application of epidural anesthetics is necessary in surgery of the caudal reproductive and gastrointestinal tracts (eg, cervical lacerations, rectal prolapse) and in cases of reproductive emergencies.[18] Analgesics can also be infused into the epidural space to alleviate pain in the hind limbs and caudal abdomen. For sheep with severely docked tails, a cranial epidural may be the only option for access to the epidural space in these animals (**Table 1**).

The lumbosacral space can be accessed by palpating the space caudal to the dorsal vertebral process of the sixth lumbar vertebrae between the wings of the ilium. Usually an 18-gauge or 20-gauge, 1.5-inch needle is sufficient. Llamas and animals with heavy body condition scores may require a 3.25-inch spinal needle for the lumbosacral space. The needle should be advanced on midline in a perpendicular manner until a "pop" is felt. Some animals may react when the epidural space is entered. A drop of lidocaine can be placed in the hub of the needle after the needle is through the skin ("hanging drop" technique). The lidocaine will be aspirated into the needle when the epidural space is entered because of the negative pressure within the epidural space. Injection into the epidural space should not have resistance. It should be noted that an epidural injection should be administered slowly over 60 to 90 seconds to prevent rapid cranial migration of the anesthetic or analgesic. It is also beneficial to keep the animal's head elevated during the injection.

The sacrococcygeal space can be accessed by "pumping" the tail up and down to identify the cranial-most moveable space. The needle is inserted at an approximately 45 angle relative to the spine. Like the lumbosacral space, using the "hanging drop" technique is helpful.

In small ruminants, the dose of lidocaine ranges between 1 mL per 15 to 50 kg of body weight[19,20] to achieve desensitization using either location. Although it is common practice to add xylazine to a lidocaine epidural in large ruminants to extend the duration of the epidural and as a method of sedation, caution should be used with

Table 1
Epidural dosing strategies for sheep, goats, and camelids

Agent	Mechanism	Dose	Note	Reference
Morphine (Preservative Free)	μ agonist	0.05–0.25 mg/kg	Mild analgesia alone; combined with bupivacaine can provide longer duration of analgesia than either agent alone. Intrathecal administration can result in respiratory depression. Note: Recommended to use preservative-free product, as regular product has been linked to pathology when administered epidural.	Sheep: Stillman et al,[55] 2019 Goats: Pablo,[23] 1993 Camelid: Martinez et al,[56] 2014
Lidocaine	Sodium channel blockade	1.2–4.8 mg/kg	Short duration of action.	Sheep: Stillman et al,[55] 2019 Goats: Dehkordi et al,[24] 2012 Camelid: Grubb et al,[27] 1993 Alpacas
Bupivacaine	Sodium channel blockade	0.5–1.2 mg/kg	Longer duration of action than lidocaine.	Sheep: Stillman et al,[55] 2019 Goats: Trim et al,[21] 1989
Xylazine	α₂ Agonist	0.05 mg/kg	Given in combination with lidocaine (4.8 mg/kg lidocaine). Caution as can be systemically absorbed.	Sheep: Stillman et al,[55] 2019

Data from Refs.[21,23,24,27,55,56]

this combination in goats, as they are especially sensitive to the effects of both xylazine and lidocaine.

Use of bupivacaine (1 mL per 4 kg of body weight) in lumbosacral epidurals in goats resulted in immediate recumbency after injection due to loss of hind limb coordination and 30% of the goats had negative central nervous system side effects following bupivacaine administration.[21] In addition, goats receiving bupivacaine lumbosacral epidurals were expectantly and unacceptably recumbent for significantly long periods of time due to the blockade of motor nerves.[22]

Morphine (0.1 mg/kg) in lumbosacral epidurals is a useful postoperative analgesic in goats that improves behavior scores and has relatively few side effects.[22,23] Clinicians should administer preservative-free formulations to prevent secondary damage to epidural structures.

In sheep and goats, the use of tramadol (1 mg/kg) with lidocaine (2.46 mg/kg) administered in the lumbosacral epidural space provided longer analgesia than lidocaine (2.86 mg/kg) alone. In addition, animals receiving lidocaine alone were severely ataxic whereas the tramadol/lidocaine combination resulted in moderate ataxia. The use of tramadol alone (1 mg/kg) resulted in a longer duration of effect but had a very slow onset of action. However, animals receiving tramadol alone were not ataxic.[24,25]

The use of lidocaine alone in the lumbosacral epidural space, intramuscular xylazine plus lidocaine in the sacrococcygeal space, or a combination of xylazine and lidocaine in the sacrococcygeal space failed to produce desensitization of the spermatic cord in alpacas undergoing castration even though cutaneous sensation was lost.[26] Similar results were observed in llamas that were administered a caudal epidural using xylazine alone (0.17 mg/kg), lidocaine alone (0.22 mg/kg), or a combination of xylazine (0.17 mg/kg) and lidocaine (0.22 mg/kg).[27] This suggests that direct infiltration of a local anesthetic is required for complete anesthesia of the testicles and spermatic cords in these species.

Epidural Catheterization

An extension of epidural anesthesia is the use of an epidural catheter for repeated drug administration. This technique is most used for analgesia of orthopedic procedures, such as pelvic limb fracture repair. Although case selection is important, epidural catheterization can provide ease of access for drug administration. Epidural catheterization should be used for *short-term* pain management, as administration can lead to inflammation. Epidural catheterization should also be limited to tractable animals that can be confined to a small space or pen in the hospital postprocedure for several days. Use of epidural catheters in nontractable animals could risk removal or damage of the catheter. A step-by-step approach for the placement of an epidural catheter in a goat before a pelvic limb fracture repair is provided in **Fig. 1**.

Regional Local Anesthesia

Benefits of local anesthesia include low cost, ease of use, and relatively low adverse effects. Local infiltration of lidocaine, bupivacaine, or mepivacaine preoperatively (ie, castration or tail docking) can improve postoperative comfort and behavior. For small ruminants, especially in the case of goats, *caution must be taken to not exceed a 10 mg/kg of lidocaine dose.* However, other anesthetics may be used if it is anticipated a longer duration of anesthesia is needed. In sheep paravertebral anesthesia, bupivacaine (45 mg) resulted in a significantly longer duration of action (303 minutes) compared with lidocaine (180 mg) alone (65 minutes).[28]

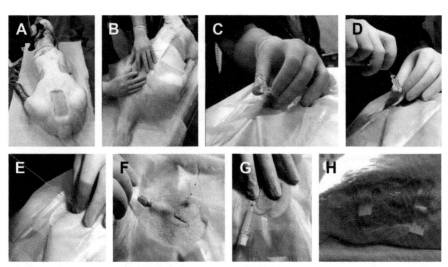

Fig. 1. Epidural catheter placement for postoperative pain management in a 4-month-old Boer Buck with a tibial fracture. (*A*) Placement of the patient in sternal positioning with wide margins clipped around the epidural space. (*B*) Placement of a sterile drape. (*C*) Advancement of the Tuohy needle until the epidural space is reached. A "pop" should be felt when the ligamentum flavum is passed. Note: This is not a hanging drop technique. (*D*) Feeding of the catheter through the Tuohy needle. (*E*) Catheter after needle removal. (*F*) Tunneling of an 18-gauge 1.5-inch needle through the skin close to the catheter at the lumbosacral space. The remaining catheter is advanced through the needle, and the needle is withdrawn. This provides extra security by the catheter being "tunneled" under the skin. (*G*) At this stage, the end cap can be placed on the catheter (*yellow cap*). (*H*) Final placement with filter port secured to cap of catheter, and protective film placed over the lumbosacral region.

Distal limb anesthesia ("Bier block") can be used in small ruminants with a modification to the technique used in large ruminants. When using this form of local anesthesia for distal limb surgery or as a diagnostic aid in lameness detection, it is often difficult to access the dorsal digital vein or the palmar (plantar) digital veins in smaller ruminants. A tourniquet should be placed above the elbow in the forelimb or above the tarsus in the hindlimb to allow for access to the cephalic or recurrent tarsal veins, respectively (**Fig. 2**). Lidocaine (2%) infused into the vein at a volume of 1 mL per 5 kg of body weight results in total limb anesthesia for as long as the tourniquet is in place and no adverse effects have been reported.[29]

The use of local anesthesia for the purposes of dehorning and disbudding has been previously reviewed.[18] Using local anesthesia for dehorning and disbudding is not only humane, but also practical, as the animal is more compliant. It is important to mention that due to the differences in anatomy, the cornual nerve block in goats requires at least 2 injection sites per horn versus one site typical of cattle.

Regional Infiltration Catheters

Regional infiltration catheters allow for release of local anesthetics into specific regions. Typically, longer-acting local anesthetics (bupivacaine, ropivacaine) are used for these techniques to reduce the risk of contamination. Although "soaker catheters" can be left in incision sites after amputations or other traumatic procedures, catheters can also be placed to allow for repeated focal nerve blocks. Bupivacaine (1 mg/kg)

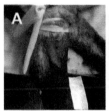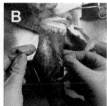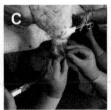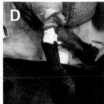

Fig. 2. Regional anesthesia in a 2-year-old Suffolk ram before removal of an interdigital mass. (*A*) A tourniquet of surgical tubing or Penrose drain is applied proximal to the targeted vein (lateral saphenous vein in this example). The skin over the vein is then clipped and prepped. Note the distention of the vein from the tourniquet. (*B*) A butterfly catheter (23 gauge in this case) is introduced into the vein until a "flash" of blood is noticed. (*C*) Lidocaine administration. (*D*) After removal of the butterfly catheter a temporary bandage of a gauze held in place with white tape. Regional anesthesia of the distal limb should occur within 5 to 10 minutes of lidocaine administration.

administered every 6 hours via a wound soaker catheter is effective in goats postoperatively.[30] Although care should be taken to not introduce foreign material into these catheters, a cross-species study identified incisional infection rates not higher than incisions that did not have wound soaker catheters applied.[30] In another example of more targeted analgesia, the pain from a mandibular fracture in an alpaca was managed by administration of a local anesthetic every 6 hours via a catheter placed in the vicinity of the mandibular foramen.[31]

TRANSDERMAL STRATEGIES
Fentanyl

Fentanyl in the transdermal delivery system can provide potent analgesia in a convenient delivery device and has been demonstrated effective in multiple orthopedic studies of sheep and goats. It is important to note that fentanyl patches are typically described as µg/h with dosing described as µg/kg/h. Patches are available in a variety of sizes, such as 1.2, 2.5, 5.0, 7.5, and 10.0 µg/h. Benefits of fentanyl patches are the provision of 72 hours of analgesia with 1 application. However, similar to the injectable formulation, practitioners should exercise caution, as the patches can provide a medium for abuse in people.

Once an appropriately sized patch is determined, the patch can be placed on the lateral or medial antebrachium following removal of hair or wool with clippers and proper cleansing of the skin (**Fig. 3**). It should be stressed that skin-patch adherence is of utmost importance. It is critical that the hair or wool be clipped and the skin cleansed and dried thoroughly before applying the patch. Failure of adherence or inability of the fentanyl to be absorbed (eg, dirty skin, excessive hair) could result in suboptimal pain control by this method.

For sheep undergoing orthopedic surgery, a dose of 2.0 µg/kg/h resulted in fentanyl reaching maximum concentrations at 12 hours and maintaining concentrations of more than 0.5 ng/mL for 40 hours.[14] Based on pharmacokinetic research, fentanyl patches should be placed at least 12 hours before initiation of pain (such as surgery).[14] Transdermal fentanyl in sheep is a superior analgesic compared with intermittent intramuscular injections of buprenorphine on the basis of reduced pain scores and reduced preanesthetic needed to achieve intubation.[32] Sheep in these studies did not show any adverse effects from the fentanyl administration.

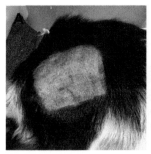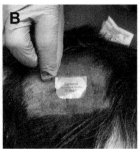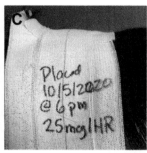

Fig. 3. Application of a fentanyl patch in a 6-month-old Nigerian Dwarf buck after surgical repair of a tibial fracture. (*A*) The patch application site is clipped with a #40 blade. After clipping, the area is lightly scrubbed for 30 seconds, then wiped with alcohol and allowed to air dry for 2 minutes.[33] (*B*) The patch is applied to the dry skin, and then held in place with a finger or palm of a hand for 30 seconds. (*C*) The patch is secured with 2 layers of adhesive bandage. At the authors' clinics, the patch is then labeled with time and date of placement as well as the strength of the patch.

For goats undergoing orthopedic surgery, transdermal fentanyl was as clinically effective as buprenorphine when evaluating postoperative pain scores.[33] However, another study reported inconsistent levels in goats.[15] In llamas, fentanyl patches resulted in steady serum concentrations without sedation.[34] It is important to mention that although no longer commercially available in the United States, a transdermal solution of fentanyl designed for small animals was reported to be unsafe in alpacas.

Adverse effects of fentanyl patch applications include tachypnea, tachycardia, respiratory depression, twitching behavior, depression, recumbency, and ataxia among others.[14,15,35,36] Clients should be warned to observe for these behaviors and take appropriate measures when removing the patch to avoid contact by wearing gloves.

Flunixin

Transdermal flunixin was recently approved in the United States for the control of pain associated with foot rot in cattle. Pharmacokinetic studies of a single dose in meat goats and alpacas demonstrated low bioavailabilities,[37,38] but more research is necessary to determine therapeutic efficacy of these formulations. It should be noted that although this product was intended for a single administration in cattle, there is only minimal accumulation in dairy cattle that have been administered multiple doses.[39] Currently there is no information to guide veterinarians on the accumulation potential in sheep, goats, and camelids.

OTHER STRATEGIES
Ultrasound-Guided Nerve Blocks

Larger nerves, such as the femoral and sciatic, as well as regions such as the psoas compartment, can be imaged via ultrasonography for local anesthetic placement. With this technique, ultrasonography is used to identify a large nerve and then local anesthetic is directed peripheral to the nerve for focused distribution. A 6- to 13-mHz linear probe has been used for identifying the sciatic and femoral nerves in sheep.[40] These blocks are typically performed under heavy sedation or anesthesia.

Ultrasound-guided nerve blocks can be performed preoperatively to decrease nociceptive windup, as well as after a painful injury. In one case series, ultrasound-guided delivery of ropivacaine was used to provide adjunctive analgesia in alpacas undergoing amputation.[41] Ropivacaine may be preferred for these procedures because of its long duration of activity and decreased tendency to block motor function compared with other local anesthetics.

Intra-articular

Intra-articular injection of a local anesthetic agent has the potential to be effective for controlling immediate postoperative pain in animals undergoing surgery of a joint. However, repeated injections are not advisable given the risk for iatrogenic infection with repeated arthrocenteses. In addition to treatment with transdermal fentanyl and phenylbutazone perioperatively, the use of intra-articular lidocaine preoperatively and intra-articular bupivacaine postoperatively significantly reduced postoperative pain in sheep undergoing stifle arthrotomy for 3 to 7 hours.[42]

Preoperative intra-articular bupivacaine in goats undergoing stifle arthrotomy reduced the amount of anesthetic required, but postoperative administration of intra-articular bupivacaine had a very short-lived effect.[43]

Acupuncture and Electroacupuncture

A nonpharmacologic intervention, acupuncture (AP) with or without the use of electrical stimulus (electroacupuncture; EAP), has become more popular in veterinary medicine. With AP, small needles are placed near specific points or traumatized structures and can have a small current applied (EAP). Acupuncture increases endogenous opioid production and regional microcirculation, as well as enhances recovery from nerve injuries. Electroacupuncture induces analgesia as well as increases beta-endorphins in sheep and decreases hypersensitivity to visceral pain in goats.[44,45] Clinical recommendations have also been made for AP and EAP in llamas and alpacas.[46] Electroacupuncture has a synergistic effect when combined with epidural nerve blocks in goats.[47] In the authors' experience, AP and EAP can be used as a minimally invasive adjunct as part of multimodal pain management. Due to the lack of a pharmacologic residue, both may be of useful benefit for food animal practice.

FUTURE DIRECTIONS FOR PAIN MANAGEMENT IN SMALL RUMINANTS

There are several new developing therapeutic strategies that may have utility for the pain management of sheep, goats, llamas, and alpacas. The liposomal encapsulation of bupivacaine has allowed for long-term release of local anesthetic from tissues and is currently being used in small animal and equine practice. The potential for durations of action of 72 to 96 hours would have considerable application for small ruminant analgesia, particularly postprocedure.

A new class of NSAIDs that function by blocking the prostaglandin receptor have recently become a staple of small animal pain management. For example, grapiprant selectively targets the prostaglandin receptor EP4 without inhibiting cyclooxygenase. This mechanism may allow for the beneficial effects of NSAIDs by downregulation of inflammatory prostaglandins without interfering with the production of beneficial prostaglandins.[48,49] However, there are currently no studies evaluating this class of prostaglandin receptor blocker in small ruminants. Finally, cannabidiol has attracted attention in small animal practice as a potential analgesic for osteoarthritis,[50] although current studies are lacking on its use in small ruminants. Although information for these therapeutics is currently limited, future studies may demonstrate utility.

UPDATES ON PAIN MANAGEMENT IN SPECIFIC CONDITIONS

A review of analgesic interventions for tail docking, castration, disbudding, dehorning, urethral obstruction, cesarean delivery, obstetrics, lameness, and rectal/vaginal prolapse was previously described.[18] The following information serves as an update to the previous review.

Amputation and Arthrodesis

Limb amputation in sheep and goats can be considered for treatment of severe orthopedic wounds, nonhealing fractures, and developmental of orthopedic diseases that cause a significant negative impact on animal welfare. Limb amputation in camelids can be less successful and is highly dependent on case selection. A consideration for pain management in orthopedic disease of the front limb is the paravertebral brachial plexus block (PBPB). To attempt this block in sheep, the scapula is shifted caudally and small amounts (0.2 mL/kg) of 0.5% bupivacaine are infiltrated around the cranial and caudal borders of the transverse process of C6.[51] When correctly performed, this technique can provide relaxation and analgesia to the limb distal to the elbow.[52] In other species, complications of the PBPB are rare but include puncture of the thoracic cavity as well as the jugular vein and axillary arteries. When this technique is used, care should be taken to implement it in a unilateral fashion to avoid complications from recovery. Ultrasound-guided nerve blocks of the brachial plexus and sciatic nerves could also be used before surgery. Postoperatively, wound soaker catheters integrated into the incision could be used to augment analgesia in small ruminants.[30]

Disbudding

Since 2013, there have been several updates to pain management for the practice of disbudding goats. The administration of isoflurane at the time of cautery disbudding has been demonstrated to reduce pain[53]; however this technique may not be applicable in all settings. Several options exist for analgesic management during disbudding. The use of local anesthetic nerve blocks as described previously in this article allows for very good anesthesia of the horn area. Use of bicarbonate to buffer the lidocaine will decrease pain during anesthesia placement. Care must be taken to not exceed the toxic dose of lidocaine, which can be very small for a young kid. In some cases, diluting the lidocaine from the standard 2% provided by the manufacturer to 1% with sterile saline may allow for more volume if needed. A ring block of lidocaine may not be sufficient by itself for pain management from cautery disbudding in goat kids.[54] The authors recommend oral meloxicam at a daily dose of 1 mg/kg for 3 to 5 days after cautery disbudding.

SUMMARY

For reasons of animal welfare as well as producer confidence, it is essential for veterinary practitioners to develop strategies for the management of pain in sheep, goats, and camelids. Through this review, we have described multiple therapeutic interventions as well as examples specific to procedures for the implementation of analgesic strategies in these species. At the least expensive end of the spectrum, oral meloxicam can be administered every 1 to 3 days depending on the target species at a cost of less than $0.20 per 50 kg body weight. For more severe pain or hospitalized cases, we have outlined the use of multimodal therapies, regional strategies, or transdermal patches that provide potent analgesia, but at greater financial expense. The goal of this article has been to provide an evidence-based, comprehensive, exploration of pain management for sheep, goats, and camelids. Individualized pain management strategies can be necessary because of the differences among cases, species, and applications.

CLINICS CARE POINTS

- Anticipation of potentially painful procedures is critical for the mitigation of pain in small ruminants.
- NSAIDs are a potent, inexpensive, and easy to administer form of analgesia for sheep, goats, llamas, and alpacas.
- Focused regional anesthesia in the form of wound soaker catheters, epidural catheters, ultrasound-guided nerve blocks, and regional limb perfusions can greatly increase the success of multimodal pain management.
- Care should be taken to obtain appropriate residue avoidance guidance for pain management in small ruminants, as almost all analgesic approaches would be considered extra-label drug use.

REFERENCES

1. George L. Pain control in food animals. In: Steffey E, editor. Recent advances in anesthetic management of large domestic animals. Ithaca (NY: International Veterinary Information Services; 2003. Available at: https://www.ivis.org/library/recent-advances-anesthetic-management-of-large-domestic-animals#in-this-book.
2. Malreddy PR, Coetzee JF, Kukanich B, et al. Pharmacokinetics and milk secretion of gabapentin and meloxicam co-administered orally in Holstein-Friesian cows. J Vet Pharmacol Ther 2012;36(1):14–20.
3. Coetzee JF, Mosher RA, Kohake LE, et al. Pharmacokinetics of oral gabapentin alone or co-administered with meloxicam in ruminant beef calves. Vet J 2011;190(1):98–102.
4. Wenger S, Hatt J-M. Oral gabapentin used to treat recurrent shoulder and neck pain in a Bactrian camel. Vet Anaesth Analg 2019;46(1):145–6.
5. Kreuder AJ, Coetzee JF, Wulf LW, et al. Bioavailability and pharmacokinetics of oral meloxicam in llamas. BMC Vet Res 2012;8(1):85.
6. Shukla M, Singh G, Sindhura BG, et al. Comparative plasma pharmacokinetics of meloxicam in sheep and goats following intravenous administration. Comp Biochem Physiol C Toxicol Pharmacol 2007;145(4):528–32.
7. Ingvast-Larsson C, Hogberg M, Mengistu U, et al. Pharmacokinetics of meloxicam in adult goats and its analgesic effect in disbudded kids. J Vet Pharmacol Ther 2011;34(1):64–9.
8. Stock ML, Coetzee JF, KuKanich B, et al. Pharmacokinetics of intravenously and orally administered meloxicam in sheep. Am J Vet Res 2013;74(5):779–83.
9. Marini D, Pippia J, Colditz IG, et al. Randomised trial of the bioavailability and efficacy of orally administered flunixin, carprofen and ketoprofen in a pain model in sheep. Aust Vet J 2015;93(8):265–70.
10. Abrahamsen EJ. Chemical restraint, anesthesia, and analgesia for camelids. Vet Clin North Am Food Anim Pract 2009;25(2):455–94.
11. Grant C, Upton RN, Kuchel TR. Efficacy of intra-muscular analgesics for acute pain in sheep. Aust Vet J 1996;73(4):129–32.
12. Fthenakis GC. Field evaluation of flunixin meglumine in the supportive treatment of ovine mastitis. J Vet Pharmacol Ther 2000;23(6):405–7.
13. Cox S, Martin-Jimenez T, van Amstel S, et al. Pharmacokinetics of intravenous and intramuscular tramadol in llamas. J Vet Pharmacol Ther 2011;34(3):259–64.

14. Ahern BJ, Soma LR, Rudy JA, et al. Pharmacokinetics of fentanyl administered transdermally and intravenously in sheep. Am J Vet Res 2010;71(10):1127–32.

15. Carroll GL, Hooper RN, Boothe DM, et al. Pharmacokinetics of fentanyl after intravenous and transdermal administration in goats. Am J Vet Res 1999;60(8): 986–91.

16. Cheng Z, McKeller Q, Nolan A. Pharmacokinetic studies of flunixin meglumine and phenylbutazone in plasma, exudate and transudate in sheep. J Vet Pharmacol Ther 1998;21(4):315–21.

17. Welsh EM, Nolan AM. Effects of non-steroidal anti-inflammatory drugs on the hyperalgesia to noxious mechanical stimulation induced by the application of a tourniquet to a forelimb of sheep. Res Vet Sci 1994;57(3):285–91.

18. Plummer PJ, Schleining JA. Assessment and management of pain in small ruminants and camelids. Vet Clin North Am Food Anim Pract 2013;29(1):185–208.

19. Ivany J, Muir W. Farm Animal Anesthesia. In: Fubini S, Ducharme N, editors. Farm animal surgery. St Louis (MO): Saunders; 2004. p. 102–3.

20. Van Metre D, editor Small Ruminant Tips. 128th Annual Meeting of the Iowa Veterinary Medical Association; 2010 September 16-17, 2010; Ames, IA.

21. Trim CM. Epidural analgesia with 0.75% bupivacaine for laparotomy in goats. J Am Vet Med Assoc 1989;194(9):1292–6.

22. Hendrickson DA, Kruse-Elliott KT, Broadstone RV. A comparison of epidural saline, morphine, and bupivacaine for pain relief after abdominal surgery in goats. Vet Surg 1996;25(1):83–7.

23. Pablo LS. Epidural morphine in goats after hindlimb orthopedic surgery. Vet Surg 1993;22(4):307–10.

24. Dehkordi SH, Bigham-Sadegh A, Gerami R. Evaluation of anti-nociceptive effect of epidural tramadol, tramadol-lidocaine and lidocaine in goats. Vet Anaesth Analg 2012;39(1):106–10.

25. Habibian S, Bigham AS, Aali E. Comparison of lidocaine, tramadol, and lidocaine-tramadol for epidural analgesia in lambs. Res Vet Sci 2011;91(3):434–8.

26. Padula AM. Clinical evaluation of caudal epidural anaesthesia for the neutering of alpacas. Vet Rec 2005;156(19):616–7.

27. Grubb TL, Riebold TW, Huber MJ. Evaluation of lidocaine, xylazine, and a combination of lidocaine and xylazine for epidural analgesia in llamas. J Am Vet Med Assoc 1993;203(10):1441–4.

28. Rostami M, Vesal N. Comparison of lidocaine, lidocaine/epinephrine or bupivacaine for thoracolumbar paravertebral anaesthesia in fat-tailed sheep. Vet Anaesth Analg 2011;38(6):598–602.

29. Babalola GO, Oke BO. Intravenous regional analgesia for surgery of the limbs in goats. Vet Q 1983;5(4):186–9.

30. Abelson AL, McCobb EC, Shaw S, et al. Use of wound soaker catheters for the administration of local anesthetic for post-operative analgesia: 56 cases. Vet Anaesth Analg 2009;36(6):597–602.

31. Stathopoulou T, Seymour C, McSloy A, et al. Pain management of a mandibular fracture in an alpaca via epidural catheter placement in the mandibular foramen. Vet Rec 2019;7(4):e000863.

32. Ahern BJ, Soma LR, Boston RC, et al. Comparison of the analgesic properties of transdermally administered fentanyl and intramuscularly administered buprenorphine during and following experimental orthopedic surgery in sheep. Am J Vet Res 2009;70(3):418–22.

33. Burke MJ, Soma LR, Boston RC, et al. Evaluation of the analgesic and pharma-cokinetic properties of transdermally administered fentanyl in goats. J Vet Emerg Crit Care 2017;27(5):539–47.

34. Grubb TL, Gold JR, Schlipf JW, et al. Assessment of serum concentrations and sedative effects of fentanyl after transdermal administration at three dosages in healthy llamas. Am J Vet Res 2005;66(5):907–9.

35. Christou C, Oliver RA, Rawlinson J, et al. Transdermal fentanyl and its use in ovine surgery. Res Vet Sci 2015;100:252–6.

36. Smith JS, Mochel JP, Borts DJ, et al. Adverse reactions to fentanyl transdermal patches in calves: a preliminary clinical and pharmacokinetic study. Vet Anaesth Analg 2018;45(4):575–80.

37. Reppert EJ, Kleinhenz MD, Montgomery SR, et al. Pharmacokinetics and phar-macodynamics of intravenous and transdermal flunixin meglumine in meat goats. J Vet Pharmacol Ther 2019;42(3):309–17.

38. Reppert EJ, Kleinhenz MD, Montgomery SR, et al. Pharmacokinetics and phar-macodynamics of intravenous and transdermal flunixin meglumine in alpacas. J Vet Pharmacol Ther 2019;42(5):572–9.

39. Kleinhenz MD, Gorden PJ, Smith JS, et al. Pharmacokinetics of multiple doses of transdermal flunixin meglumine in adult Holstein dairy cows. J Vet Pharmacol Ther 2018;41(3):490–3.

40. Waag S, Stoffel MH, Spadavecchia C, et al. Ultrasound-guided block of sciatic and femoral nerves: an anatomical study. Lab Anim 2014;48(2):97–104.

41. Foster A, McSloy A, Monticelli P. Ultrasound-guided psoas compartment and sciatic nerve blocks for pain management of hind limb procedures in the alpaca (Vicugna pacos). Open Vet J 2020;10(2):120–7.

42. Shafford HL, Hellyer PW, Turner AS. Intra-articular lidocaine plus bupivacaine in sheep undergoing stifle arthrotomy. Vet Anaesth Analg 2004;31(1):20–6.

43. Krohm P, Levionnois O, Ganster M, et al. Antinociceptive activity of pre- versus post-operative intra-articular bupivacaine in goats undergoing stifle arthrotomy. Vet Anaesth Analg 2011;38(4):363–73.

44. Bossut DF, Stromberg MW, Malven PV. Electroacupuncture-induced analgesia in sheep: measurement of cutaneous pain thresholds and plasma concentrations of prolactin and beta-endorphin immunoreactivity. Am J Vet Res 1986;47(3):669–76.

45. Shah MK, Ding Y, Wan J, et al. Electroacupuncture intervention of visceral hyper-sensitivity is involved in PAR-2-activation and CGRP-release in the spinal cord. Sci Rep 2020;10(1):11188.

46. Robinson NG, Holt TN. Acupuncture in the camelid. llama and alpaca care. St. Louis (MO): Elsevier; 2014. p. 628–48.

47. Cui LY, Guo NN, Li YL, et al. Analgesic and physiological effect of electroacu-puncture combined with epidural lidocaine in goats. Vet Anaesth Analg 2017; 44(4):959–67.

48. Rausch-Derra LC, Rhodes L, Freshwater L, et al. Pharmacokinetic comparison of oral tablet and suspension formulations of grapiprant, a novel therapeutic for the pain and inflammation of osteoarthritis in dogs. J Vet Pharmacol Ther 2016;39(6): 566–71.

49. de Salazar Alcalá AG, Gioda L, Dehman A, et al. Assessment of the efficacy of firocoxib (Previcox®) and grapiprant (Galliprant®) in an induced model of acute arthritis in dogs. BMC Vet Res 2019;15(1):309.

50. Brioschi FA, Di Cesare F, Gioeni D, et al. Oral transmucosal cannabidiol oil formu-lation as part of a multimodal analgesic regimen: effects on pain relief and quality

of life improvement in dogs affected by spontaneous osteoarthritis. Animals 2020; 10(9):1505.

51. Rodrigo-Mocholí D, Schauvliege S. Paravertebral brachial plexus blockade as part of a balanced anaesthesia in a sheep undergoing thoracic limb amputation. Vet Anaesth Analg 2016;43(2):239–40.

52. Michielsen A, Schauvliege S. Plexus brachialis block as part of balanced analgesia in a sheep undergoing arthrodesis of the carpus. Vet Anaesth Analg 2019;46(5):710–1.

53. Hempstead MN, Waas JR, Stewart M, et al. Effect of isoflurane alone or in combination with meloxicam on the behavior and physiology of goat kids following cautery disbudding. J Dairy Sci 2018;101(4):3193–204.

54. Hempstead MN, Lindquist TM, Shearer JK, et al. Acute cortisol and behavior of dairy goat kids administered local anesthesia, topical anesthesia or systemic analgesia prior to cautery disbudding. Physiol Behav 2020;222:112942.

55. Stillman MW, Whittaker AL. Use and efficacy of analgesic agents in sheep (Ovis aries) used in biomedical research. J Am Assoc Lab Anim Sci 2019;58(6): 755–66.

56. Martínez M, Murison PJ, Murrell J. Possible delayed respiratory depression following intrathecal injection of morphine and bupivacaine in an alpaca. J Vet Emerg Crit Care 2014;24(4):450–4.

Evaluating the Welfare of Small Ruminants
Practical Management Advice

Paul J. Plummer, PhD, DVM*, Melissa N. Hempstead, PhD,
Jan K. Shearer, DVM, MS, Taylor M. Lindquist, BS

KEYWORDS

- Sheep • Goat • Animal-based indicator • Management • Husbandry
- Small ruminant welfare • Welfare indicators • Welfare assessment

KEY POINTS

- Although animal welfare cannot be measured directly, a variety of welfare indicators can reflect welfare status.
- Useful indicators of welfare include body condition, mastitis, claw overgrowth, lameness, and the human–animal relationship.
- With knowledge and careful identification of indicators of welfare, practitioners can work together with producers to improve the welfare of sheep and goats.

INTRODUCTION

Public concern for high standards of animal production has resulted in an increased demand for animals that are raised in a manner that encompasses good health, food safety, and respect for animal welfare. Animal welfare (or well-being) is difficult to define because there are multiple viewpoints; however, in this article we define good welfare as an animal in a state where its nutritional, environmental, health, behavioral, and mental (ie, affective state) needs are met.[1] High standards of welfare are vital for improved animal performance with higher product quality and profit. As a consequence, good animal welfare benefits not only animals, but producers as well and practitioners by reflection.

Animal welfare cannot be directly measured; however, it can be evaluated using a multifactorial approach. Quantifying multiple variables will provide an accurate

Conflicts of interest: The authors have no commercial or financial conflicts of interest to report.
Funding: The authors gratefully acknowledge funding on this topic from the United States Department of Agriculture (USDA) through the National Institute for Food and Agriculture (NIFA) (grant number 2018-67015-28136).
Department of Veterinary Diagnostic and Production Animal Medicine, College of Veterinary Medicine, Iowa State University, 2426 Lloyd Vet Med Center, Ames, IA 50011, USA
* Corresponding author.
E-mail address: pplummer@iastate.edu

reflection of the current welfare status. Useful welfare indicators are valid (meaning they evaluate what they are meant to), reliable (meaning they are consistent over time), and feasible (meaning they are simple and practical to use on the farm).[2] To achieve accurate evidence-based information from welfare assessment, indicators of welfare should focus on the animal, resources, and management (**Table 1**).

On-farm welfare assessment has certain benefits, including the potential for the early identification of welfare issues, quantification of the impact of husbandry practices (eg, disbudding, castration, hoof trimming, tail docking), examination of the influence of resources on individual animals (eg, diet, housing), and welfare audits or certification program.[3] A welfare assessment is made by a second-party assessor such as a herd veterinarian. An evaluation is performed to identify the major issues or problems associated with a herd or flock and to offer suggestions for improvement. In distinction, a welfare audit is performed by a third-party auditor who evaluates and

Table 1
Summary of the key animal-, management- and resource-based indicators of small ruminant on-farm welfare assessment

On-Farm Welfare Assessment Summary		
Animal-Based Indicators	**Management-Based Indicators**	**Resource-Based Indicators**
Focused Directly on the Animals	**Protocols Used by Animal Managers**	**Resources Available to Animals**
Nutrition	Evaluate management	Evaluate resources available
BCS	practices	Quantity and quality of food
Queuing behavior at	SOPs for	Space per goat in lying areas
the feed bunk	Disbudding	Stocking density of pens
Environment and housing	Castration	Outdoor spaces
Thermal stress (extreme	Hoof trimming	Enrichment
temperatures)	Tail docking	Sheltered areas from
Animal cleanliness/	Environment cleanliness	weather extremes
hygiene	Feed distribution, quality	
Health	and amount	
Mastitis	Water	
Fecal soiling	Health records	
Cutaneous lesions	Vaccination and	
Ocular and nasal	deworming protocols	
discharge	Records of veterinary	
Tail docking	treatment	
Lameness	Pain relief usage	
Claw overgrowth	Humane euthanasia	
Scurs/horns (disbudding)	practices	
Behavior	Protocols for	
Human–animal	euthanizing animals	
relationship	Methods and anatomic	
Human approach tests	sites	
Stereotypic behavior	Carcass disposal	
Positive affective state	Nonambulatory animal	
Synchronized feeding	care	
Expression of natural	Pen management	
behaviors	Sufficient and clean	
	bedding	
	Cleanliness of water	
	troughs and feeders	
	Walkways and alleyways	

determines whether a farm meets a set standard and who does not offer advice. The Animal Welfare Indicators program was designed to evaluate the welfare of production animals (eg, sheep, goats, horses, donkeys, and turkeys).[4,5] Until such programs, assessment protocols for these species was limited. Certification programs to evaluate sheep and goat welfare on commercial farms do exist in the United States. Examples of these include American Humane Certified, Certified Animal Welfare Approved, Food Alliance, and Certified Humane.

Together with a knowledge and awareness of the useful welfare indicators and the effective identification of welfare issues on farms, practitioners can aid animal managers to develop a management plan that can ensure a high standard of welfare for small ruminants. This article discusses the key welfare issues for sheep and goats and gives practical management advice, including identification, prevention, and treatment (where necessary).

ANIMAL-BASED INDICATORS OF WELFARE

Animal-based welfare indicators such as body condition, disease state, or flight distance (ie, fear of humans) can indicate the performance or outcome within a husbandry system[6]; these indicators provide a more accurate picture of the welfare state of the animals than indicators that are concerned with management or resources, because they focus directly on the animal.[7] The following animal-based indicators of welfare will be organized into the following categories: nutrition, environment, health, behavior, and affective state.

Nutrition

Body condition scoring (BCS) evaluates the amount of muscling and fat development and is useful for monitoring changes in body fat reserves.[8] Visually observing the rump region of dairy goats for obvious overweight or underweight animals can be used for those without a thick hair coat.[9] Between the hip and pin bones, an overweight animal will generally have a convex shape, whereas an underweight animal will have a concave shape. However, more detailed BCS is performed by palpation of the lumbar area, sternum, or breastbone and the ribs and intercostal spaces (**Figs. 1** and **2**). For sheep and goats, a numerical rating scale of 5 points is commonly used.[10,11] However, the use of a 3-point scale focused on identifying obviously fat, thin, and normal animals is useful for on-farm assessment because it improves reliability (between and within observers). This simplified assessment scoring is important for all welfare indicators and allows for a quicker assessment without the need to restrain and touch each animal.[12,13] A low BCS is observed when energy expenditure exceeds nutritional status owing to decreased intake, which may reflect an inadequate feed supply (or disease) or increased energy output.[3] Conversely, a high BCS can indicate overfeeding or excessive confinement that limits exercise.[3] Both extreme conditions impact health, production, and welfare.

Feeding behavior at the feed bunk can be monitored to determine the number of animals queuing (lining up) behind one another over a period of time. Queuing behavior can reflect inadequate space for the animals at the feed bunk or an uneven distribution of feed in the bunk. Small ruminants are gregarious and tend to perform activities, such as feeding and drinking, at the same time as others[14]; their welfare may be negatively impacted if they are prevented from performing activities with their pen mates. Sheep spend less time feeding when the feed space is decreased from 1 sheep per feed space to 3 sheep per feed space, and spend more time queuing for a feed space.[15] A study of dairy goat farms in Portugal reported that queuing for feed and water were associated

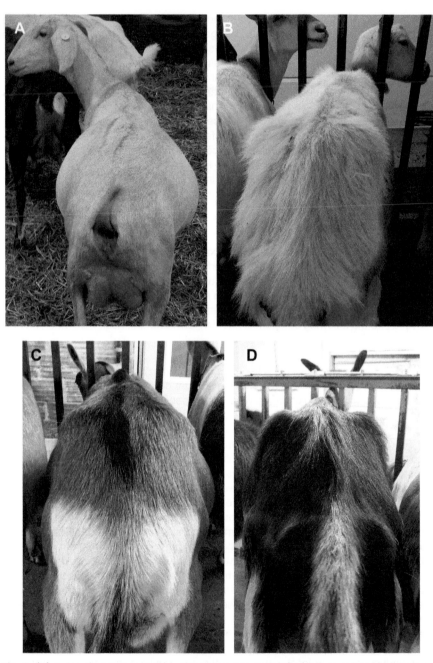

Fig. 1. (*A*) A doe that is overweight. She is carrying excess fleshing over her hip bones and thurl area. (*B*) A doe that is underweight. She has very little fleshing over her hip bone and thurl area. (*C* and *D*) Does that are in good body condition. There is sufficient fleshing over their hip bones and thurl area.

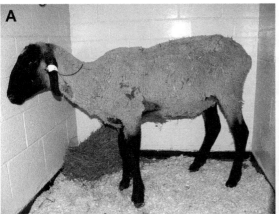
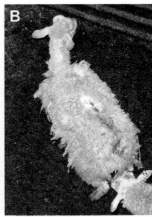

Fig. 2. Examples of low BCS ewes. (*A*) There is very little fleshing along the spine, hips, thurl, and shoulder area. (*B*) The ewe seems to have little fleshing over her shoulder, spine, and rump, even with the wool. (*Courtesy of* P. Menzies, DVM, Guelph, Canada.)

and that both were more prevalent in farms with more than 100 goats.[16] Furthermore, the amount of time spent queuing increases and feeding decreases with increased animal-to-feed space ratio[17] and with associated increased aggression, which may result in injuries.[18] Low-ranking animals may be outcompeted by higher ranking animals and, therefore, prevented from accessing feed spaces.[17] These animals may then have a lower body condition owing to a decreased opportunity to feed.

Extension of the feed bunk or the addition of free-standing feeders or decreasing the stocking density may decrease the amount of queuing behavior observed and ensure all animals have equal access to feed. Proper feed bunk design should allow for animals to stand during feeding, whereas poorly designed feeders may result in kneeling because the feed may be too low (or the pen floor too high).

Environment and Housing

Thermal stress

Thermal stress, which includes prolonged exposure to excessively high or low temperatures, can have negative impacts on animal welfare, health, and production. Although sheep and goats are generally considered to be resistant to climatic extremes, especially high temperatures, their physiology and production performance can be negatively affected. An animal experiencing heat stress (**Fig. 3**) is typically characterized by an elevated respiration rate, signs of panting, increased water intake, and decreased feed intake and milk production.[19,20] Furthermore, milk from heat-stressed goats has different coagulation properties to milk from goats under thermoneutral conditions, and this difference may negatively impact cheese making.[20] Additionally, nutritional strategies that include the use of a high-energy diet, protein with low rumen degradability, alteration of feeding time to periods of the day when temperatures are less extreme, and the provision of dietary supplementation can decrease the negative effects of heat stress on physiologic responses.[21,22]

Compared with sheep, goats are more susceptible to low temperatures owing to the obvious differences in the amount of fleece they carry.[23] The thermoneutral zones typically range from $-12°C$ to $32°C$ for sheep and $6°C$ to $27°C$ for goats. Goats typically spend less time outdoors (than indoors) when the air temperature is decreasing. The

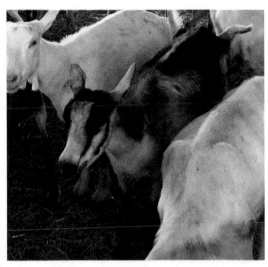

Fig. 3. An example of an animal experiencing thermal stress (eg, open-mouthed breathing or panting). The ears are also angled back and the head is dropped lower than the shoulders.

negative effect of a low outdoor temperature may be decreased in the short term with a roof covering the outdoor area.[24] In contrast, the amount of time sheep spend outdoors seems to be unaffected by environmental factors.[23] Low air temperatures, together with wind and/or rain, will increase heat loss; therefore, this environmental condition will trigger physiologic and behavioral responses to decrease heat loss.[25] Such responses include the bristling of hair along the back (ie, horripilation), shivering, huddling, and a cramped posture where the head and neck are lowered (**Fig. 4**)[24,26]; however, it is important to note also that some animals that undergo agonistic confrontations (fighting) with others or are suffering from an illness may present similarly. Appropriate housing designed to minimize drafts (eg, insulation, heating, cross-wind ventilation, ceiling vents, electric fans) or extra provision of feed can decrease the effects of thermal stress.[22]

Hygiene
Animal cleanliness is an important indicator of welfare in cattle.[27] Poor hygiene associated with a dirty environment can increase the risk of mastitis and can be assessed

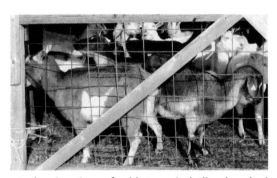

Fig. 4. Multiple goats showing signs of cold stress. including hunched posture, huddling behavior, and horripilation (piloerection).

by hygiene scoring.[28] Hygiene scoring generally uses a 3-point scale to rank the fecal soiling present on the rump and legs of the goat or sheep (see the section on Health for a discussion on fecal soiling). A key issue affecting lactating dairy goats on 24 United Kingdom farms was udder and teat cleanliness.[29]

Goats generally show a clear preference for dry, clean bedding.[2] There is limited research available on the effect of cleanliness on goat welfare, but coat cleanliness is a useful indicator of welfare in sheep.[30] The presence of dirty sides, limbs, and udders may indicate inadequate management of bedding.[3]

Health

Mastitis

Mastitis is a painful condition in lactating animals. In sheep and goats, mastitis negatively impacts health, production, and welfare.[31] Clinical symptoms of acute mastitis include inflammation and increased heat in the udder, hyperemia of the udder skin, hardening, and secretions that contain flakes or clots.[32] However, in sheep or goats in large herds, individual examination may not always be possible. Therefore, the feasible assessment of mastitis of the herd includes evaluating the udder asymmetry of goats (which may indicate a previous bout of mastitis) or observations of fibrotic lesions on sheep udders (**Fig. 5**).[16,33] Of course, there are slight udder asymmetries that occur naturally and may not necessarily be associated with mastitis; therefore, only exaggerated differences between udders should be assessed. The risk of mastitis can be minimized by isolating affected animals and the culling of those with chronic symptoms. Other tactics to minimize mastitis are a high standard of routine milking hygiene, including single-use wipes between animals; postmilking teat dips; sanitation of the milking system; and the use of gloves by staff during milking. Additionally, bacteria in the environment can be decreased by regular freshening of the bedding and treatment of affected animals. Pain associated with mastitis can be decreased by the

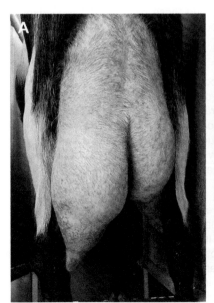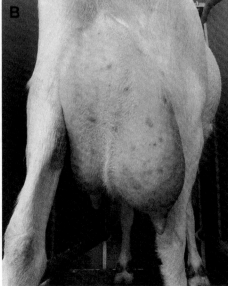

Fig. 5. Two examples (*A* and *B*) of goats showing signs of udder asymmetry (1 side of the udder is 25% larger than the other).

administration of nonsteroidal anti-inflammatory drugs in combination with broad-spectrum antimicrobials.

Altered fecal consistency
Fecal soiling occurs when fecal material becomes attached to the hair or wool around the tail and anus area. Generally, fecal soiling is more problematic for sheep than goats, owing to loose moist feces that can stick to the wool and dry without falling off. These are commonly termed *dags* in Australia and New Zealand.[34] Dags increase the risk of cutaneous myiasis or flystrike, which is a significant welfare concern in sheep.[35,36] Fecal soiling can indicate a nutritional imbalance or endoparasites in goats.[2]

Skin lesions and trauma
The prevalence of cutaneous lesions and masses (including damaged skin and swellings) or abscesses in sheep and goat herds can be an indicator of poor health.[10,29] During previous welfare assessments of sheep and goats, lesions or abscesses may result from injuries or sunburn,[10] infection,[11] and diseases such as caseous lymphadenitis.[16,37] Caseous lymphadenitis is caused by *Corynebacterium pseudotuberculosis* and is prevalent in US herds and flocks. Treatment approaches vary based on the herd or flock status for disease and the desires of the producers. In farms where the disease is not endemic, the identification of a potential sentinel lesion should result in consideration of isolation and culling. However, in endemic farms treatment generally focuses on decreasing environmental contamination and includes drainage and disposal of the abscess material. Vaccinations are available and decrease the number of external abscesses observed in a herd; however, they generally fail to provide sterilizing immunity.[38] For a comprehensive explanation of caseous lymphadenitis see the review by Windsor.[37] For sheep, causal factors of caseous lymphadenitis may be related to age (ie, increased prevalence for sheep more than 1 year of age), increased duration with other sheep shortly after shearing, and dips for ectoparasites.[37] Additionally, lesions or abscesses on goats including those of caseous lymphadenitis, may result from heat stress, inappropriate housing conditions, or injuries caused by other animals with horns or scurs.[2]

Irritated mucous membranes
Ocular and nasal discharge may indicate a poor environment that has excessive particulate matter in the air, high ammonia levels, or disease states (eg, infection) and can be observed clearly without the need for restraint.[29] Ocular and nasal discharge was reported in 1.9% and 5.7%, respectively, of goats on 30 Italian farms[16] and 9.0% and 4.5%, respectively, of goats on 30 Portuguese farms.[12] Increased ventilation, if possible, or decreased stocking density may improve the air quality and resultant ocular and nasal discharge, if disease states are not the cause.

Tail docking
The tails of sheep are routinely docked to decrease the incidence of flystrike,[39] but animals with excessively short-docked tails have a greater risk of rectal prolapse (**Fig. 6**),[40] flystrike,[41] and bacterial arthritis.[42] Importantly, unlike in some companion animal species where tail docking is purely cosmetic, failure to dock wool sheep tails correctly can result in welfare concerns. A recent Australian study reported that 85.7% of sheep (5318 of 6200) had excessively shortened tails.[10] Excessively short tail docks are also a problem in the United States, especially in lambs raised for exhibition, where there is a belief that short docks provide a better side profile for the judges. The ideal tail length includes coverage of the anus and vulva (**Fig. 7**). Therefore, the identification

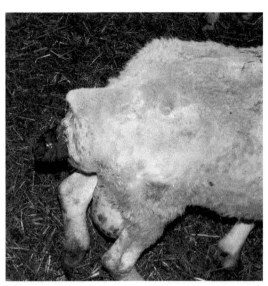

Fig. 6. An example of a rectal prolapse in a sheep with a short-docked tail. (*Courtesy of* P. Menzies, DVM, Guelph, Canada.)

of sheep within a herd that have excessively short-docked tails can indicate a problem with the efficacy of the tail docking procedure and highlight the notion that producers may require further training.[10] Both the American Veterinary Medical Association and the American Association of Small Ruminant Practitioners have position statements

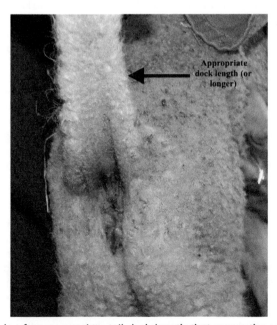

Fig. 7. An example of an appropriate tail dock length that covers the anus and vulva on ewes and anus on rams/wethers. (*Courtesy of* P. Menzies, DVM, Guelph, Canada.)

reflecting the need for adequate tail length to minimize welfare concerns. It is generally accepted that tail docking causes pain (see the review by Sutherland and Tucker[39]), and therefore the provision of pain mitigation strategies such as nonsteroidal anti-inflammatory drugs should be considered.[43]

Lameness and foot care

Lameness is an important behavioral indicator of pain that impedes a normal walking gait and this is a serious welfare issue for both sheep and goats.[44,45] Lameness can be caused by claw overgrowth (with or without deformation) or diseases that affect the claw, skin, or joints, such as interdigital dermatitis and foot rot in sheep or caprine arthritis-encephalitis in goats.[45–47] Gait scoring systems to detect the prevalence and degree of lameness use either a 4-point[11,30] or 5-point scoring system.[48,49] Most scoring systems require a definite limp to be observed to classify an animal as lame; however, gait scoring individual animals may be difficult because of the level of training required and management and resource differences across farms.[48] Therefore, the identification of animals at the herd level with severe lameness may be more practical for evaluating welfare status. An alternative to using a numerical scale to lameness score goats, uses a modified visual analogue scale, which can improve reliability.[50] The site where lameness scoring is carried out can impact the level of lameness detected. Estimates of lameness are often lower when evaluated in pens that have soft bedding,[16] compared with observations of goats exiting the parlor, where flooring is usually concrete.[29] Lameness rates may be higher (or more apparent) when walking on hard surfaces.[29] Treatment for lameness depends on the outcome of physical examination, but usually includes hoof trimming (described elsewhere in this article), foot baths with treatment added (eg, zinc sulfate), or antimicrobial treatment.

Claw overgrowth can cause impeded locomotion with an irregular gait that may result in long-term unfixable damage to the bones in the foot and lower leg. Overgrown claws are generally associated with a lack of wear of the hooves or insufficient hoof trimming. Excessive claw growth (where the hoof resembles an elf shoe; **Fig. 8**) may be easier to identify without restraint of individual animals; however, mild and moderate claw overgrowth can be evaluated during milking, where the hoof is on a flat surface (ie, without bedding).[29] An abundance of overgrown hooves indicates the need for more regular hoof trimming or the provision of areas of hard flooring in the pens. In severe and prolonged cases of lameness, small ruminants are also prone to start walking on their knees (**Fig. 9**). In cases where animals are walking on their knees, the animals can rapidly develop tendon contracture resulting in a poor long-term prognosis. When performing welfare assessments, the recognition of animals walking on their knees should raise concerns and prompt a further evaluation of lameness.

Disbudding

Disbudding is a common husbandry practice on dairy goat farms and in some cases other goat operations, and it is usually performed with a hot cautery iron. Anecdotally, some producers believe that the practice is not painful because goat kids seem to rapidly return to performance of normal behaviors after disbudding (eg, feeding). However, there is a large body of evidence available highlighting the pain associated with cautery disbudding and support for the use of pain mitigation strategies to improve goat kid welfare.[51–55] If disbudding is not performed correctly (ie, disbudded at an age where the horn buds are large), then incomplete horn growth or scurs may result (**Fig. 10**).[46] Scurs can become stuck in housing structures and break off or grow

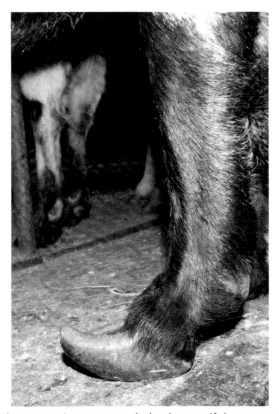

Fig. 8. A goat with extreme claw overgrowth that has an elf shoe appearance.

toward the head or eyes, both resulting in pain and injuries.[2] Horned and hornless goats should not be housed together because there can be increased aggression, which may be directed toward those without horns, and this behavior may lead to injuries.[56] The number of animals with scurs and horns can reflect problems with disbudding efficacy. Ideally, kids should be disbudded at less than a week of age or once the horn buds are palpable. Kids should have some form of analgesia administered. Oral meloxicam is readily available, economically feasible (less than $0.10 per kid), easily administered, and has been repeatedly shown to provide analgesic benefit.[43,53,54,57]

Behavior

The human–animal relationship is vitally important, because animal managers have a key role in sustaining the health, production, and welfare of the animals in their care. A comprehensive review of the human–animal relationship in farmed species was published by Waiblinger and colleagues.[58] Fear of humans, often caused by negative handling, can decrease milk yield or let-down in dairy goats; gentle handling of lambs during rearing can increase weight gains.[59,60] Sheep that are fearful of humans owing to limited (or negative) human contact and handling may be more challenging to manage during transport and in preslaughter periods.[61] It is possible to assess the human–animal relationship of commercial sheep and goats by using human approach tests. These tests include monitoring the minimum distance between an approaching

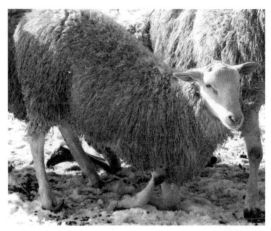

Fig. 9. Example of an animal maneuvering around on its knees owing to overgrowth of the back claws.

familiar human and animal or also a latency to approach test, which measures the time taken for an animal to approach and contact an unfamiliar human in their pen.[62] Goats that are more fearful of humans owing to negative or rough handling are more likely to have a larger flight zone or distance or a greater latency to approach time than animals that have been positively or gently handled.[63] Additionally, sheep that received gentle

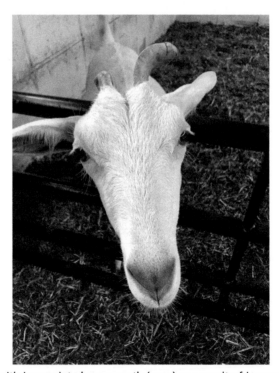

Fig. 10. A goat with incomplete horn growth (scurs) as a result of incomplete disbudding.

handling had a lower flight distance than those that received rough handling.[64] It is important to note that animals that are difficult to handle will increase the difficulty of administration of veterinary treatment, if required.

Abnormal or stereotypic behavior, termed "stereotypy," is characterized by repetitive behaviors that serve no obvious goal or function. This behavior is a useful indicator of mental well-being. Stereotypies generally result from deficient environmental conditions that do not adequately stimulate the animal. In confined environments, sheep can perform oral (repetitive licking, chewing, and mouthing pen fixtures) and locomotor (rearing, butting, route tracing, and weaving) stereotypies.[65] In addition, sheep confined to the indoors carry out fleece-pulling behavior, particularly when housed at high stocking densities.[65] Some goat breeds display self-suckling or inter-suckling when fed a low-fiber diet.[66] Additionally, dairy goats on commercial farms in the United Kingdom have been reported to display abnormal oral behaviors directed at the bars of fences or walls of the pens.[29]

Affective State

Many of the indicators of welfare set out in this article have focused on negative welfare states (eg, poor body condition, lameness, and fear). However, an important consideration for welfare assessment is to evaluate positive welfare (eg, pleasure), in addition to the negative experiences or sensations. Evaluation of positive animal welfare includes an assessment of animal feelings or affective state (ie, internal state). Animals that are provided with the opportunities to synchronize their feeding may indicate positive welfare; feed behavior synchronization is an adaptive behavior that is beneficial for (1) providing information about the food source, (2) allowing more time to graze, and (3) for animals on pasture, there is a decreased risk of predation in feeding behavior of synchronized animals.[67] The ability to express behaviors that an animal would be able to do so in a natural environment, and interact with others resulting in exploration, foraging, hunting, bonding, or other social behaviors (eg, play, allogrooming, positive parent–offspring interactions) may reflect positive welfare.[67] A comprehensive review of positive indicators of welfare for ruminants was published by Mattiello and colleagues.[67]

MANAGEMENT-BASED INDICATORS

Management-based indicators assess how animals are managed by stock handlers and these indicators can be collected in an objective manner. Examples of management practices that can be evaluated include disbudding, castration, and/or tail docking; environmental cleanliness; feed distribution, including quality and amount; and regular veterinary care. Poor management can impact negatively on animal welfare and may result in aggressive or fearful animals, and this can cause increase difficulty of handling or mustering.

For multiple reasons, sheep and goats may require euthanasia. These reasons may include disease or injury that cannot be treated practically or an excess of male neonates in a dairy herd. Euthanasia is derived from the Greek terms *eu* and *thanatos*, which means "good death" and describes the ending of an animals' life with minimal pain and distress.[68] The key objective of euthanasia is to cause an immediate loss of consciousness that remains until death. For this to occur, the cerebral hemispheres and brainstem (including the midbrain, pons, and medulla oblongata) must be damaged. Suitable forms of euthanasia for adult sheep and goats include a lethal overdose of barbiturates, gunshot, and penetrating or nonpenetrating captive bolt devices.[68] The use of barbiturates causes a smooth transition to unconsciousness and death, although they can only be administered by a licensed veterinarian, which can increase the costs associated with euthanasia.[68] Physical methods of euthanasia that include gunshot and captive bolt devices (penetrating or nonpenetrating) cause an immediate loss of consciousness and death; however, the efficacy of these devices depends on the anatomic location and the directional aim used.[69] Gunshot may put the operator or bystanders at risk because the bullet may travel through the skull and ricochet off solid surfaces. Controlled blunt force trauma using nonpenetrating captive bolt devices deliver a consistent force and cause rapid loss of consciousness and death in goat kids up to 3 weeks of age.[70–72] Note that the target location for adult sheep and goats is similar between species (**Fig. 11**). The recommendation for euthanizing neonates is to use a nonpenetrating captive bolt (or penetrating captive bolt if this can be done without risk of injury to the operator; **Fig. 12**), which should be accompanied by an adjunctive method to ensure death. Examples of appropriate adjunctive methods to follow the use of the captive bolt include intravenous injection of potassium chloride or exsanguination.

There is limited information available on the care, handling, and transport of nonambulatory sheep and goats; however, there is a considerable amount of information available on nonambulatory cattle. Generally, nonambulatory or "downer" cattle are referred to as those that are unable to stand after 24 hours of recumbency.[73] Causes of nonambulatory animals include and are not limited to injuries, metabolic disorders, and infectious or toxic diseases. The primary response is to physically examine the animal, which will help to make a diagnosis. Treatment and care of nonambulatory animals should aim to correct the primary cause of recumbency, while minimizing secondary nerve and muscle damage.[73] Nonambulatory animals should be sheltered from inclement weather and segregated from healthy animals that might cause further injury to the downer animal. Additionally, they should have direct access to feed and water from their position; the provision of feed and water in the pen is not useful if the animal cannot move to be able to access it. Medical treatment should be used to mediate dehydration, inflammation, infection, and metabolic derangements.[73] At a minimum, downer animals should be assessed every 12 hours. If aggressive medical treatment and supportive care fail to result in measurable improvement within 24 hours, euthanasia should be considered. Animals that are improving should continue to be reassessed for progress every 12 hours with euthanasia considered

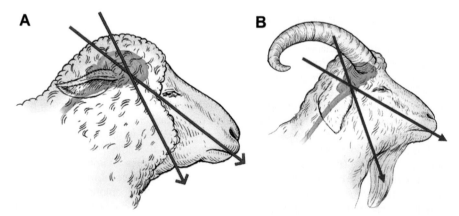

Fig. 11. The correct anatomic location in sheep (A) and goats (B) for captive bolt placements for euthanasia. (*Courtesy of* J. Shearer, DVM, Ames, IA.)

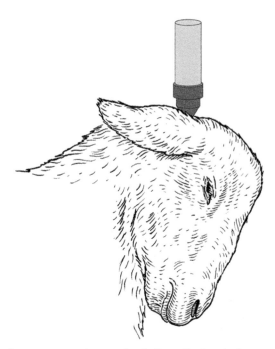

Fig. 12. Position of a nonpenetrating captive bolt on the head of a neonatal kid with the chin tucked into the chest, to expose the occipital protuberance. (*Data from* Grist A, Lines JA, Knowles TG, et al. Use of a non-penetrating captive bolt for euthanasia of neonate goats. *Animals.* 2018;8(4):58 and Sutherland MA, Watson TJ, Johnson CB, et al. Evaluation of the efficacy of a non-penetrating captive bolt to euthanase neonatal goats up to 48 hours of age. *Anim Welfare* 2016;25(4):471-479.)

if progress stalls out or is lost. It is completely unacceptable to take a "wait and see if they get better" approach to downer animals that are unable to stand. If a complete physical examination, treatment, and supportive care are not feasible, these animals should be euthanized (**Box 1**).

Common bedding materials such as straw, corn stalks, or wood chip/saw dust may not allow for regular hoof wear, compared with harder surfaces (eg, concrete). However, sufficient bedding is required for comfort around resting and patches of bare floor in the lying areas should be avoided. Additionally, the cleanliness of the bedding can affect lying behavior and can be assessed visually from outside of the pen. Ideally, sheep and goats should be given the opportunity to use both soft and hard surfaces.

Further management-based indicators that can be assessed include the cleanliness of the water troughs or feeders, access ways, and the milking parlor; vaccination or deworming program; the level of record keeping; and procedures for protection from inclement weather or pain relief use. These management-based indicators could be discussed with the producer during regular visits or a phone call.

RESOURCE-BASED INDICATORS

Resource-based indicators can be assessed objectively and are concerned with the resources available to the animal; these indicators include the quantity and quality of the feed and water supply, space per goat in the lying areas, outdoor spaces,

---

Box 1
Components of care for recumbent/"downer" small ruminants

- Provide clean feed and water that are easily accessible to the downer animal.
- Provide deep bedding to protect the downer animal from myonecrosis.
- Avoid dragging or pulling the animal; consider using slings to help move the animal when needed.
- Regularly observe the animals.
- Shift the animal from side to side to maintain even blood flow in the tissues.
- Observe urination and defecation, remove feces and wet bedding.
- Monitor air temperature and adjust environment as necessary to help prevent the down animal from getting too hot or too cold.
- Monitor body temperature.

---

and any other resource of value to an animal. The assessment of stocking density and shelter from extreme climates can be reliable measures of welfare for both sheep and goats.[3] It has been suggested that a stocking density of less than 2 m^2 (21.5 ft^2) may increase mastitis prevalence and reduce milk yield in sheep.[74] Furthermore, goats spent less time feeding in pens stocked at 1 m^2/goat (10.7 ft^2/goat) compared with 2 m^2/goat (21.5 ft^2/goat), which demonstrates decreased production efficiency.[17] Further research on stocking densities and the effect on animal welfare are required.

It is vital that a water source is available, especially in the extensive environments that small ruminants (ie, sheep) are often farmed. Waterers should be checked to ensure that they are clean, in good working order, and that multiple waterers are available (when needed) to decrease crowding.[10]

ANIMAL CRUELTY, ABUSE, AND NEGLECT

Cruelty to animals, abuse, and neglect are terms that are often used interchangeably; however, it is important to note their distinction. Animal cruelty is generally defined as any act by intention (or neglect) that causes unnecessary pain, distress, suffering, or death. Animal abuse is willfully failing to provide care or causing harm and implies maltreatment regardless of the intent, whereas animal neglect denotes a lack of care whereby the basic necessities of life are not provided (eg, an adequate amount of food, shelter, water, and veterinary care). Neglect is most commonly investigated by animal protection authorities.[75]

Based on their knowledge and expertise, a veterinary practitioner may be called on to assist with investigations into animal cruelty, abuse, or neglect. These cases are often difficult to deal with emotionally and can have legal consequences, which should be considered before agreeing to participate in the process. However, in some states it may be required by law to report any evidence of animal cruelty, abuse, or neglect. For detailed information on practical guidance for veterinary response to cruelty, abuse, and neglect, including laws and regulations for each state, see the American Veterinary Medical Association document prepared by Arkow and colleagues.[75] It is important to note the progress in the recognition of animal maltreatment that has been made. First, a relatively new and emerging field of veterinary forensics has been developed to provide training in clinical identification of conditions usually associated with animal abuse.[76] Second, considering the link between animal abuse and domestic violence, various laws have been enacted granting veterinarians with absolute or limited immunity for reporting suspected family violence.[75]

There is no one clear indicator of animal cruelty, abuse, or neglect, but rather multiple indictors as outlined within this article. An example from sheep and goat production may include poor body condition and the lack of feed readily available or evidence of a management plan and veterinary treatment. Any form of animal cruelty, abuse, or neglect is not acceptable, and veterinarians have a pivotal role in identification of potential maltreatment, which should be raised to the appropriate agency. Despite the difficulties these kinds of situations present, veterinarians are a key advocate for animals and optimal animal welfare should be their highest priority.

SUMMATION OF INDICATORS OF WELFARE

Once a variety of indicators of welfare have been evaluated, and any areas for concern have been highlighted, conclusions on the welfare status of the animals should be made. However, it is important that follow-up visits are conducted to ensure that what was observed on the farm on 1 day was not an isolated event. For example, if fresh bedding was not added to the pen owing to inclement weather and the animals displayed poor hygiene, this situation does not necessarily mean that the animals are experiencing poor welfare. On a subsequent visit, the animals may have clean bedding and good hygiene. However, if over a period of time an animals' body condition remains poor and there has been no effort to improve its condition by providing more feed or administering treatment for a disease, then this may equate to poor welfare and require outside intervention. A further issue to reflect on is whether there are multiple animals with compromised welfare. If a single goat had severely overgrown hooves and was lame as a consequence, this animal may have simply been missed at the time of hoof trimming. In comparison, a herd of lame goats with overgrown hooves does indicate welfare compromise.

In cases where farms have elected to participate in third-party auditing, the results of the audit are objectively compared with the standard set out by the certification program and the farm is certified or deemed to be in noncompliance. However, in cases where farms are not part of a certification program, there are presently no industry standards on which to compare sheep or goat welfare. Therefore, it is incumbent on the practitioner to work with the producer to build consensus and improvement. Some industries are working on benchmarking projects that would further allow practitioners to compare the results of an operation to peers.

It is vital to maintain an open and fluid communication with the producer on key findings on observations of welfare assessment to ensure willingness and compliance. In some cases, it might be beneficial to provide information in the form of a brief report where the information can be presented visually as well as verbally. Visual feedback can effectively highlight areas of positive welfare and areas that can be improved.

SUMMARY

The indicators of welfare highlighted in this article can be (1) used without the requirement for animal restraint, (2) conducted in the home pen (which both can decrease stress), and (3) used to observe multiple animals efficiently. It is vital to remember that the first step of improving the welfare of sheep and goats is to accurately identify areas of welfare compromise. Practitioners can play a key role in aiding animal managers to identify areas of potential welfare compromise and implement suitable interventions. With the knowledge and careful identification of indicators of welfare, practitioners can work together with producers to develop a management plan that can ensure proper (1) nutrition, environment, and health to allow for natural behaviors and a positive affective state of sheep and goats, (2) animal management, and (3) allocation of adequate resources to improve the welfare of sheep and goats.

CLINICS CARE POINTS

- External or independent welfare assessment from welfare auditors is recommended to identify deficiencies in animal management.
- Animal welfare cannot be directly measured; however, it can be evaluated using a multifactorial approach and quantifying multiple variables to provide an accurate reflection of the current welfare status.
- Focus on animal-related indicators of welfare because they most accurately reflect animal welfare status.
- A reasonable clinical working definition good animal welfare as an animal in a state where its nutritional, environmental, health, behavioral, and mental (ie, affective state) needs are met.
- Management-based indicators assess how animals are managed by stock handlers and can be collected in an objective manner.
- Examples of management practices that can be evaluated include disbudding, castration or tail docking, environmental cleanliness, feed distribution including quality and amount, and regular veterinary care.
- Resource-based indicators can be assessed objectively and are concerned with the resources available to the animal; these indicators include the quantity and quality of the feed and water supply, space per goat in the lying areas, outdoor spaces and any other resource of value to an animal.
- Animal cruelty is generally defined as any act by intention (or neglect) that causes unnecessary pain, distress, suffering, or death.
- Animal abuse is willfully failing to provide care or causing harm and implies maltreatment regardless of the intent.
- Animal neglect denotes a lack of care whereby the basic necessities of life are not provided (eg, adequate amount of food, shelter, water, and veterinary care).

REFERENCES

1. Mellor DJ, Reid CSW. Concepts of animal well-being and predicting the impact of procedures on experimental animals. In: Baker RM, Jenkin G, Mellor DJ, editors. Improving the well-being of animals in the research environment. Adelaide (Australia): ANZCART; 1993. p. 3–18.
2. Battini M, Vieira A, Barbieri S, et al. Invited review: animal-based indicators for on-farm welfare assessment for dairy goats. J Dairy Sci 2014;97(11):6625–48.
3. Caroprese M, Casamassima D, Rassu SPG, et al. Monitoring the on-farm welfare of sheep and goats. Ital J Anim Sci 2009;8:343–54.
4. The Euorpean Animal Welfare Indicators Project. AWIN welfare assessment protocol for goats. Online Report. 2015. Available at: https://air.unimi.it/retrieve/handle/2434/269102/384790/AWINProtocolGoats.pdf. Accessed June 9, 2020.
5. The Euorpean Animal Welfare Indicators Project. AWIN welfare assessment protocol for sheep. Online Report. 2015. Available at: http://uni-sz.bg/truni11/wp-content/uploads/biblioteka/file/TUNI10015667(1).pdf. Accessed June 9, 2020.

6. Main DCJ, Kent JP, Wemelsfelder F, et al. Applications for methods of on-farm welfare assessment. Anim Welfare 2003;12(4):523–8.

7. Stilwell G. Small ruminants' welfare assessment—Dairy goat as an example. Small Rumin Res 2016;142:51–4.

8. Ferguson JD, Azzaro G, Licitra G. Body condition assessment using digital images. J Dairy Sci 2006;89(10):3833–41.

9. Vieira A, Brandão S, Monteiro A, et al. Development and validation of a visual body condition scoring system for dairy goats with picture-based training. J Dairy Sci 2015;98(9):6597–608.

10. Munoz CA, Campbell AJD, Hemsworth PH, et al. Evaluating the welfare of extensively managed sheep. PLoS One 2019;14(6):e0218603.

11. Muri K, Stubsjoen SM, Valle PS. Development and testing of an on-farm welfare assessment protocol for dairy goats. Anim Welfare 2013;22(3):385–400.

12. Can E, Vieira A, Battini M, et al. On-farm welfare assessment of dairy goat farms using animal-based indicators: the example of 30 commercial farms in Portugal. Acta Agric Scand A Anim Sci 2016;66(1):43–55.

13. Phythian CJ, Michalopoulou E, Jones PH, et al. Validating indicators of sheep welfare through a consensus of expert opinion. Animal 2011;5(6):943–52.

14. Nielsen BL, de Jong IC, De Vries TJ. The Use of Feeding Behaviour in the Assessment of Animal Welfare. In: Phillips CJC, editor. Nutrition and the welfare of farm animals. Cham (Switzerland): Springer International Publishing; 2016. p. 59–84.

15. Bøe KE, Andersen IL. Competition, activity budget and feed intake of ewes when reducing the feeding space. Appl Anim Behav Sci 2010;125(3–4):109–14.

16. Battini M, Barbieri S, Vieira A, et al. Results of testing the prototype of the AWIN welfare assessment protocol for dairy goats in 30 intensive farms in Northern Italy. Ital J Anim Sci 2016;15(2):283–93.

17. Loretz C, Wechsler B, Hauser R, et al. A comparison of space requirements of horned and hornless goats at the feed barrier and in the lying area. Appl Anim Behav Sci 2004;87(3–4):275–83.

18. Jørgensen GHM, Andersen IL, Bøe KE. Feed intake and social interactions in dairy goats—The effects of feeding space and type of roughage. Appl Anim Behav Sci 2007;107(3):239–51.

19. Contreras-Jodar A, Nayan NH, Hamzaoui S, et al. Heat stress modifies the lactational performances and the urinary metabolomic profile related to gastrointestinal microbiota of dairy goats. PLoS One 2019;14(2):e0202457.

20. Salama AAK, Caja G, Hamzaoui S, et al. Different levels of response to heat stress in dairy goats. Small Rumin Res 2014;121(1):73–9.

21. Chauhan SS, Celi P, Leury BJ, et al. Dietary antioxidants at supranutritional doses improve oxidative status and reduce the negative effects of heat stress in sheep. J Anim Sci 2014;92(8):3364–74.

22. Sevi A, Caroprese M. Impact of heat stress on milk production, immunity and udder health in sheep: a critical review. Small Rumin Res 2012;107(1):1–7.

23. Jørgensen GHM, Bøe KE. Outdoor yards for sheep during winter – Effects of feed location, roof and weather factors on resting and activity. Can J Anim Sci 2011; 91(2):213–20.

24. Bøe KE, Ehrlenbruch R. Thermoregulatory behavior of dairy goats at low temperatures and the use of outdoor yards. Can J Anim Sci 2013;93(1):35–41.

25. Curtis SE. Environmental management in animal agriculture. Ames (IA): Iowa State University Press; 1983.

26. Battini M, Barbieri S, Waiblinger S, et al. Validity and feasibility of Human-Animal Relationship tests for on-farm welfare assessment in dairy goats. Appl Anim Behav Sci 2016;178:32–9.

27. Sant'Anna AC, Paranhos da Costa MJR. The relationship between dairy cow hygiene and somatic cell count in milk. J Dairy Sci 2011;94(8):3835–44.

28. Schreiner DA, Ruegg PL. Relationship between udder and leg hygiene scores and subclinical mastitis. J Dairy Sci 2003;86(11):3460–5.

29. Anzuino K, Bell NJ, Bazeley KJ, et al. Assessment of welfare on 24 commercial UK dairy goat farms based on direct observations. Vet Rec 2010;167(20):774–80.

30. Munoz C, Campbell A, Hemsworth P, et al. Animal-based measures to assess the welfare of extensively managed ewes. Animals (Basel) 2017;8(1):2.

31. McLennan KM, Rebelo CJB, Corke MJ, et al. Development of a facial expression scale using footrot and mastitis as models of pain in sheep. Appl Anim Behav Sci 2016;176:19–26.

32. Mavrogianni VS, Fthenakis GC, Burriel AR, et al. Experimentally induced teat stenosis in dairy ewes: clinical, pathological and ultrasonographic features. J Comp Pathol 2004;130(1):70–4.

33. Munoz C, Campbell A, Barber S, et al. Using longitudinal assessment on extensively managed ewes to quantify welfare compromise and risks. Animals 2018; 8(1):8.

34. Scholtz AJ, Cloete SWP, Cloete JJE, et al. Divergent selection for reproduction affects dag score, breech wrinkle score and crutching time in Merinos South African. J Anim Sci 2012;42:274–9.

35. Phillips CJC. A review of mulesing and other methods to control flystrike (cutaneous myiasis) in sheep. Anim Welfare 2009;18(2):113–21.

36. Leathwick DM, Atkinson DS. Dagginess and flystrike in lambs grazed on Lotus corniculatus or ryegrass. Proceedings of the New Zealand Society of Animal Production. Hamilton, NZ, 1995. p. 55.

37. Windsor PA. Control of caseous lymphadenitis. Vet Clin North Am Food Anim Pract 2011;27(1):193–202.

38. Menzies PI, Muckle CA, Brogden KA, et al. A field trial to evaluate a whole cell vaccine for the prevention of caseous lymphadenitis in sheep and goat flocks. Can J Vet Res 1991;55(4):362–6.

39. Sutherland MA, Tucker CB. The long and short of it: a review of tail docking in farm animals. Appl Anim Behav Sci 2011;135(3):179–91.

40. Thomas DL, Waldron DF, Lowe GD, et al. Length of docked tail and the incidence of rectal prolapse in lambs. J Anim Sci 2003;81(11):2725–32.

41. Fisher MW, Gregory NG, Kent JE, et al. Justifying the appropriate length for docking lambs' tails - a review of the literature. Proceedings of the New Zealand Society of Animal Production; Jan, 2004; Hamilton.

42. Lloyd J, Kessell A, Barchia I, et al. Docked tail length is a risk factor for bacterial arthritis in lambs. Small Rumin Res 2016;144:17–22.

43. Small A, Belson S, Holm M, et al. Efficacy of a buccal meloxicam formulation for pain relief in Merino lambs undergoing knife castration and tail docking in a randomised field trial. Aust Vet J 2014;92(10):381–8.

44. Ley SJ, Waterman AE, Livingston A. A field study of the effect of lameness on mechanical nociceptive thresholds in sheep. Vet Rec 1995;137(4):85–7.

45. Hill NP, Murphy PE, Nelson AJ, et al. Lameness and foot lesions in adult British dairy goats. Vet Rec 1997;141(16):412–6.

46. Smith MC, Sherman DM. Fundamentals of goat practice. In: Smith MC, Sherman DM, editors. Goat medicine. 2nd edition. Ames (IA): Wiley-Blackwell; 2009. p. 3–20.

47. Winter AC. Lameness in sheep. Small Rumin Res 2008;76(1):149–53.

48. Deeming LE, Beausoleil NJ, Stafford KJ, et al. Technical note: the development of a reliable 5-point gait scoring system for use in dairy goats. J Dairy Sci 2018; 101(5):4491–7.

49. Welsh EM, Gettinby G, Nolan AM. Comparison of a visual analogue scale and a numerical rating scale for assessment of lameness, using sheep as a model. Am J Vet Res 1993;54(6):976–83.

50. Vieira A, Oliveira MD, Nunes T, et al. Making the case for developing alternative lameness scoring systems for dairy goats. Appl Anim Behav Sci 2015;171: 94–100.

51. Ajuda I, Battini M, Mattiello S, et al. Evaluation of pain mitigation strategies in goat kids after cautery disbudding. Animals 2020;10(2):277.

52. Alvarez L, De Luna JB, Gamboa D, et al. Cortisol and pain-related behavior in dis-budded goat kids with and without cornual nerve block. Physiol Behav 2015; 138(0):58–61.

53. Hempstead MN, Waas JR, Stewart M, et al. Effect of isoflurane alone or in com-bination with meloxicam on the behavior and physiology of goat kids following cautery disbudding. J Dairy Sci 2018;101(4):3193–204.

54. Ingvast-Larsson C, Hogberg M, Mengistu U, et al. Pharmacokinetics of meloxi-cam in adult goats and its analgesic effect in disbudded kids. J Vet Pharmacol Ther 2011;34(1):64–9.

55. Nfor ON, Chan JPW, Kere M, et al. Disbudding pain: the benefits of disbudding goat kids with dexmedetomidine hydrochloride. Small Rumin Res 2016;139:60–6.

56. Waiblinger S, Schmied-Wagner C, Mersmann D, et al. Social behaviour and in-juries in horned and hornless dairy goats. Proceedings of the XVth International Congress of the International Society for Animal Hygiene; 2011; Vienna, Austria.

57. Paull DR, Small AH, Lee C, et al. Evaluating a novel analgesic strategy for ring castration of ram lambs. Vet Anaesth Analg 2012;39(5):539–49.

58. Waiblinger S, Boivin X, Pedersen V, et al. Assessing the human–animal relation-ship in farmed species: a critical review. Appl Anim Behav Sci 2006;101(3): 185–242.

59. Lyons DM. Individual differences in temperament of dairy goats and the inhibition of milk ejection. Appl Anim Behav Sci 1989;22(3):269–82.

60. Napolitano F, Caroprese M, Girolami A, et al. Effects of early maternal separation of lambs and rearing with minimal and maximal human contact on meat quality. Meat Sci 2006;72(4):635–40.

61. Goddard P, Waterhouse T, Dwyer C, et al. The perception of the welfare of sheep in extensive systems. Small Rumin Res 2006;62(3):215–25.

62. Forkman B, Boissy A, Meunier-Salaün MC, et al. A critical review of fear tests used on cattle, pigs, sheep, poultry and horses. Physiol Behav 2007;92(3): 340–74.

63. Jackson KMA, Hackett D. A note: the effects of human handling on heart girth, behaviour and milk quality in dairy goats. Appl Anim Behav Sci 2007;108(3): 332–6.

64. Hargreaves AL, Hutson GD. The effect of gentling on heart rate, flight distance and aversion of sheep to a handling procedure. Appl Anim Behav Sci 1990; 26(3):243–52.

65. Richmond SE, Wemelsfelder F, de Heredia IB, et al. Evaluation of animal-based indicators to be used in a welfare assessment protocol for sheep. Front Vet Sci 2017;4:210.
66. Martínez-de la Puente J, Moreno-Indias I, Morales-Delanuez A, et al. Effects of feeding management and time of day on the occurrence of self-suckling in dairy goats. Vet Rec 2011;168(14):378.
67. Mattiello S, Battini M, De Rosa G, et al. How Can We Assess Positive Welfare in Ruminants? Animals 2019;9(10):758.
68. AVMA. In: AVMA Guidelines for the euthanasia of animals, 2020. Schaumburg, IL: American Veterinary Medical Association; 2020. Available at: https://www.avma.org/sites/default/files/2020-01/2020-Euthanasia-Final-1-17-20.pdf. Accessed June 9, 2020.
69. Plummer PJ, Shearer JK, Kleinhenz KE, et al. Determination of anatomic landmarks for optimal placement in captive-bolt euthanasia of goats. Am J Vet Res 2018;79(3):276–81.
70. Grist A, Lines JA, Knowles TG, et al. Use of a non-penetrating captive bolt for euthanasia of neonate goats. Animals 2018;8(4):58.
71. Sutherland MA, Watson TJ, Johnson CB, et al. Evaluation of the efficacy of a non-penetrating captive bolt to euthanase neonatal goats up to 48 hours of age. Anim Welfare 2016;25(4):471–9.
72. Sutherland MA, Watson TJ, Millman ST. Technical contribution: evaluation of the efficacy of a non-penetrating captive bolt to euthanase dairy goat kids up to 30 days of age. Anim Welfare 2017;26(3):277–80.
73. Stull CL, Payne MA, Berry SL, et al. A review of the causes, prevention, and welfare of nonambulatory cattle. J Am Vet Med Assoc 2007;231(2):227–34.
74. Sevi A, Massa S, Annicchiarico G, et al. Effect of stocking density on ewes' milk yield, udder health and microenvironment. J Dairy Res 1999;66(4):489–99.
75. Arkow P, Boyden P, Patterson-Kane E. Practical guidance for the effective response by veterinarians to suspected animal cruelty, abuse and neglect. Schaumburg, IL. Available at: https://ebusiness.avma.org/Files/ProductDownloads/AVMA%20Suspected%20Animal%20Cruelty.pdf. American Veterinary Medical Association. Accessed January 12, 2021.
76. Parry NMA, Stoll A. The rise of veterinary forensics. Forensic Sci Int 2020;306: 110069.

Abdominal Imaging in Small Ruminants: Liver, Spleen, Gastrointestinal Tract, and Lymph Nodes

Susanne M. Stieger-Vanegas, Dr med vet, PhD*,
Erica McKenzie, BSc, BVMS, PhD

KEYWORDS

- Computed tomography • Goat • Radiography • Sheep • Ultrasound

KEY POINTS

- Ultrasound is a quick, noninvasive method of assessing small ruminants with abdominal disease.
- Transcutaneous ultrasound provides information about amount and type of peritoneal fluid, liver and spleen parenchyma, gallbladder, rumen and intestinal content and motility, intestinal wall thickness, and abdominal lymph nodes.
- Contrast-enhanced computed tomography is an excellent technique to obtain summation-free images of the abdomen, providing detailed information about disease of the parenchymal abdominal organs and gastrointestinal structures.

INTRODUCTION

Small ruminants commonly present with abdominal disease, especially involving the urinary, reproductive, and gastrointestinal tracts. Abdominal imaging is often an essential procedure in the clinical decision-making process because it can be challenging to definitively relate abdominal disease to a specific organ or organ system from history and physical examination alone. Furthermore, small ruminants are becoming popular pets. This has resulted in more small ruminants undergoing abdominal imaging, and more advanced techniques such as computed tomography (CT) being used more frequently for comprehensive evaluation.

Clinical evaluation of the small ruminant abdomen can be challenging because palpation can be limited by their size and rumen content and is frequently confined to the caudal abdomen. The use of plain radiography, contrast radiography, ultrasound, or combinations have been reported for evaluation of suspected reproductive,

Department of Clinical Sciences, Carlson College of Veterinary Medicine, Oregon State University, Magruder Hall, 700 Southwest 30th Street, Corvallis, OR 97331, USA
* Corresponding author.
E-mail address: Susanne.stieger@oregonstate.edu

Vet Clin Food Anim 37 (2021) 55–74
https://doi.org/10.1016/j.cvfa.2020.10.001
0749-0720/21/© 2020 Elsevier Inc. All rights reserved.
vetfood.theclinics.com

gastrointestinal, and urinary tract disease. However, radiography is often limited by difficulty achieving adequate penetration of the abdomen in these species. Contrast radiography for evaluation of the gastrointestinal tract has now been largely replaced by ultrasonography or, when available, CT.

EXAMINATION TECHNIQUE

Before performing any imaging study in a small ruminant, the wool or fiber should be brushed to remove superficial debris, which can create artifacts (**Fig. 1**) in radiographic or CT studies. For ultrasound, the fiber or wool can be split apart or clipped to access the skin, which is moistened with gel or alcohol. Ultrasound and radiography are often performed in standing animals or can be performed with the animal typically in lateral or ventral recumbency. Radiography and ultrasound can be performed in manually restrained animals; however, sedation may be required. For an abdominal CT study, depending on the scanner available and the expected length of the study, sedation or anesthesia is usually required unless the animal is obtunded. In addition, an intravenous catheter should be placed to provide access for contrast administration, which allows better evaluation of the parenchymal organs in CT, and potentially for emergency drug administration. Without intravenous contrast agent administration, normal and abnormal tissue often have a very low difference in attenuation on CT and cannot be readily differentiated. In contrast-enhanced CT, abnormal tissue might be distinguished from normal surrounding tissues by the difference in contrast enhancement pattern and behavior. In addition, contrast-enhanced CT also allows evaluation of vascular structures and performance of timed studies, providing information about various abdominal vessels and organs.

PERITONEAL CAVITY
Neonates and Juvenile Animals

Neonates and very young animals lack intraperitoneal fat, and the fat that is present (brown fat) has a higher water content making identification and differentiation of

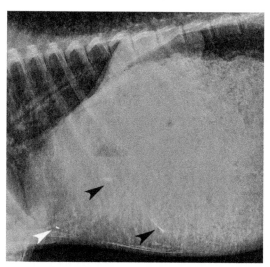

Fig. 1. Lateral abdominal radiograph of a 4-month-old lamb, demonstrating wool artifact and metal objects in the ventral aspect of the reticulum (*white arrowhead*) and rumen (*black arrowhead*).

abdominal organs difficult using radiography. It is important to differentiate normally reduced serosal detail in young animals from excessive peritoneal fluid (**Fig. 2**). Ultrasound is an excellent technique to evaluate the entire abdomen of young animals, including the umbilicus.

Body Condition

In animals with a large amount of peritoneal fat, such as mature dwarf breeds or Boer goats, reduced penetration of the radiographic beam may occur, resulting in increased scatter and lack of contrast between abdominal organs. Abdominal ultrasound also may be more challenging; organs may be harder to scan in their entirety and the liver or pancreas may appear subjectively increased in echogenicity because of apposition with hypoechoic intra-abdominal fat.

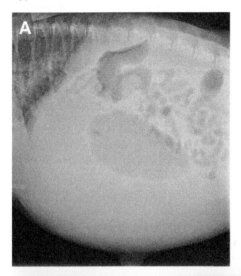

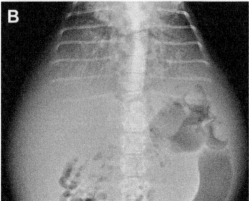

Fig. 2. Lateral (*A*) and ventrodorsal (*B*) abdominal radiographs of a 2-week-old kid with respiratory distress and abdominal enlargement. The cardiac silhouette (not visible) was severely enlarged. A large amount of peritoneal fluid is displacing the gas-filled gastrointestinal tract dorsally in the lateral view and centrally in the ventrodorsal view. A diffuse unstructured interstitial lung pattern is noted in the dorsal aspects of the caudal lung lobes due to cardiogenic edema. Necropsy revealed a complex cardiac abnormality causing right-sided and left-sided heart failure.

Peritoneal Disease

Reduced peritoneal detail

A wide range of physiologic and pathologic conditions, including young age, emaciation, increased peritoneal fluid, and carcinomatosis can reduce peritoneal detail in all imaging modalities. Ultrasound or CT can help differentiate etiologies and facilitate guided sampling of abdominal fluid or lesions.

Peritoneal fluid

Peritoneal fluid causes reduced serosal detail on radiography and CT (see **Fig. 2**), independent of the nature of the fluid (eg, transudate, exudate, urine, bile). If a small amount is present, wispy soft tissue attenuation of the abdomen resulting in reduced definition of abdominal organs may be noted on radiographs or CT images; however, large amounts of fluid can cause the abdomen to appear uniform in soft tissue opacity and displacement of the intestinal tract by the fluid frequently occurs (see **Fig. 2**). Furthermore, when radiographs are obtained in standing animals, a horizontal fluid line may be noted exterior to intestinal structures (**Fig. 3**). In addition, distension of

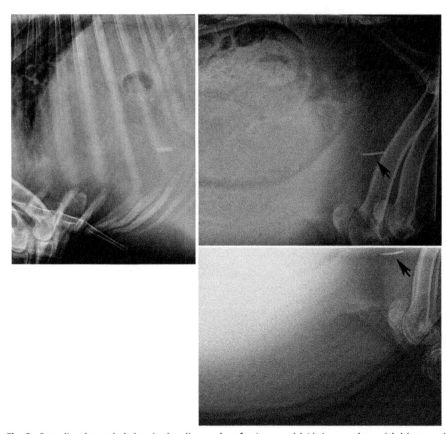

Fig. 3. Standing lateral abdominal radiographs of a 4-year-old Alpine wether with bloat and inappetence for 3 days. A large amount of soft tissue attenuating material is evident in the ventral abdomen. The urinary bladder is ill-defined, and summating with this area is a small amount of granular mineral-attenuating material (*black arrow*). Urinary bladder rupture secondary to obstructive urolithiasis was confirmed at necropsy.

the abdomen, including ventral displacement of the abdominal wall, is often present; however, this also can occur in obese animals. Carcinomatosis related to metastatic seeding of tumor cells throughout the peritoneal cavity can also cause increased peritoneal fluid, and nodules or masses.[1,2] Ultrasound is more sensitive than radiography for detecting small amounts of peritoneal fluid, or an irregular peritoneal surface or peritoneal nodules. Scant quantities of anechoic fluid are normal in most species. Peritoneal fluid can easily be detected with the animal standing or in lateral recumbency; common sites where fluid accumulates include between the liver lobes and at the cranioventral aspect of the urinary bladder, where an anechoic triangle can be seen. Ultrasonography often permits determination of fluid quality; transudate or modified transudates are commonly anechoic, and exudates frequently appear echogenic in nature. Ultrasound cannot differentiate between septic or nonseptic peritonitis, and if there is concern for a septic process, ultrasound-guided fluid sampling and analysis should be performed.

Peritoneal gas (pneumoperitoneum)

Peritoneal gas is often iatrogenic, secondary to abdominocentesis or surgical procedures, and can likely persist for 1 month or more postsurgery. Pathologic causes of peritoneal gas include penetrating injury to the abdomen (**Fig. 4**), and rupture or perforation of the gastrointestinal tract. Recognition of peritoneal gas in the absence of a prior interventional procedure comprises a surgical emergency and it is therefore critical to recognize. In standing patients, gas usually rises to the highest aspect of the

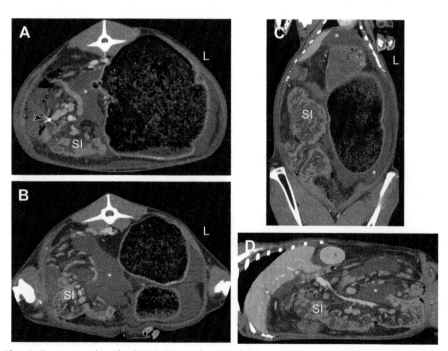

Fig. 4. Transverse (*A, B*), dorsal (*C*), and sagittal (*D*) contrast-enhanced CT images of the abdomen of a 1.5-year-old Anglo-Nubian doe with history of tachypnea and abdominal distension. Excessive peritoneal fluid (*asterisk*) containing small gas bubbles is evident displacing the intestinal tract centrally and dorsally. A metallic ballistic object (*arrowhead*) is present in the mid-right cranial abdomen. Findings are consistent with ballistic injury, pneumoperitoneum, and septic peritonitis. L, left; SI, small intestine.

abdomen and can be located close to the spine. In laterally recumbent patients, gas usually rises to the area of the costal arch. Small quantities of air may be noted in dorsally recumbent patients, where a horizontal lateral radiograph is obtained, and gas may be noted along the inner (peritoneal) aspect of the ventral abdominal wall. Ultrasound is a sensitive method for detection of small amounts of gas, which are usually noted as a hyperechoic band or pinpoint area with reverberation artifacts. However, ultrasound is operator-dependent, and small quantities of gas may be missed with lack of operator experience. In addition, peritoneal gas should not be confused with the normal lung, which also creates reverberation artifacts that may partially reduce the ability to visualize cranial abdominal organs.

Hernias and diaphragmatic/abdominal wall rupture

Hernias often arise as congenital defects in the peritoneal lining and boundaries of the peritoneal cavity, and commonly include the diaphragm, abdominal wall including umbilicus, and inguinal, perineal, and scrotal areas.[3–5] Traumatic events can lead to acquired rupture of the diaphragm, and trauma or surgical incision dehiscence to defects of the abdominal wall in mature animals.

Radiography and ultrasound are often the first modalities used to evaluate a hernia or rupture for displacement or compromise of abdominal organs (**Figs. 5** and **6**). Diaphragmatic hernias are rare in small ruminants but have been reported secondary to trauma in goats, and as a potentially congenital phenomenon in sheep.[4–6] On radiographs or CT, abnormal cranial displacement of abdominal organs may be noted (see **Fig. 5**). If a diaphragmatic hernia or rupture is suspected, radiography or CT provide more information than ultrasound, because reverberation artifacts from air-filled lung tissue limit evaluation of the entire diaphragm by ultrasound.

Radiography and CT also can be used to evaluate abdominal wall hernias and ruptures; however, ultrasound is often preferred because it is more readily available than CT and offers superior evaluation of soft tissues than radiography. Both ultrasound and CT allow evaluation of defects in the abdominal wall in addition to evaluation of displaced organs and secondary effects such as increased peritoneal fluid. Using ultrasound or CT, separation of the peritoneum and muscular aspect of the abdominal

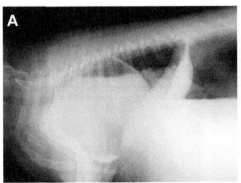
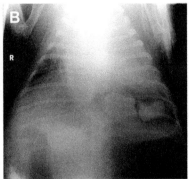

Fig. 5. Lateral (*A*) and ventrodorsal (*B*) radiographs of the caudal thorax and cranial abdomen of an 8-month-old sheep with a 1-month history of respiratory distress. Summating with the left caudoventral thorax and extending into the left cranial abdomen, there is a large, round soft tissue attenuating structure with a large dorsal gas cap. The left diaphragmatic crus is not identified. The cardiac silhouette and lungs are right laterally displaced, and the left lung is diffusely soft tissue attenuating. Diaphragmatic hernia or rupture with cranial displacement of the reticulum is suspected.

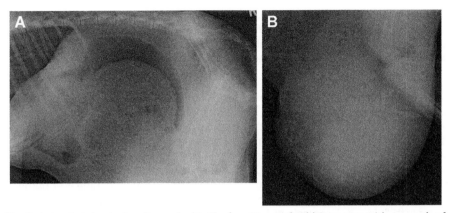

Fig. 6. Lateral abdominal radiographs (*A, B*) of an 11-month-old Soay ewe with 1 month of weight loss, and abdominal and mammary distension. A large defect in the abdominal wall is evident with displacement of the caudoventral aspect of the rumen and the gravid uterus ventrally into the defect. There are no radiographic signs of fetal death, and the 2 fetuses had normal heart rates on percutaneous ultrasound.

wall can be detected; in addition, displacement of peritoneal fat and organs may be present.[3] Ultrasound and contrast-enhanced CT can provide additional information about the viability of intestines and the urinary bladder if incarceration of these organs is suspected.

PARENCHYMAL ABDOMINAL ORGANS AND DISEASE
Liver

In ruminants, the liver is positioned predominately right of midline due to location of the voluminous rumen in the mid-to-left cranial abdomen. Compared with other domestic species, the liver has minimal lobation; however, a right, left, quadrate, and caudate lobe are described. The caudate process is relatively large in ruminating species, extending beyond the margin of the right liver lobe, and together with the right liver lobe contains the renal fossa in which the cranial aspect of the right kidney resides.[7,8] The gallbladder of small ruminants has a narrow pear shape and is located adjacent to the visceral surface of the liver and connected to the liver by connective tissue.[7]

Radiography provides very limited information about the liver. Ultrasound is most commonly used for through evaluation of the liver. The liver can be viewed from the right seventh to ninth intercostal space (ICS); in some goats, the cranial aspect can be seen in the right 5th to 6th ICS and the most caudal extent in the right 10th to 12th ICS.[8] Some aspects of the liver also can be seen with the transducer positioned caudal to the xiphoid. The portal vein is more ventrally positioned than the caudal vena cava and can be seen in most of the liver. The caudal vena cava can usually be seen only in the 11th to 12th ICS and has a triangular cross-section.[8] The hepatic veins are largest cranially and decrease in size caudally. The portal vein divides into its branches at the porta hepatis and the branches decrease in diameter from caudal to cranial, and have a thin, hyperechoic wall. The liver shows a coarse echotexture, uniform midlevel echogenicity, and is hypoechoic relative to the splenic parenchyma. The normal biliary ducts are sonographically unidentifiable. The gallbladder usually can be seen from the 9th to 10th ICS and has a thin hyperechoic wall and anechoic luminal content. It ranges from 0.8 to 3.0 cm wide and 2.3 to 6.2 cm long, based on values obtained in Saanen goats[9]; values for smaller breeds are not reported. In some goats, the gallbladder extends ventrally beyond the liver margin.[8,10] On CT images, the entire liver is visible located in the cranial abdomen (see **Fig. 4**) and shows uniform contrast enhancement after intravenous, iodinated contrast agent injection. Depending on the delay after contrast administration, the individual vascular structures of the liver can be imaged.

Imaging liver disease

Common ultrasonographic findings in small ruminants with liver disease include diffuse changes related to hepatitis, fibrosis, lipidosis, and neoplasia, such as lymphoma or carcinoma, or focal parenchymal changes such as abscessation, granuloma, neoplasia, and cystic lesions, including congenital liver cysts or those secondary to *Echinococcus granulosus*.[11,12] In hepatitis, increased liver size may be noted, and the parenchyma may be diffusely decreased in echogenicity; similar changes may be noted with lymphoma. In liver fibrosis, rounding of the liver borders and increased echogenicity of the parenchyma may be noted; similar changes can occur with lipidosis. Neoplasia of the liver is rare in small ruminants; however, lymphoma can cause diffusely reduced liver echogenicity or multinodular changes; carcinoma also can cause diffuse nodular changes of the liver parenchyma.[13] However, diffuse changes occur with a wide range of diseases, and as such, are usually nonspecific and ultrasound-guided fine needle aspirates or biopsies should be obtained.

Localized hepatic lesions are rare in small ruminants and can include abscess formation, which might be seen as a cavitary lesion with central hypoechogenicity, or cysts secondary to parasitism, which might be noted as thin-walled, cavitary lesions with central an-echogenicity.[11] In both scenarios, distal enhancement of the lesion is noted. Gas also may be noted in the liver secondary to parasite migration (**Fig. 7**) or inflammation. Focal neoplasia of the liver can create a focal area of heterogeneous echogenicity.[13] Mineralizations such as choleliths are sonographically easily identifiable by their hyperechogenicity, distinct surface reflection, and acoustic shadowing. When biliary obstruction is present, for example, secondary to choleliths, enlargement of the biliary tree can be noted. In these cases, the enlarged biliary ducts can be differentiated from vascular structures by their lack of Doppler signal.

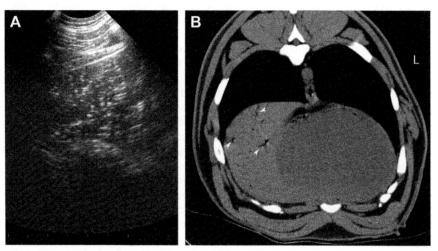

Fig. 7. Ultrasound (*A*) and transverse non–contrast-enhanced, soft tissue window CT (*B*) images of a 2-year-old Boer buck with abdominal pain. (*A*) Multiple hyperechoic foci with incomplete reverberation artifacts are noted in the liver. (*B*) Gas tracking (*arrowhead*) through the liver parenchyma is noted. L, left.

Effective evaluation of the liver also can be achieved by CT but requires administration of intravenous contrast agent to allow assessment of both the parenchyma and its vascular structures. The use of CT has been described for the evaluation of Echinococcosis in sheep, in which cysts were noted as small, round-to-ovoid variably sized hypoattenuating structures in the liver parenchyma. In later stages of disease, thickening and mineralization of the cyst walls were noted.[14]

Spleen

The spleen has a platelike shape in goats and a more triangular to trapezoid shape in sheep. The spleen is located left and dorsal to the rumen and caudal to the diaphragm at the level of the 10th to 13th rib. Sonographically, the spleen typically can be scanned in the dorsal aspect of the 10th ICS to caudal of the last left rib.[15] The splenic parenchyma has a uniform echogenicity and is mildly hyperechoic relative to the liver. The splenic capsule is a thin hyperechoic linear area. Sonographically, diffuse or focal changes of the spleen may be noted. Moderate, diffuse splenomegaly is often a nonspecific finding. Masses of the spleen related to splenic neoplasia and rarely abscessation are described and can have a similar appearance as described in the liver.

GASTROINTESTINAL TRACT DISEASE AND IMAGING
Stomach

The stomach is the largest and most distensible aspect of the gastrointestinal tract and is located caudal to the diaphragm in the left cranial to mid-abdomen. In small ruminants, the stomach is composed of the reticulum, rumen, omasum, and abomasum. There is a sphincter on each end of the stomach; at the caudal end of the esophagus and orad in the stomach is the cardia, and aborad is the pylorus at the interface of the abomasum to duodenum. The rumen is the largest compartment and is internally lined by diffuse papillae. In young animals, the rumen is smaller and increases in size as the animal consumes fibrous feed. The reticulum is located at the cranioventral aspect of the rumen ventral to the esophagus; the ventral aspect of the reticulum has a triangular shape. The reticulum is typically where foreign objects, including wires and nails, lodge. The omasum is located aborad to the rumen and has many folds or layers of tissue, sometimes described as similar in appearance to the pages of a book. The abomasum is aborad to the omasum and is the acid-secreting compartment. The abomasum extends at the caudoventral aspect of the rumen from left lateral to right lateral in the mid-abdomen.

On radiographs, the rumen occupies much of the left cranial to mid-abdomen, and the reticulum lies dorsal to the caudal aspect of the manubrium, in the cranioventral abdomen. The normal rumen is usually filled with fluid, fibrous material, and gas, and the luminal material has a layered appearance. The omasum and abomasum are often not distinguishable on radiography. Contrast radiography of the gastrointestinal tract of goats is reported; however, is rarely used and likely replaced by ultrasound.[16] Ultrasound and CT of the reticulum and rumen have been described.[8,17,18] The reticulum has a crescent to triangular shape and its serosal margin is smoothly outlined; the individual wall layers may be difficult to see and this might be dependent on the frequency used for ultrasound scanning. The rumen is examined in the left 8th to 12th ICS and the flank area; cranially the rumen will not always be visible due to summation with lung. The rumen wall is thinnest dorsally adjacent to the gas cap ranging in thickness from 0.1 to 0.4 cm and ventrally next to the rumen fiber mat measures 0.2 to 0.8 cm; however, measurements are reported only in Saanen goats.[17,18]

Imaging of Gastric Disease

Increase in ruminal size

Rumen acidosis secondary to excessive consumption of readily fermentable carbohydrates can cause rumen enlargement, which may be appreciable on radiographs and ultrasound.[18,19] Similarly, rumen bloat or large amounts of foreign material can cause a prominent increase in size (**Fig. 8**).

Traumatic reticuloperitonitis

Traumatic reticuloperitonitis rarely occurs in goats and sheep[20]; on ultrasound, thickening of the reticulum wall and a luminal hyperechoic and strongly shadowing foreign body may be noted. In addition, in cases of perforation, echogenic fluid may be noted adjacent to the serosal margin of the reticulum, suggesting focal inflammation (abscessation).

Abomasal impaction

Impaction has been described in small ruminants fed poor-quality roughage or secondary to foreign body obstruction. Imaging reports are lacking; however, an enlarged abomasum is present in these animals, which could be detected on radiographs and CT.

Inflammation of the gastric wall

Inflammation of the gastric wall is most likely to occur in the abomasum (see **Fig. 9**); currently imaging reports are lacking. Abomasitis is reported secondary to rumen acidosis, and parasitism with organisms including *Eimeria gilruthi* and *Haemonchus contortus*. *Clostridium perfringens* can cause abomasitis, particularly in neonatal lambs and kids.

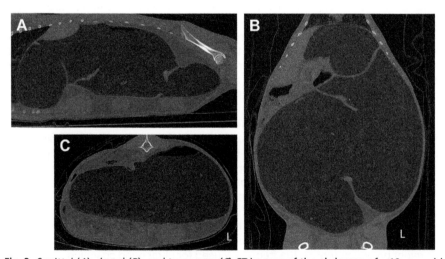

Fig. 8. Sagittal (*A*), dorsal (*B*), and transverse (*C*) CT images of the abdomen of a 10-year-old Nigerian dwarf wether with 6-month history of decreased appetite, weight loss, and waxing and waning lethargy. The rumen is severely enlarged, extending from the diaphragm to the pelvis, displacing other abdominal organs. Abnormal material is present in the rumen with a lack of normal ruminal feed material and layering. A rumenotomy was performed, and multiple plastic bags and twine were removed.

Foreign body

Gastrointestinal foreign bodies are less frequent than in cattle, but can include plastic bags (**Fig. 9**), cloth, rope, metal, and leather.[21] In addition, phytobezoars can occur in the rumen and are frequently asymptomatic until they occlude the small intestine (**Fig. 10**) or spiral colon.[22,23]

Neoplasia of the gastric wall

Tumors of the stomach are rarely reported in small ruminants. Gastrointestinal stromal tumor originating from the rumen was reported postmortem in one goat; no imaging was performed.[24]

Small Intestine

The small intestine consists of the duodenum, jejunum, and ileum. The proximal aspect of the descending duodenum adjacent to the pylorus is normally mildly wide and then narrows rapidly. The descending duodenum is in the right dorsal abdomen and parallels the abdominal wall. The jejunum has a long mesentery and limited fixation; in the cranial abdomen, the jejunum is located right of the rumen and extends through the mid-abdomen until the cranial pelvic canal. The ileum is located between the jejunum and colon and enters the colon next to the cecum; sonographically, the ileum and jejunum cannot be differentiated. The jejunum and ileum wall range on ultrasound from 0.8 to 2.1 mm in Saanen goats.[25]

Imaging of Small Intestinal Disease

Inflammatory disorders of the small intestine

Imaging reports in small ruminants are lacking; however, like other species, severe enteritis such as associated with coccidiosis or *Clostridium perfringens* can induce

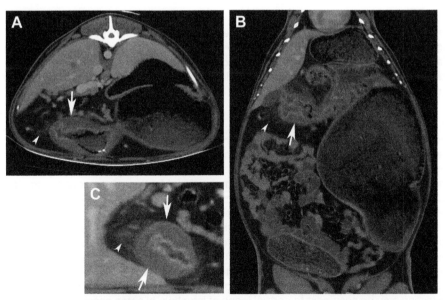

Fig. 9. Transverse (*A*), dorsal (*B*), and sagittal (*C*) contrast-enhanced CT images of the cranial abdomen of a 5-year-old Nigerian Dwarf doe with a history of inappetence. Diffuse, circumferential thickening of the abomasum near the pylorus (*white arrow*) with adjacent stranding of the fat (*arrowhead*) is evident. Biopsy of the abomasum and adjacent fat revealed abomasitis and steatitis.

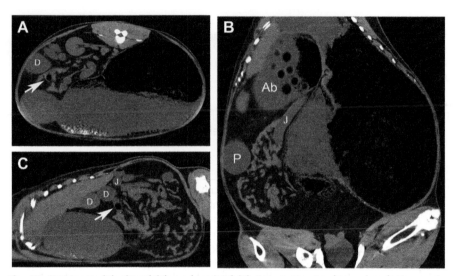

Fig. 10. Transverse (*A*), dorsal (*B*), and sagittal (*C*) non–contrast-enhanced, soft tissue window, CT images of the abdomen of a 1.3-year-old Boer doe with a history of bloat and colic. In the abomasum (Ab) there are multiple centrally hypoattenuating and peripherally soft tissue attenuating structures. The pylorus (P) and duodenum (D) are distended. The proximal jejunum (J) is fluid distended until the site of a single, round, centrally hypoattenuating and peripherally soft tissue attenuating structure (*white arrow* on [*C*]) causing luminal obstruction. Immediately caudal to this structure the aborad jejunum is empty. At exploratory laparotomy, 1 trichobezoar was removed from the jejunum and at least 9 from the abomasum.

increased intestinal wall thickness with preservation of wall architecture. Definition of individual wall layers may be reduced. However, in mild to moderate disease, the small intestines might appear normal. In addition, inflammatory changes of the intestinal tract can have similar imaging characteristics to diffuse neoplasia and it can be difficult to differentiate the definitive cause based on imaging alone.

Small intestinal obstruction

Radiographic changes noted with small intestinal obstruction depend on the extent and chronicity of the obstruction. Common causes of small intestinal obstruction include foreign bodies, intussusception, bezoars, and, less commonly, intestinal neoplasia or a mass causing intestinal compression. Metal or mineral opaque foreign bodies are often prominent on radiographs (see **Fig. 1**); however, soft tissue attenuating foreign bodies may be easily missed. In addition, nonmetallic foreign bodies also can summate with feed material in the rumen and can therefore be difficult to detect. The most common radiographic signs of small intestinal mechanical obstruction include intestinal distension, and variation in appearance. In radiographs obtained in standing animals, frequently fluid-gas interfaces at variable levels throughout the intestinal tract are noted. Similarly, on ultrasound, distended loops of poorly motile small intestine may be seen next to normal loops of intestine. In some cases, foreign material might be evident as a hyperechoic structure with complete or incomplete acoustic shadowing. Sonographically, intussusception has a characteristic pattern consisting of a series of hyperechoic and hypoechoic concentric rings with a central hyperechoic area on transverse images ("target" or "onion ring" sign). On longitudinal ultrasound images, a similar pattern of hyperechoic and hypoechoic lines maybe noted, in addition to circumferential inward folding of the intestine at the site of the intussusception. CT also can be used to identify the precise location and type of foreign body (see **Fig. 10**; **Fig. 11**) and can help to differentiate an obstructive lesion caused by a luminal foreign body from an obstructive lesion caused by an inflammatory or neoplastic process.

Pancreas

The pancreas is bilobed and located in the right craniodorsal abdomen of goats.[26] The large right lobe extends along the medial aspect of the descending duodenum caudally. Only a small aspect of the pancreas can be noted sonographically at the medial aspect of the descending duodenum, dorsolateral to the right of the rumen. Using CT, the entire pancreas can be identified, and the normal pancreas is similar to other species in that it is hypointense to the liver and spleen in precontrast images and uniformly contrast enhancing on postcontrast images. On postcontrast images, the pancreas is mildly hypoattenuating to the spleen (**Fig. 12**). Pancreatic disease is rare in small ruminants. Congenital cystic lesions, and pancreatic insulinoma in combination with cholecystic adenocarcinoma have been reported postmortem in goats with no preceding imaging.

Large Intestine

The large intestine consists of the cecum, colon, and rectum. The colon consists of the ascending, spiral, and descending colon. The cecum is a short tubular structure at the junction of the colon and ileum. The cecum is caudally directed and can extend into the cranial pelvic canal. The initial ascending colon is relatively wide and narrows into the spiral colon, followed by the descending colon and rectum. On radiography,

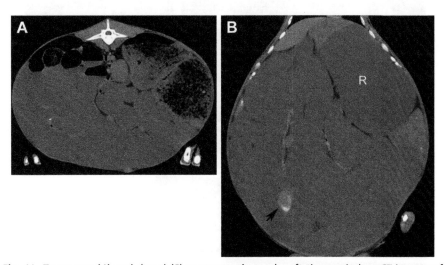

Fig. 11. Transverse (A) and dorsal (B) contrast-enhanced, soft tissue window CT images of the abdomen of a 4-month old Merino ram with a 3-day history of lethargy and inappetence. Diffuse fluid distension of the small intestines is evident. A large amount of fluid and small amount of fibrous material is noted in the rumen (R). In one loop of distal intestine, mineral attenuating fibrous material (*black arrow*) is noted. At exploratory laparotomy, the ram had a partial distal jejunal obstruction with fibrous plant material.

the spiral colon may be identified by its centrifugal and centripetal arrangement; however, usually only the descending colon and rectum can be reliably identified because of their location and fecal content. On ultrasound, the spiral colon has a characteristic centripetal and centrifugal arrangement and can be seen near the right abdominal wall. On ultrasound, only the colon wall adjacent to the transducer can be identified, the opposite wall is frequently obscured by artifacts caused by intraluminal gas and fecal material. Spiral colon wall thickness on ultrasound ranges from 1.0 to 2.6 mm and the cecum wall from 1.8 to 4.1 mm.[27]

Imaging of Large Intestinal Disease

Large intestinal obstruction
Large intestinal obstruction most commonly occurs in the interface of the ascending to spiral colon or in the spiral colon. On radiography, the location of obstruction can be difficult to diagnose; however, an obstructive pattern with distended loops of intestine may be noted. Non–contrast-enhanced CT can be very useful for detection of bezoars in the spiral colon and can assist with planning the optimal surgical approach. Ultrasound can confirm distension of the spiral colon; however, reliable identification of the cause of obstruction is challenging.

Colonic volvulus
Intestinal volvulus is rare but has been reported in a pygmy goat.[28] Any aspect of the colon can be involved in a volvulus. Radiographically, these cases are challenging to

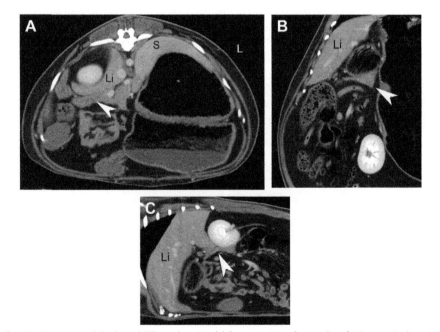

Fig. 12. Transverse (*A*), dorsal (*B*), and sagittal (*C*), contrast-enhanced, soft tissue window, CT images of the cranial abdomen of a 10-year old ewe. The normal pancreas (*white arrowhead*) can be seen at the caudal aspect of the liver (Li) in the right cranial abdomen, ventral to the right kidney and extending toward the right lateral aspect of the rumen at the caudodorsal aspect of the omasum. In (*A*), the pancreas is mildly less contrast enhancing compared with the spleen. L, left.

diagnose but severe gas distension of the colon may be noted (**Fig. 13**) and is also appreciable on CT (**Fig. 14**).

Atresia ani/recti/coli

Atresia ani has been reported in goats and sheep[29–31] and must be differentiated from other causes of ileus and abdominal pain. On radiographs, diffuse gas distension or accumulated fecal matter in some aspect of the colon may be noted (**Fig. 15**). When atresia recti or coli is suspected, retrograde infusion of a positive contrast agent such as barium sulfate can help to outline the defect and demonstrate lack of communication with the rest of the intestinal tract. Furthermore, abdominal CT can also outline the defect, identify additional anomalies, and aids in surgical planning.

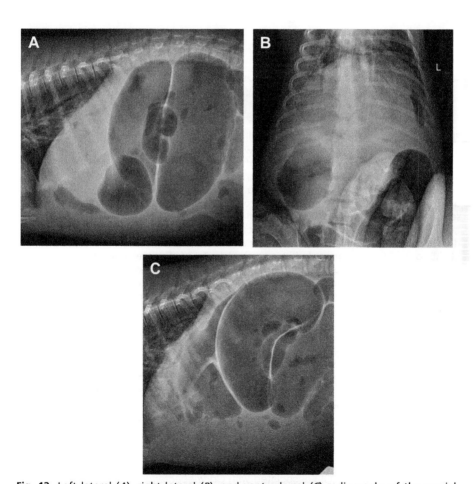

Fig. 13. Left lateral (*A*), right lateral (*B*), and ventrodorsal (*C*) radiographs of the cranial abdomen of a 16-day old lamb with persistent bloat. Severe gas dilation of the large intestines is evident, and multiple small intestinal loops contain gas and fluid and are of relatively normal diameter. An interstitial to alveolar lung pattern is evident in the right and ventral lungs, most consistent with pneumonia and atelectasis. At necropsy, mesenteric root torsion with torsion of the cecum was identified. L, left.

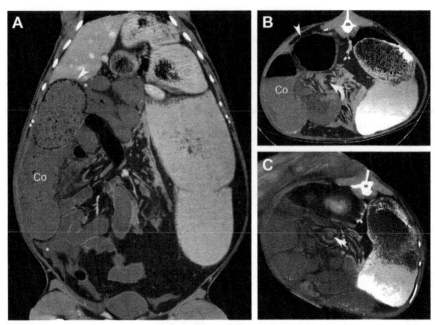

Fig. 14. Dorsal (*A*), transverse (*B*), and oblique (*C*) soft tissue window CT images of the abdomen of a 1.5-year-old Saanen doe with inappetence and reduced defecation for 9 days. Images were obtained 90 seconds after intravenous injection of iodinated contrast agent and approximately 2 hours after orogastric administration of iodinated contrast agent. A small amount of free peritoneal fluid (*asterisk*) is evident. In the most dorsal aspect of the right cranial abdomen adjacent to the diaphragm, a severely dilated, twisted segment of ascending colon (Co) and cecum containing fluid and soft tissue attenuating fiberlike material is present. (*A*) A small amount of gas is noted in the wall of the severely dilated ascending colon and cecum (*white arrowhead*). (*B* and *C*) A "swirl sign" is noted at the root of the mesentery (*white arrow*). Volvulus of the ascending colon and cecum with severe secondary dilation of the small intestine was confirmed on exploratory laparotomy. The pneumatosis (gas within the intestinal wall) of the ascending colon and cecum evident on CT suggests severe ischemia and intestinal necrosis secondary to severe, sustained volvulus.

ABDOMINAL LYMPH NODES

Most abdominal lymph nodes are inaccessible using ultrasound in mature small ruminants but are visible in young animals. On ultrasound, lymph nodes have medium echogenicity of the parenchyma and usually a hyperechoic center (**Fig. 16**). On CT, abdominal lymph nodes are easily identified, assessed, and measured.

Caseous Lymphadenitis

Caseous lymphadenitis (CL) associated with *Corynebacterium pseudotuberculosis* is a chronic, contagious disease causing internal and external abscesses. External abscesses commonly form in and around peripheral lymph nodes, and internal abscesses form within internal lymph nodes and organs. External CL is more common in goats. In one goat, radiography and CT findings included enlarged lymph nodes and a pulmonary mass with an irregular, layered appearance.[32] In a hospital case,

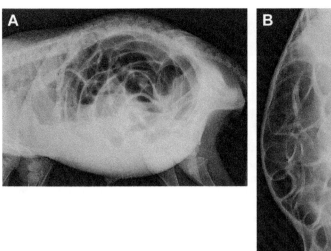
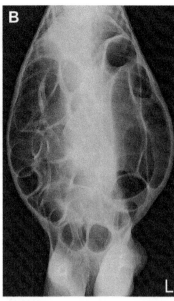

Fig. 15. Lateral (A) and ventrodorsal (B) radiographs of the abdomen of an 8-day-old lamb with abdominal distension and absent defecation despite a normal-appearing anus. The entire gastrointestinal tract is severely gas distended. The centripetal and centrifugal loops of the spiral colon are readily discerned in the lateral view. No gas is noted in the region of the rectum. Atresia recti was confirmed on necropsy.

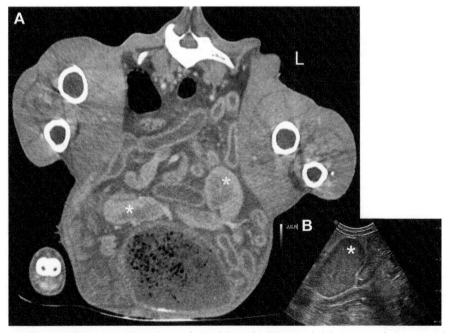

Fig. 16. Transverse contrast-enhanced CT (A) and ultrasound (B) image of the caudal abdomen. Severely enlarged jejunal lymph nodes (*asterisk*) are noted. Ultrasound-guided fine-needle aspirates were inconclusive, suggesting either reactive inflammation or small cell lymphoma.

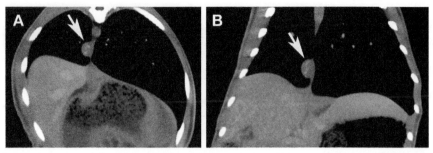

Fig. 17. Transverse (*A*) and dorsal (*B*) soft tissue window CT images obtained after intravenous iodinated contrast agent injection in a 5-year-old Nigerian dwarf buck with a history of chronic weight loss, and more recent intermittent regurgitation in the prior 2 days. In the caudal mediastinum, a small ovoid, centrally heterogeneously contrast-enhancing mass is noted next to the esophagus (*arrows*). A similar lesion was also noted in the superficial soft tissues of the distal cervical region and was aspirated. Cytology was consistent with an inflammatory process and culture revealed *Corynebacterium pseudotuberculosis* consistent with CL.

enlargement of the caudal mediastinal lymph nodes adjacent to the esophagus was visible on CT (**Fig. 17**).

SUMMARY

Medical imaging contributes substantially to the clinical evaluation of small ruminants with abdominal disease. Ultrasound is an excellent modality to evaluate a wide range of abdominal diseases, despite the limitations encountered because of ingesta and gas in the gastrointestinal tract. CT offers advantages that often circumvent the limitations of radiography and ultrasound and has a wide range of applications in small ruminants with abdominal disease.

CLINICS CARE POINTS

- Radiography can provide a good overview of the gastrointestinal tract; however, ultrasound is needed to evaluate the walls and motility of the gastrointestinal tract and to permit evaluation of the intra-abdominal parenchymal organs.
- When available, contrast-enhanced CT is an excellent technique to evaluate the entire gastrointestinal tract and to permit evaluation of the intra-abdominal parenchymal organs.
- Ultrasound is strongly operator-dependent; however, familiarity with common disorders, and clinical experience in interpreting studies is critical for all imaging modalities.

DISCLOSURE

The authors have nothing to disclose.

REFERENCES

1. Memon MA, Schelling SH, Sherman DM. Mucinous adenocarcinoma of the ovary as a cause of ascites in a goat. J Am Vet Med Assoc 1995;206(3):362–4.

2. Braun U, Irmer M, Steininger K, et al. Ultrasonographic findings in a goat with ascites due to a mesothelioma. Schweiz Arch Tierheilkd 2009;151(8):397–400.
3. Sadan M. Superficial swellings in sheep (Ovis aries) and goats (Capra hircus): clinical and ultrasonographic findings. J Vet Med Sci 2019;81(9):1326–33.
4. Tafti AK. Diaphragmatic hernia in a goat. Aust Vet J 1998;76(3):166.
5. Narayanan MK. Diaphragmatic hernia in a kid – first case reported. Isr J Vet Med 2014;69(3):146–50.
6. Al-Sobayil FA, Ahmed AF. Surgical treatment for different forms of hernias in sheep and goats. J Vet Sci 2007;8(2):185–91.
7. Schummer A, Habermehl KH. Anhangsdruesen des darmes. In: Schummer A, Nickel R, editors. Lehrbuch der Anatomie der Haustiere, vol II. Berlin (Germany): Parey; 1987. p. 189–94.
8. Kandeel A, Omar M, Mekkawy N, et al. Anatomical and ultrasonographic study of the stomach and liver in sheep and goats. Iraqi J Vet Sci 2009;23(Suppl II):181–91.
9. Braun U, Irmer M, Augsburger H, et al. Computed tomography of the abdomen in Saanen goats: I. Reticulum, rumen and omasum. Schweiz Arch Tierheilkd 2011; 153(7):307–13.
10. Braun U, Jacquat D, Steininger K. Ultrasonographic examination of the abdomen of the goat. II. Liver, spleen, urinary tract and greater omentum. Schweiz Arch Tierheilkd 2013;155(3):185–95.
11. Guarnera EA, Zanzottera EM, Pereyra H, et al. Ultrasonographic diagnosis of ovine cystic echinococcosis. Vet Radiol Ultrasound 2001;42(4):352–4.
12. Krotec K, Meyer BS, Freeman W, et al. Congenital cystic disease of the liver, pancreas, and kidney in a nubian goat (Capra hircus). Vet Pathol 1996;33(6): 708–10.
13. Trösch L, Krügger S, Grest R, et al. Sonographic findings in two miniature goats with metastatic bile duct carcinoma. Schweiz Arch Tierheilkd 2015;157(9):513–8.
14. Mao R, Qi H, Pei L, et al. CT scanning in identification of sheep cystic echinococcosis. Biomed Res Int 2017;2017:4639202.
15. Braun U, Steininger K. Ultrasonographic examination of the spleen in 30 goats. Schweiz Arch Tierheilkd 2010;152(10):477–81.
16. Cegarra IJ, Lewis RE. Contrast study of the gastrointestinal tract in the goat (Capra hircus). Am J Vet Res 1977;38(8):1121–8.
17. Braun U, Jacquat D. Ultrasonography of the reticulum in 30 healthy Saanen goats. Acta Vet Scand 2011;53(1):19.
18. Braun U, Jacquat D, Hässig M. Ultrasonography of the rumen in 30 Saanen goats. Schweiz Arch Tierheilkd 2011;153(9):393–9.
19. Braun U, Jacquat D, Steininger K. Ultrasonographic examination of the abdomen of the goat. I. Reticulum, rumen, omasum, abomasum and intestines. Schweiz Arch Tierheilkd 2013;155(3):173–84.
20. Çevik A, Timurkaan N, Yilmaz F. Traumatic reticulopericarditis in a goat. F Ü Sağ Bil Vet Derg 2010;24(2):103–5.
21. Sheferaw D, Gebru F, Asrat M, et al. Ingestion of indigestible foreign materials by free grazing ruminants in Amhara Region, Ethiopia. Trop Anim Health Prod 2014; 46(1):247–50.
22. Hollins J. Multiple phytobezoars in sibling goats. Vet Rec 2016;178(13):323–4.
23. Sherman DM. Duodenal obstruction by a phytobezoar in a goat. J Am Vet Med Assoc 1981;178(2):139–40.
24. Pesato ME, Boyle AG, Fecteau ME, et al. Gastrointestinal spindle cell tumor of the rumen with metastasis to the liver in a goat. J Vet Diagn Invest 2018;30(3):451–4.

25. Braun U, Steininger K, Tschuor A, et al. Ultrasonographic examination of the small intestine, large intestine and greater omentum in 30 Saanen goats. Vet J 2011; 189(3):330–5.

26. Smith MC, Sherman DM. Goat medicine. 2nd edition. Hoboken (NJ): Wiley-Blackwell; 1994.

27. Bayne JE, Edmondson MA. Diseases of the gastrointestinal system. In: Pugh D, Baird N, Edmondson M, et al, editors. Sheep, goat, and cervid medicine. 3rd edition. St. Louis (MO): Elsevier; 2020. p. 63–96.

28. Wagener MG, Grimm LM, Koch W, et al. Volvulus of the spiral colon in a pygmy goat buck. Tierarztl Prax 2019;47(1):49–54.

29. Al-Ani FK, Khamas WA, Al-Qudah KM, et al. Occurrence of congenital anomalies in Shami breed goats: 211 cases investigated in 19 herds. Small Rumin Res 1998;28(3):225–32.

30. Hemant K, Sharma AK, Dass LL, et al. Atresia ani with scrotal anomaly in a Goat. Vet World 2009;2(2):68.

31. Dennis SM, Leipold HW. Atresia ani in sheep. Vet Rec 1972;91(9):219–22.

32. Vilaplana Grosso F, Tinkler S, Sola M, et al. Radiographic and computed tomographic appearance of caseous lymphadenitis in a goat. Vet Radiol Ultrasound 2020;61(1):e6–11.

Imaging of the Urinary and Reproductive Tract in Small Ruminants

Susanne M. Stieger-Vanegas, Dr med vet, PhD*,
Erica McKenzie, BSc, BVMS, PhD

KEYWORDS

- Abdomen • Computed tomography • Goat • Radiography • Sheep • Ultrasound

KEY POINTS

- Ultrasound examination can be a quick, noninvasive tool to provide information about the reproductive tract, kidneys, urinary bladder, and penile urethra contents.
- Evaluation of small ruminants with signs of urinary obstruction can be performed by radiography in areas where calcium carbonate stones are prevalent, and by ultrasound examination in areas where nonradiopaque stone types predominate.
- Contrast-enhanced computed tomography scans provide a detailed anatomic depiction of the genitourinary system and functional information regarding the renal system.

INTRODUCTION

Point-of-care ultrasound examination has evolved as an invaluable tool in the diagnostic evaluation of animals with abdominal disease. The lack of ionizing radiation, noninvasiveness, portability, and ease of use has made ultrasound examination an invaluable first-line modality in the diagnostic assessment of small ruminants with suspected urinary or reproductive disease. Several steps should be considered in preparation for performing and imaging procedure (**Box 1**).

Radiography can provide an excellent overview of the abdomen and provides information about urinary stones, as well as the size, age, viability, and number of fetuses. Excretory urography has rarely been performed in small ruminants but is also superseded by ultrasound or contrast-enhanced computed tomography (CT). CT urography is like excretory urography in that excretion of intravenously injected iodinated contrast medium allows visualization of the renal parenchyma and the renal collecting system. Additionally, contrast-enhanced CT scans can be useful for reproductive

Department of Clinical Sciences, Carlson College of Veterinary Medicine, Oregon State University, Magruder Hall, 700 Southwest 30th Street, Corvallis, OR 97331, USA
* Corresponding author.
E-mail address: Susanne.stieger@oregonstate.edu

Vet Clin Food Anim 37 (2021) 75–92
https://doi.org/10.1016/j.cvfa.2020.10.002
0749-0720/21/© 2020 Elsevier Inc. All rights reserved.
vetfood.theclinics.com

Box 1
Preparation and general ideas for performing imaging of the urinary and reproductive tract in small ruminants

- Brushing the fiber or wool can reduce artifacts on radiographs and computed tomography images
- Position the animal comfortably and use appropriate sedation or anesthesia if needed
- Use appropriate ultrasound transducers and machine presettings for examination
- For ultrasound examinations, either split the fiber or wool to access the skin, or clip the fiber or wool to achieve optimal contact with the transducer
- All imaging modalities benefit from a standardized approach and protocol to ensure a complete examination is performed.
- For computed tomography examination, an intravenous catheter should be placed to allow iodinated contrast agent administration thereby allowing easier differentiation of the various organs from each other and timed studies for evaluation of the kidneys, renal pelvis, and ureters.

---

lesions involving and located within the pelvic canal, because this area can be challenging to evaluate in its entirety via transabdominal and transrectal ultrasound techniques.

RETROPERITONEAL SPACE
Normal Retroperitoneum

The retroperitoneum is the space in the dorsal abdomen not covered by peritoneum, in which the retroperitoneal organs reside, including the kidneys, ureters, adrenal glands, aorta, caudal vena cava, tributary vessels, and the lumbar aortic, renal, medial iliac, hypogastric, and sacral lymph nodes. The retroperitoneum is cranially connected with the mediastinum and caudally with the pelvic canal, and disease processes can extend from one of these spaces unhindered into the other (**Fig. 1**).

Retroperitoneal Disease

Retroperitoneal fluid
Retroperitoneal fluid accumulation commonly develops after trauma to the retroperitoneal space and its organs. Causes include hemorrhage from the kidneys, rupture of ureters with urine leakage, acute renal failure causing perirenal edema, or rarely retroperitoneal metastatic disease. Retroperitoneal fluid causes a loss of visualization of the normal organs of the retroperitoneal space, specifically the kidneys and major vessels. If small quantities are present, a mottled appearance of the retroperitoneal space including the retroperitoneal fat may be noted.

Retroperitoneal gas
Pneumoretroperitoneum can be caused by traumatic injury to the retroperitoneal space, or from gas extending from a pneumomediastinum, or pelvic canal injury into the retroperitoneal space. Retroperitoneal gas results in increased definition of the retroperitoneal organs on radiographs (see **Fig. 1**). On ultrasound imaging, reverberation artifacts can be noted adjacent to the retroperitoneal organs. CT is an excellent technique to identify retroperitoneal gas and can help with tracking

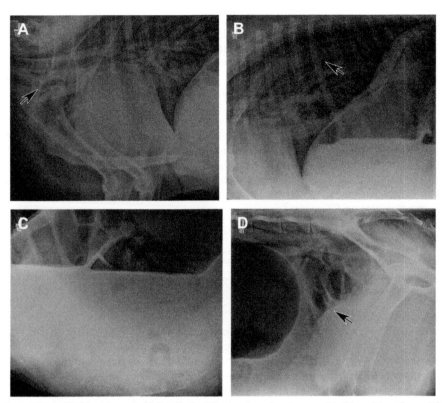

Fig. 1. Lateral thoracic and abdominal radiographs of a 5-year-old Shropshire ewe with inappetence. The ewe had been orally medicated (drenched) the previous 2 days by the owner, with violent coughing reported after 1 treatment. Large amounts of air are evident along the soft tissues of the neck, extending into the mediastinum (*A,B*) and retroperitoneal space (*C, D*) and enhancing visualization of structures in these regions (*black arrows*). Pneumomediastinum with gas extension into the retroperitoneum secondary to a tracheal defect or severe coughing from inadvertent aspiration was suspected.

perforating injuries or foreign bodies and evaluating the extent of retroperitoneal injury.

URINARY TRACT DISEASE AND IMAGING
Kidneys and Ureters

In small ruminants, the left kidney is displaced medially by the dorsal sac of the rumen and located on midline or to the right of midline, and caudal to the right kidney. In smaller animals, both kidneys may be visible on radiographs. The right kidney has been reported to measure approximately 2.1 to 2.6 times the length of the second lumbar vertebral body on radiographs.[1] On CT scans, the kidneys range in size up to nearly 3 times the lumbar vertebrae.[2] The right kidney is accessible to ultrasound examination caudal to the last rib in the right dorsolateral abdomen.[3] In small or thin animals, the left kidney can also be seen from the right or from ventral in the abdomen. Both kidneys are ovoid and have a hyperechoic cortex and hypoechoic medulla. The renal pelvis is anechoic and surrounded by a thin hyperechoic rim. The kidneys in Saanen goats range from 6.4 to 9.7 cm long and 3.1 to 5.6 cm wide. The renal cortices range in thickness from 0.4 to 1.4 cm.[4] The proximal aspect of the right ureter is visible by ultrasound examination; however, the mid-to-distal ureter is normally not visible unless enlarged.[5] CT is an excellent technique to evaluate the morphometry of the kidneys and ureters and is likely replacing the use of excretory urography.[2,6,7] Both kidneys can be seen on survey, excretory urography and contrast-enhanced CT images. Iodinated contrast agents are filtered through the kidneys and therefore, enhancement of the renal cortices and in later images, of the renal pelvis and ureters, can be viewed. On excretory urography as well as contrast-enhanced CT scans, both kidneys show parenchymal enhancement on venous phase images and renal pelvis enhancement on delayed venous phase images. On delayed contrast-enhanced CT images, the ureters can be followed from the renal pelvis to the papillae at the urinary bladder. Dilation of the ureters or ectopic location of the ureters regarding the urinary bladder can also be identified on delayed images. The normal ureters measure up to 0.2 cm diameter on CT scans.[2]

Imaging of Renal Disease

Except for obstructive urolithiasis, renal disease is infrequently encountered in small ruminants; however, renal insufficiency, nephritis, pyelonephritis, and mineralization of the kidneys can occur.

Renal insufficiency

Renal insufficiency can be acute or chronic and can result from hemodynamic insults or a wide range of toxic compounds, including heavy metals, chemicals, plant or fungal toxins, and nephrotoxic drugs. Specific infectious diseases such as leptospirosis can cause renal failure, as can pregnancy toxemia and other nutritional or metabolic disorders. Clinical renal disease is uncommon in goats. At slaughter, 0.8% of goat and 1.2% of sheep kidneys were condemned; interstitial nephritis was diagnosed by histopathology in approximately 70% of condemned kidneys. None of the classic imaging techniques including radiography, ultrasound imaging, and CT scans can provide quantitative information about renal function; however, a contrast-enhanced CT scan can provide qualitative information about renal function. Currently used CT contrast agents all contain iodine, which is filtered through the kidneys. Prolonged contrast enhancement of the kidneys may be noted in acute renal failure. In acute renal failure, on ultrasound imaging, a small amount of anechoic fluid might be noted in the retroperitoneal space and on radiography, reduced definition of the kidneys and small strands of soft tissue attenuation may be noted in the retroperitoneal area. In chronic renal failure, decreased size and irregularity of one or both kidneys may be noted on radiographs, ultrasound imaging, or CT scans.

Renal enlargement

An increase in renal size can be noted with primary or metastatic neoplasia, renal cysts, abscesses, hydronephrosis, acute nephritis, and other disorders. Renal trauma can cause an abnormal shape of 1 or both kidneys and increased size secondary to intracapsular hemorrhage and retroperitoneal fluid. If mass lesions are noted in the kidneys during imaging, ultrasound-guided fine needle aspirates may help to differentiate between various etiologies. On radiographs, detection of mass lesions of the kidneys can be challenging owing to summation with normal structures. On excretory urography, solid and cystic lesions both can cause contrast-sparing lesions in the kidneys. Ultrasound imaging can differentiate between a cystic and parenchymal lesion and can additionally be used to perform guided aspirates. On ultrasound examination, cystic lesions will be anechoic and show distal enhancement, whereas parenchymal lesions will be hypoechoic to hyperechoic with no distal enhancement. On contrast-enhanced CT scans, the enhancement behavior of the lesion and the attenuation of the lesion can be measured. Fluid-containing lesions are often hypoattenuating to normal renal parenchyma, will range in Hounsfield units close to 0, and will have no contrast enhancement, whereas parenchymal lesions can be hypoattenuating to iso-attenuating to renal parenchyma and will usually show mild to moderate contrast enhancement. Polycystic kidney disease is one of the congenital renal diseases reported in sheep and goats causing renal enlargement and which can have negative effects on breeding programs if not detected early. Furthermore, animals with polycystic kidney disease can also have cystic lesions in other organs, including the liver and pancreas.[8–12]

Renal agenesis
Failure of one or both kidneys to develop is reported in sheep.[9] Renal agenesis can be challenging to diagnose on radiography. Ultrasound examination can readily identify the absence of one or both kidneys, especially in young animals. Similarly, CT imaging is an excellent technique to evaluate the presence and morphometrics of the kidneys.

Pyelonephritis
On imaging, pyelonephritis can cause mild dilation of the renal pelvis and proximal ureter, and blunting of the renal papillae. Renal size is often normal or mildly increased in acute disease and decreased in chronic disease. On ultrasound examination, enlargement of the renal pelvis by anechoic or echogenic fluid is noted and, depending on the extent of renal pelvis dilation, the cortex of the kidney may be decreased in width.

Hydronephrosis
Hydronephrosis represents unilateral or bilateral enlargement of the renal pelvis secondary to urine retention. In small ruminants, it is most commonly secondary to obstruction by ureteroliths. On radiographs, smoothly outlined and enlarged kidneys may be noted. On ultrasound and CT imaging, increased width of the renal pelvis and dilation of the renal recesses can be noted (**Figs. 2–4**). On ultrasound examination, the renal pelvis is distended with anechoic fluid and if infection or hemorrhage is present, dilation with echogenic urine may be noted.

Renal mineralization
Renal mineralization can represent mineralization of the renal parenchyma (dystrophic mineralization) or mineral within the renal pelvis (nephrolithiasis). Rarely, diffuse mineralization of the renal parenchyma may occur, such as with ethylene glycol toxicity,[13] which has been noted in other species on radiographs. On radiographs, dystrophic mineralization and nephrolithiasis may be noted, but often cannot be differentiated when it is focal (**Fig. 5**). On ultrasound examination, the mineralized material may be localized to the renal pelvis and may be accompanied by dilation of the renal pelvis. The mineralized material will be hyperechoic and demonstrate complete acoustic shadowing. Renal mineralization and diffuse renal enlargement have been described in an experimental ultrasound study of Barki sheep consuming salinated water over a 9-month period.[14]

Ureteral calculi
Ureteral calculi are very challenging to diagnose on radiographs owing to summation with surrounding organs; however, if retroperitoneal mineralizations caudal to the kidneys are noted, ultrasound examination of that area may provide additional information. The normal ureter is sonographically only seen close to the kidneys;

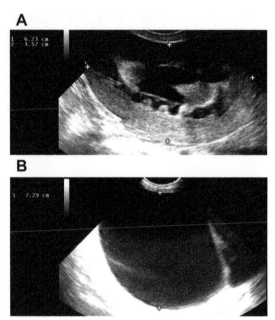

Fig. 2. Ultrasound images of the right kidney (*A*) and urinary bladder (*B*) of a 5-year-old Pygmy wether with a 3-day history of possible constipation and urine dribbling. The kidney is normal in size, but the renal pelvis is dilated with anechoic fluid. The urinary bladder is moderately distended. No urinary bladder stones were identified. A single urethral stone was subsequently identified as the cause of the obstruction and was surgically removed.

however, if ureteral dilation secondary to obstruction is present, the ureter may be identified on ultrasound imaging at more distant locations. Mineralized material in the ureters will be hyperechoic and show complete acoustic shadowing. Excretory urography can be used to evaluate the ureters in goats and sheep; however, in large individuals, summation with material in the gastrointestinal tract and lack of adequate penetration can limit the diagnostic value of the study. A contrast-enhanced CT scan with delayed postcontrast administration phases is an excellent technique to evaluate the ureters. In obstructed male goats and in female small ruminants with uterine masses, secondary dilation of the ureters has been observed on CT scans (see **Fig. 3**).

Ectopic ureters

This is a rare congenital disorder where one or both ureters terminate caudal to the ureteral papillae in the trigone area.[15] It may be detected sonographically by lack of visualization of normal ureteral papillae in the urinary bladder and an ability to track the ureters into the pelvic canal adjacent to the urethra. Ultrasonographically, the point of termination of the ureters may not always be defined owing to their intrapelvic location; however, in delayed venous phase CT images, the entire length of the ureters can be identified.

Urinary Bladder and Urethra

The urinary bladder is often visible on plain radiographs of small ruminants owing to its tear drop to ovoid shape and its soft tissue attenuation, which contrasts with the

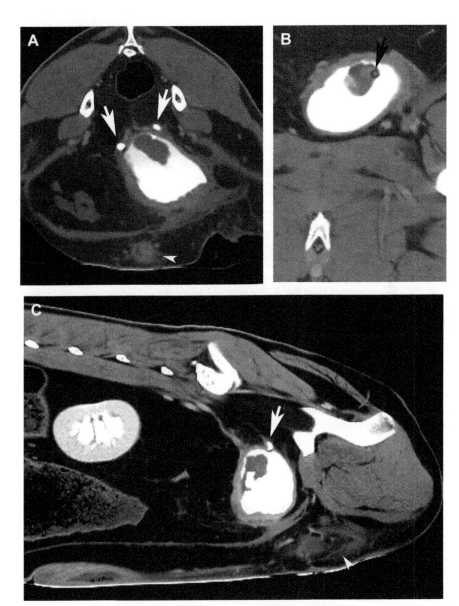

Fig. 3. Transverse (*A*), dorsal (*B*) and sagittal (*C*) soft tissue window CT images of the caudal abdomen of a 7-year-old Nigerian Dwarf goat wether obtained after a 5-minute delay after injection of intravenous iodinated contrast agent. Tube cystostomy and urethrotomy had been performed 7 days prior and it had been observed that the tube did not seem patent and that the patient had developed ventral abdominal edema and a swollen prepuce. (*A*) The distal ureters (*white arrows*) at their insertion into the urinary bladder are mildly enlarged (the right ureter more than the left). (*B*) Dorsally within the bladder lumen, extending from the dorsocaudal urinary bladder wall toward the trigone area and adjacent to the cystostomy tube tip (*black arrow*) is a mildly hypoattenuating filling defect consistent with a hematoma. The bladder wall is diffusely and mildly thickened. Mild peritoneal fluid is noted. Mild wispy subcutaneous fat is noted surrounding the urethra (*arrowhead*). (*C*) The right kidney is normal in size and contrast enhancement, with very mild hydronephrosis.

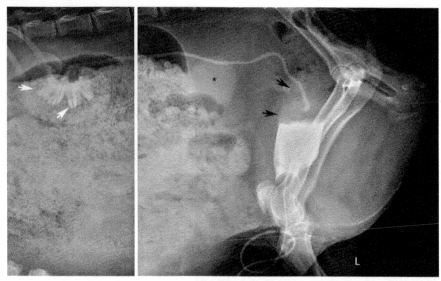

Fig. 4. Lateral abdominal radiographs with normograde cystography of the 7-year-old Nigerian dwarf goat wether from **Fig. 3**. The wether had a tube cystostomy and urethrotomy 8 days prior to address obstructive urolithiasis. Contrast agent from a contrast-enhanced CT study performed 1 day prior (see **Fig. 3**) can be seen remaining in the mildly dilated right renal pelvis and recesses (*white arrows*) and mildly dilated right ureter. The right ureter is entering the urinary bladder in the trigone area and is segmentally wide. Similar to the CT study, a contrast sparing area is evident in the caudal aspect of the urinary bladder including the trigone area (*black arrows*), which did not fill with contrast in sequential images and is consistent with the hematoma noted on CT scan. The left kidney (*asterisk*) shows a mild amount of diffuse contrast enhancement, but no hydronephrosis. Findings from both studies are consistent with mild right hydronephrosis and hydroureter secondary to development of a urinary bladder hematoma associated with tube cystostomy and urethrotomy.

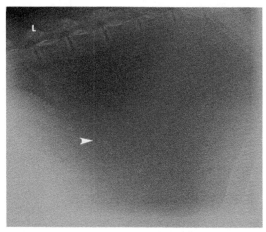

Fig. 5. Lateral radiograph of the mid-to-caudal abdomen of a 6-year-old Saanen buck with a history of urolithiasis. A small mineral attenuation is evident in the left kidney (*white arrow*).

peritoneal fat and fat in the pelvic canal. The urinary bladder can easily be evaluated using ultrasound imaging and has a thin echogenic wall and normally anechoic content. Depending on the filling status, normal bladder wall thickness may vary, being mildly thicker when empty than distended. Normal wall thickness on ultrasound is between 0.8 to 2.3 mm in Saanen goats[16] and is expected to be similar in other sheep and goat breeds. In sheep it has been reported that when the bladder extends more than 10 cm cranially to the pelvic brim, it is abnormally distended, which is commonly caused by obstructive urolithiasis.[17]

The extrapelvic portion of the urethra is similar in opacity to the surrounding soft tissue on radiographs, but is easily accessible using ultrasound imaging. It is preferable to use a linear probe with a high frequency to obtain good near-field resolution; however, ultrasound examination of the urethra can also be successfully performed with a convex or rectal probe. The urethra is very superficial, and the lumen is often small and not visible. The urethral wall is of medium echogenicity and the urethral lumen, when visible, usually contains anechoic urine; the urethra can be followed from the ischial arch to the tip.[4,18] When the urethral lumen is readily visible on ultrasound examination, it is usually secondary to obstructive urolithiasis or other obstructive processes causing urethral dilation.[18]

In the female small ruminant, the urethra and urinary bladder can also be evaluated with retrograde cystography; however, in the male animal, challenges performing urinary catheterization related to the urethral process and sigmoid flexure usually prevent retrograde urethrography. Retrograde cystography can be performed with thin angiographic catheters, but is a challenging technique and only successful in approximately 50% of the bucks in which it is attempted.[19] Normograde urethrography has been described in animals with a tube cystostomy.[20]

Imaging of Disease of the Urinary Bladder and Urethra

Obstructive urolithiasis

Urolithiasis is the presence of urinary stones (uroliths) within the urinary tract, including the ureters, urinary bladder, and urethra. Clinical signs usually manifest when uroliths obstruct the urinary tract resulting in urine retention, bladder distention, pain, and possible urethral and bladder rupture.[21] Urolithiasis occurs in a variety of breeds and most frequently in castrated male goats. Urolithiasis represents a nutritional disorder; most often it is linked to dietary factors. Radiographs of the caudal abdomen frequently obtained in lateral recumbency and including the urethra can provide valuable information for surgical planning. Some uroliths can be detected with radiography (**Figs. 6** and **7**) including struvite, calcium oxalate, calcium phosphate, calcium carbonate, and silicate, although some are radiolucent, including cysteine, urate, and xanthine stones. Independent of their mineral composition, uroliths can be identified using ultrasound imaging, on which they are hyperechoic with acoustic shadowing (**Fig. 8**). Unenhanced CT scans can identify most uroliths, including those that are soft tissue attenuating (nonradiopaque) on conventional radiographs.[22] Treatment of obstructive urolithiasis varies depending on the severity of the condition. In some cases, adequate pain relief may relax the musculature enough to permit spontaneous relief of the obstruction. In other cases, surgical interventions such as urethral process amputation, urethrotomy, or tube cystostomy is needed to alleviate the obstruction.[23] The extent of surgical intervention increases if the bladder has been ruptured (**Fig. 7**). Imaging can assist in planning appropriate surgical intervention and determining if there are additional stones in the bladder, and the number of stones contributing to obstruction.

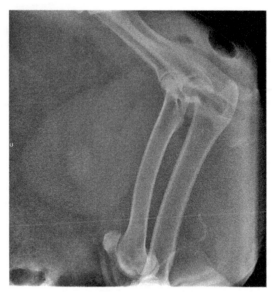

Fig. 6. Lateral radiograph of the caudal abdomen of a 5-year old Anglo-Nubian wether with a history of urinary obstruction; image obtained with the animal in lateral recumbency. Urethral process amputation did not resolve obstruction. Multiple mineral attenuating stones are present in the central aspect of the urinary bladder and penile urethra.

Urethral stenosis

Normograde cystography (see **Fig. 9**) can be used evaluate the urethra for areas of stenosis. Contrast-enhanced CT scans provide limited evaluation of the urethra for stenosis because unless the urethral lumen is filled with urine or contrast agent, it is

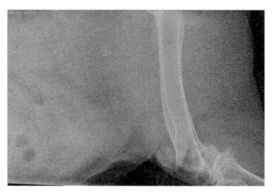

Fig. 7. Lateral radiograph of the caudal abdomen of a 4-year-old Boer buck with signs of partial urethral blockage, inappetance and recumbency. In the central aspect of the urinary bladder, numerous round mineral opacities are noted. Similar small round mineral opacities are present summating outside the urinary bladder with the caudal abdomen. The caudal abdominal serosal and retroperitoneal detail is reduced. Findings are consistent with cystolithiasis and urinary bladder rupture with secondary uroperitoneum, and uroliths free within the abdominal cavity.

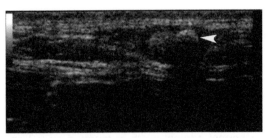

Fig. 8. Ultrasound image of the penile urethra of 2-year-old Nigerian Dwarf wether with a 2-day history of possible urinary obstruction. A round, hyperechoic, distally shadowing structure is noted in the penile urethra (*arrowhead*), consistent with a urethrolith.

usually small and the walls are collapsed. Normograde cystography or retrograde urethrography CT scans could be used to evaluate the urethra for regions of stenosis.

Cystitis
Inflammation of the urinary bladder can occur as a singular lesion or can extend into the ureters and kidneys, causing secondary pyelonephritis. Bacterial colonization of the mucosal lining of the bladder usually follows some form of trauma and typically presents as hematuria (blood in the urine) and pyuria (white cells in the urine). Bacterial culture of urine samples facilitates appropriate antibiotic selection. Inflammation of the bladder wall causes thickening of the wall, usually most visible at the cranioventral aspect of the bladder. It is important to remember that, if the urinary bladder is incompletely filled, the wall will be thicker when measured by any imaging technique.

Urinary bladder neoplasia
Urinary bladder neoplasia is rare in small ruminants, and leiomyoma of the bladder wall has been described elsewhere.[24,25]

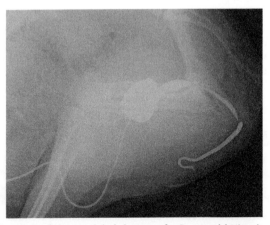

Fig. 9. Lateral radiograph of the caudal abdomen of a 3-year old Nigerian Dwarf buck with a previous history of urolithiasis demonstrating a positive contrast normograde cystogram performed via cystostomy tube. Focal stenosis of the proximal urethra is evident at the level of the ischial arch, most compatible with a urethral mucosal flap at this level. No obstructing stones are evident.

ADRENAL GLANDS

The adrenal glands are located at the craniomedial aspect of the kidneys in the cranial retroperitoneum. The left adrenal lies lateral to the abdominal aorta cranial to the left renal artery (**Fig. 10**); the right adrenal is located at the dorsolateral aspect of the caudal vena cava at the caudal aspect of the liver. On ultrasound examination, the normal adrenal glands are often not visible, except in young or very small animals. These glands have a hyperechoic medulla relative to the hypoechoic cortex. There are no established criteria for normal adrenal size in small ruminants using ultrasound imaging. The normal adrenal width is reported as 0.9 cm on CT scans of Saanen goats.[2] Mass lesions may be recognized in the adrenal glands and can be unilateral, including functional and nonfunctional adrenal tumors.[24] Bilateral change usually represents hyperplasia and rarely metastasis. Adrenal tumors are rarely described, and the few reports include multiple benign hyperplastic nodules and pheochromocytoma in a goat with 2 other tumors.[24] In 1 wether, adrenal hyperplasia resulted in the onset of lactation for many years[26] A CT scan can identify adrenal enlargement (see **Fig. 10**) and allows for the evaluation of vascular invasion by an adrenal tumor.

REPRODUCTIVE TRACT

The uterus is dorsal to the urinary bladder and ventral to the colon. The 2 uterine horns are located on either side of the urinary bladder and have a curved to curled appearance, which is more pronounced than in cows. The caudal parts of the uterine horns are for a short distance externally fused into a double tube. The ovaries are relatively small and ovoid to round and measure approximately 10 × 15 mm on ultrasound examination. Although transabdominal ultrasound imaging is technically easier to perform, evaluation of the female reproductive system, including the nonpregnant and early pregnant uterus, may require transrectal ultrasound examination owing to partial location within the osseous pelvic canal. Therefore, the transrectal technique is the method of choice for ultrasound examination of nonpregnant and early pregnant females.[27] Transabdominal ultrasound imaging can be used for diagnosing pregnancy from day 25 to 30 of pregnancy onward, and transrectal ultrasound from days 24 to 34. After day 60, transabdominal scanning is usually necessary to identify pregnancy and to permit visualization of the entire uterus, and pregnancy is usually readily detectable at this time and onward because of the obvious presence of intrauterine fluid, fetal structures, and the semicircular placentomes.[17,28] Fetal counting is often most readily

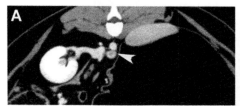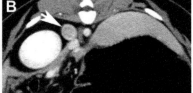

Fig. 10. Transverse soft tissue window images obtained after intravenous iodinated contrast agent injection in a 3-year-old Nigerian Dwarf wether with a history of a buck-like behavior. An androgen-producing tumor of the right adrenal gland (adrenal cortical tumor) was suspected. (A) The left adrenal gland (*arrowhead*) is normal in size and shows a normal central hypoenhancing and peripheral moderately contrast enhancing pattern. (B) The right adrenal gland (*arrow*) is enlarged and shows centrally heterogeneous contrast enhancement.

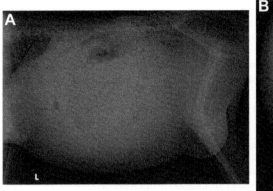
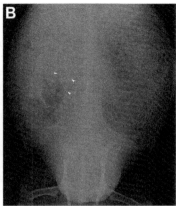

Fig. 11. Lateral (*A*) and ventrodorsal (*B*) abdominal radiographs of a 10-month-old Nigerian Dwarf doe pregnant at unknown gestational stage after accidental breeding. One fetus is visible, in which the distal phalanges are mineral attenuating, and incisors and molars of the mandibles (*arrow heads*) of the fetus are also identifiable. There are no signs of fetal death.

achieved transabdominally between days 40 and 70 of gestation, with the probe angled from the right caudoventral flank region caudally toward the urinary bladder. Radiography can be performed to evaluate for mineralized fetuses or signs of fetal death, and to accurately count fetuses in late pregnancy (**Figs. 11** and **12**).

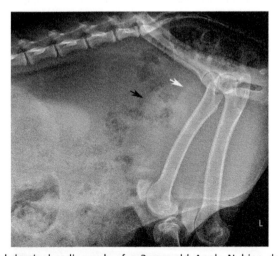

Fig. 12. Lateral abdominal radiograph of a 2-year-old Anglo-Nubian doe. In the caudal abdomen, there are 2 rounded, 1 large and 1 medium sized, well-defined soft tissue attenuating structures that summate with each other. The more craniodorsally positioned structure (*black arrow*) is suspected to be the uterus and the more ventrocaudally positioned structure (*white arrow*) is suspected to be the urinary bladder. This finding is consistent with uterine enlargement and possible pregnancy, although no mineral-attenuating fetal structures are evident.

Endometritis and Metritis

Endometritis refers to inflammation or infection of the uterine lining and metritis when the uterine wall is affected; both conditions are uncommon in small ruminants. They can result from postpartum infections, retained placenta, retained fetuses, and dystocia. Metritis can lead to septicemia and death if left untreated. Ultrasound examination is useful to identify abnormal post partum uterine involution and the accumulation of excessive echogenic fluid within the uterine lumen.[29] Retained fetuses or parts of a fetus can be noted on radiography, ultrasound imaging, or CT scans (**Figs. 13** and **14**).

Hydrometra and Pseudopregnancy

Goats are renowned for this unusual condition during which persistence of a corpus luteum promotes the accumulation and retention of occasionally large volumes of aseptic, mucoid fluid within the uterine lumen. Before day 40 of potential pregnancy, it may be impossible to distinguish hydrometra from a viable pregnancy, but as true pregnancy or pseudopregnancy develop, the 2 conditions will become readily distinguishable on ultrasound examination after day 40 through the presence or absence of the characteristic placentomes and fetal structures that denote pregnancy. These are absent in the pseudopregnant animal and multiple thin walled chambers containing anechoic fluid are visualized, which represent transverse imaging through dilated and curved uterine horns.

Neoplasia of the Female Reproductive Tract

A limited number of tumors of the reproductive system have been reported in does and ewes. Both an ovarian granulosa cell tumor[30] and mucinous adenocarcinoma metastasized to regional tissue, including the uterus and peritoneum.[31] Although there are few reports of uterine tumors, they are being increasingly recognized as an

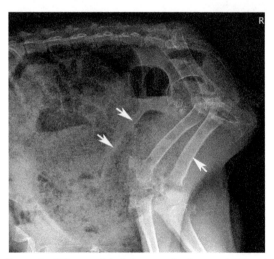

Fig. 13. Lateral radiograph of the caudal abdomen of a 4-year-old Nigerian Dwarf doe with a history of a large ventral abdominal swelling after kidding 1 month prior. A retained fetal head is noted in the cranial aspect of the pelvic canal. The uterus is enlarged (*white arrows*) and contains gas and heterogenous soft tissue attenuating material. Findings are consistent with retained fetus and pyometra.

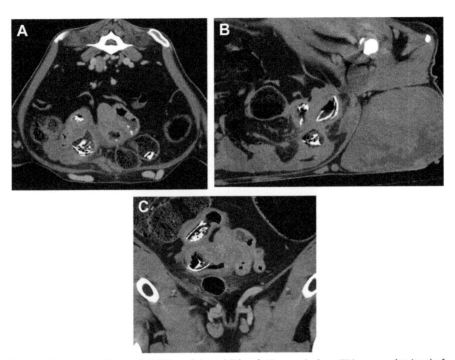

Fig. 14. Transverse (*A*), sagittal (*B*), and dorsal (*C*) soft tissue window CT images obtained after intravenous iodinated contrast agent injection in a 5-year-old Alpine goat with brown vulvar discharge and suspected rectovaginal fistula. The goat had kidded 3 months prior. The uterus is diffusely and moderately enlarged (*white arrow*) and contains numerous, well-defined, angular, and variably shaped bone fragments. Additionally, there is a marked amount of heterogenous soft tissue material and gas within the uterus. The peritoneal fat surrounding the uterine horns has a striated soft tissue attenuation. Findings are consistent with a retained, decomposing fetus and accompanying severe pyometra and regional peritonitis. No rectovaginal fistula was identified.

important disease in mature does. Reported uterine tumors include leiomyoma leiomyosarcoma, leiomyofibroma, adenocarcinoma, fibroid, and fibroma.[32]

Vaginal Prolapse

Vaginal prolapse is particularly common in sheep in late gestation. Multiple management factors contribute to this disorder, including short tail docking. Prolapse involves folding and eversion of the ventral floor of the vaginal vault, which can range in severity and persistence. The urinary bladder, intestinal loops, and occasionally even the uterus can move into the prolapse, complicating management. Replacement before 24 hours is associated with a good prognosis. Prolapses that have been present for more than 36 hours, and with extensive damage, are typically amputated.[30,33] Ultrasound imaging can assist in successful management by identifying the presence of the bladder, intestines, or uterus in the prolapse. In a study in sheep, the urinary bladder was displaced and visible on ultrasound examination as an anechoic structure in the prolapse in 41.6% of affected animals. In another 25% of cases, 1 uterine horn was also present within the prolapse appearing as an anechoic circular structure surrounded by a hyperechoic wall.[30] The bladder can be decompressed by ultrasound-guided aspiration before attempting reduction of the prolapse.

Uterine Torsion

Uterine torsion is a challenging diagnosis in small ruminants because per rectum palpation of uterine position is restricted by their small size. Ultrasound imaging can identify uterine wall edema as a supporting sign, reflected by wall measurements exceeding 10 mm (normally ≤5 mm). Additionally, contrast-enhanced CT scans could be used to evaluate the uterine vessels and blood supply to the uterine wall. It would be expected in a torsion that the vessels would be rotated ("swirl sign") similarly to what is noted with torsion of the mesenteric root or intestines.

SUMMARY

Ultrasound imaging is often the initial modality of choice in the evaluation of small ruminants with genitourinary disease. Radiography can be an important in areas where radiopaque uroliths are common, to determine the site and severity of disease and to assist with treatment planning but has less value in areas where nonradiopaque stones are prevalent. CT urography is a promising diagnostic technique allowing comprehensive evaluation of the urinary tract in small ruminants. Contrast-enhanced CT scans combine the diagnostic capabilities of excretory urography with CT imaging and has the potential to be used as the primary imaging modality for evaluation of genitourinary conditions in small ruminants.

CLINICS CARE POINTS

- Ultrasound imaging is an essential technique in the diagnostic assessment of small ruminants with genitourinary disease, facilitating the diagnosis of a wide range of reproductive and urinary disorders

- Urinary tract disease is one of the most common presenting abdominal complaints of small ruminants. Radiography is an excellent imaging choice in regions where stones are commonly radiopaque; otherwise, ultrasound imaging is the more appropriate selection for initial imaging.

- Contrast-enhanced CT scans offer excellent morphometric and functional information about the kidneys and collecting system

DISCLOSURE

The authors have nothing to disclose.

REFERENCES

1. Ragab G, Seif M, Hagag U. Radiologic and ultrasonographic studies of kidneys in goat. J Vet Med Res 2010;20:30–7.
2. Braun U, Irmer M, Augsburger H, et al. Computed tomography of the abdomen in Saanen goats: III. kidneys, ureters and urinary bladder. Schweiz Arch Tierheilkd 2011;153(7):321–9.
3. Scott P. Practical use of ultrasound scan in small ruminant medicine and surgery. Vet Clin North Am Food Anim Pract 2016;32(1):181–205.
4. Steininger K, Braun U. Ultrasonography of the urinary tract in 29 female Saanen goats. Schweiz Arch Tierheilkd 2012;154(2):67–74.

5. Braun U, Schefer U, Gerber D. Ultrasonography of the urinary tract of female sheep. Am J Vet Res 1992;53(10):1734–9.

6. Cegarra IJ, Lewis RE. Excretory urography in the goat (Capra hircus). Am J Vet Res 1977;38(8):1129–32.

7. Verma MK, Purohit S, Gowtham A, et al. Excretory urographic and ultrasonographic studies of urinary system in goats (Capra hircus). Rumin Sci 2017;6(1): 177–84.

8. Johnstone AC, Davidson BI, Roe AR, et al. Congenital polycystic kidney disease in lambs. N Z Vet J 2005;53(5):307–14.

9. Dennis SM. Urogenital defects in sheep. Vet Rec 1979;105(15):344–7.

10. Jones TO, Clegg FG, Morgan G, et al. A vertically transmitted cystic renal dysplasia of lambs. Vet Rec 1990;127(17):421–4.

11. Steffen F, Tontis A. Clinical findings and pathology of congenital polycystic renal disease in the goat. Tierarztl Prax 1996;24(5):453–8 [in German].

12. Newman SJ, Leichner T, Crisman M, et al. Congenital cystic disease of the liver and kidney in a pygmy goat. J Vet Diagn Invest 2000;12(4):374–8.

13. Boermans HJ, Ruegg PL, Leach M. Ethylene glycol toxicosis in a pygmy goat. J Am Vet Med Assoc 1988;193(6):694–6.

14. Ghanem M, Zeineldin M, Eissa A, et al. The effects of saline water consumption on the ultrasonographic and histopathological appearance of the kidney and liver in Barki sheep. J Vet Med Sci 2018;80(5):741–8.

15. Scarratt WK, Lombard CW, Buergelt CD. Ventricular septal defects in two goats. Cornell Vet 1984;74(2):136–45.

16. Braun U, Jacquat D, Steininger K. Ultrasonographic examination of the abdomen of the goat. I. Reticulum, rumen, omasum, abomasum and intestines. Schweiz Arch Tierheilkd 2013;155(3):173–84.

17. Scott P. Abdominal ultrasonography as an adjunct to clinical examination in sheep. Small Rumin Res 2017;152:132–43.

18. Al Lugami A, von Pückler K, Wehrend A, et al. Sonography of the distal urethra in lambs. Acta Vet Scand 2017;59(1):16.

19. Reppert EJ, Streeter RN, Simpson KM, et al. Retrograde catheterization of the urinary bladder in healthy male goats by use of angiographic catheters. Am J Vet Res 2016;77(11):1295–9.

20. Palmer JL, Dykes NL, Love K, et al. Contrast radiography of the lower urinary tract in the management of obstructive urolithiasis in small ruminants and swine. Vet Radiol Ultrasound 1998;39(3):175–80.

21. Kannan KV, Lawrence KE. Obstructive urolithiasis in a Saanen goat in New Zealand, resulting in a ruptured bladder. N Z Vet J 2010;58(5):269–71.

22. Andrabi Y, Patino M, Das CJ, et al. Advances in CT imaging for urolithiasis. Indian J Urol 2015;31(3):185–93.

23. Fortier LA, Gregg AJ, Erb HN, et al. Caprine obstructive urolithiasis: requirement for 2nd surgical intervention and mortality after percutaneous tube cystostomy, surgical tube cystostomy, or urinary bladder marsupialization. Vet Surg 2004; 33(6):661–7.

24. Lairmore MD, Knight AP, DeMartini JC. Three primary neoplasms in a goat: hepatocellular carcinoma, phaeochromocytoma and leiomyoma. J Comp Pathol 1987; 97(3):267–71.

25. Timurkaan N, Yener Z, Ycjksel H. Leiomyoma of the urinary bladder in a goat. Aust Vet J 2001;79(10):708–9.

26. Löfstedt RM, Laarveld B, Ihle SL. Adrenal neoplasia causing lactation in a castrated male goat. J Vet Intern Med 1994;8(5):382–4.

27. Gonzalez-Bulnes A, Pallares P, Vazquez MI. Ultrasonographic imaging in small ruminant reproduction. Reprod Domest Anim 2010;45(Suppl 2):9–20.
28. Scott P. Practical Use of ultrasound scan in small ruminant medicine and surgery. Vet Clin North Am Food Anim Pract 2016;32(1):181–205.
29. Hesselink JW, Taverne MA. Ultrasonography of the uterus of the goat. Vet Q 1994; 16(1):41–5.
30. Smith MC, Sherman DM. Goat medicine. 2nd edition. Hoboken (NJ): Wiley-Blackwell; 1994.
31. Memon MA, Schelling SH, Sherman DM. Mucinous adenocarcinoma of the ovary as a cause of ascites in a goat. J Am Vet Med Assoc 1995;206(3):362–4.
32. Linton JK, Heller MC, Bender SJ, et al. Neoplasia of the tubular genital tract in 42 goats. J Am Vet Med Assoc 2020;256(7):808–13.
33. Scott PR, Gessert ME. Ultrasonographic examination of 12 ovine vaginal prolapses. Vet J 1998;155(3):323–4.

Management of Urologic Conditions in Small Ruminants

Clare M. Scully, MA, DVM, MS

KEYWORDS

- Small ruminant • Obstructive urolithiasis • Ulcerative posthitis • Vulvitis
- Urinary tract infection

KEY POINTS

- The most common urinary tract diseases in small ruminants are related to management practices.
- Urologic conditions in small ruminants affect males more than females primarily due to anatomic differences.
- As more goats and sheep are kept as pets, there is an increasing number of patients that present for urologic conditions.

INTRODUCTION

Small ruminants are a unique food production species because a significant number are also kept as pets, used as breeding animals, or to produce milk for a single family. Small ruminant owners have a strong emotional attachment to their animals and are more likely to bring them to the veterinarian to be treated for certain medical disorders. This additional emotional value of the animal has brought about the need to revisit the approach and management of urologic conditions in these small ruminants that may have previously warranted culling from the herd without significant efforts in treatment. The most common urologic condition seen in these animals is obstructive urolithiasis. However, posthitis, vulvitis, and urinary tract infections are being seen more commonly and should not be neglected.

OBSTRUCTIVE UROLITHIASIS

Obstructive urolithiasis is the most common urinary tract disease in small ruminants and can be the direct result of certain management practices.[1] As more goats and sheep are kept as pets, an increasing number of patients present for urolithiasis.

Department of Veterinary Clinical Sciences, Louisiana State University School of Veterinary Medicine, Skip Bertman Drive, Baton Rouge, LA 70803, USA
E-mail address: cscully@lsu.edu

Vet Clin Food Anim 37 (2021) 93–104
https://doi.org/10.1016/j.cvfa.2020.10.003
0749-0720/21/© 2020 Elsevier Inc. All rights reserved.

These small ruminants are typically purchased with little direction or instruction regarding appropriate care, such as age at castration, nutrition, and general husbandry practices. These elements can play a large role in the development of urinary tract diseases.[2] Because duration of clinical signs and how quickly the animal responds to treatment administered determines prognosis, it is important that owners are capable of recognizing early signs of disease, as this can be a life-threatening condition.[3,4] For successful resolution, the problem must be recognized and treated early in the disease course, before complications such as urethral necrosis/rupture, bladder leakage/rupture, or hydronephrosis develop.[1]

Obstructive urolithiasis is primarily a disease of males due to their unique anatomy. Obstructive urolithiasis is rarely seen in females.[5] This is especially common in castrated males and even more common in males that are castrated at an early age.[6,7] Urethral development depends on testosterone. Therefore, if the source of testosterone is removed before the urethra has matured, the urethral diameter will not fully develop and the penile-preputial attachment may be retained (eg, persistent frenulum).[8] The long, convoluted urethra (made narrow from early castration), the sigmoid flexure, and the urethral process provide several potential sites of urethral obstruction with a single large stone or many small, sandlike stones. Anatomically, the most common sites for a urolith to obstruct are the urethral process and the distal sigmoid flexure. Three clinical manifestations or syndromes exist following blockage of the urethra with a stone: partial or complete urethral obstruction; urethral rupture; and bladder rupture. Two or all three of these clinical manifestations can exist simultaneously. Prolonged partial obstruction or complete urethral obstruction can lead to hydroureter, hydronephrosis, bladder wall damage, and urethral strictures.[9]

In addition to the anatomic factors that predispose small ruminants to urethral obstruction, numerous predisposing dietary factors can also contribute to urolith formation. Awareness of these risk factors can aid in prevention. The composition of the obstructive uroliths is commonly struvite and/or calcium phosphate, and this highly depends on diet. Diets that are high in calcium (Ca), magnesium (Mg), and/or phosphorus (P) result in an altered Ca:P ratio and can result in stone formation.[10] Pelleted concentrate diets and diets deficient in vitamin A are also risk factors. Small ruminants can also develop calcium carbonate and calcium oxalate uroliths.[11,12] Forages and concentrates containing legumes, oxalates, sweet potatoes, dock, apple, and pigweed have been shown to contribute toward formation of these crystals.[12]

Nondietary predisposing factors that contribute to urolith development include increased urine concentration, urine stasis, increased urine pH, increased mineral excretion, desquamated epithelial cells, urinary tract infections, and increased urinary mucoproteins.[13] Most urinary calculi will form more readily in alkaline urine. In small ruminants, factors that predispose to an alkaline urine pH include an herbivore diet, diets that are high in protein, and urinary tract infections.[14] Water intake may be the single most important factor in prevention of urolithiasis.[6,15] Clean, fresh water needs to be available all year long. A good rule of thumb to provide to producers is, "if you are not willing to drink the water in their troughs neither should they." Addition of supplements (eg, salt or mineral block) and exercise can also help encourage water consumption.

Many times, these small ruminants may present for straining (often mistaken by producers and pet owners as constipation) (**Fig. 1**). On physical examination, depending on duration of symptoms and pain level, the heart and respiratory rates are frequently increased. The animal may be anorectic, exhibit a mild bloat, and be lethargic. Many times, they act colicky with stretching, treading, kicking at their belly, and vocalization/ lip curling. On abdominal palpation/ultrasound, a large distended bladder is noted

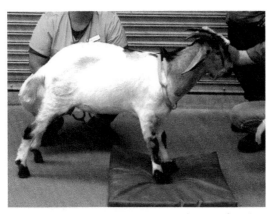

Fig. 1. Straining stance usually seen on presentation, often confused with constipation.

(**Fig. 2**).[16,17] When examining the prepuce, blood or crystals may be observed or palpated on the preputial hairs as well as a mild urethral swelling at site of obstruction. A concurrent preputial and/or rectal prolapse may also be presented due to the degree of straining. If the obstruction is left unattended, it will result in a ruptured urethra, allowing urine to accumulate in the subcutaneous tissues and pool ventrally and/or a ruptured bladder with development of uroperitoneum.[10]

When attempting to make a diagnosis of and prognosis for obstructive urolithiasis, the animal's value, both economic and emotional, as well as his unique anatomic structures must be taken into consideration.[18] Clinical signs associated with a ruptured urethra include ventral and preputial edema, signs of uremia, and in chronic cases, hyperemic skin and edematous subcutaneous tissues begin to slough. Clinical signs associated with a ruptured bladder include gradual abdominal distension, signs of uremia, and an acute reduction in pain.

During the physical examination, the perineal area should be observed for the presence of focal swelling. Aspirated subcutaneous fluid would smell as urine if heated. Palpating pulsations of the urethra below the anus without urination indicate urethral obstruction.[19] Based on physical examination findings, an ultrasonographic examination of the urogenital tract should be performed to assess bladder and urethral

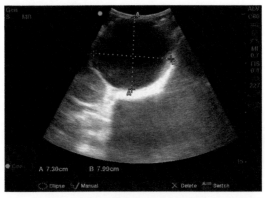

Fig. 2. Typical ultrasound image of the bladder in a blocked small ruminant.

distention. Abdominal ultrasonography would show large amounts of free fluid that (if aspirated) would smell as urine. Fluid accumulation in the renal pelvis indicates hydronephrosis should be documented as well as evidence for the site of urethral obstruction.[1]

If a urine sample can be collected, it should be inspected for viscosity (it should be watery); color (it should be a light straw to amber in color); clarity (it should be transparent); and odor (it should lack a strong ammonia smell).[20] Initial assessment should include a minimum hematological database that assesses hydration, electrolytes, and renal enzymes. Goats with uroliths have higher blood urea nitrogen (BUN), creatinine, total CO_2, potassium (K), glucose concentrations and lower phosphorus (P), sodium (Na), and chloride (Cl) concentrations.[7] These abnormalities should be corrected when considering medical or surgical options.

Surgical treatment options depend on where the stone is lodged, type of stone, and the intended use of the animal. A tube cystotomy will preserve breeding ability, keep the animal continent, and is most successful when the cause of the blockage is struvite stones/sludge. Calcium carbonate stones are often identified during this initial surgery or with postop radiographs (**Fig. 3**) and will not resolve with a simple tube cystotomy or dietary changes. A further surgical procedure may be necessary to resolve calcium carbonate stones such as a urethrostomy. A tube cystotomy diverts urine while allowing urethral swelling to subside so that uroliths can pass. It also allows for removal of other stones from the bladder as well as retro and antegrade flushing of the urethra. However, urethral rupture is still possible. In order to ensure a successful outcome, the cystotomy tube should be left open until urine is noted at the tip of the prepuce (**Fig. 4**) At this point, the tube can be closed and the animal is challenged under continual supervision to see if they can urinate normally. This process can take up to 10 days, and the animal should be maintained on broad-spectrum antibiotics, flunixin meglumine (1.1 mg/kg intravenously [IV]), morphine (0.1–0.4 mg/kg), phenazopyridine (5 mg/kg PO), or N-butylscopolammonium bromide (0.3 mg/kg IV) to relax the urethra, and urinary acidifiers.[21] If successful, the patient should remain on urine acidifiers and a reduced concentrate diet for the rest of its life. Reobstruction is a common complication of this procedure especially if management conditions do not change.

If tube cystotomy is unsuccessful and a follow-up procedure is needed, or if breeding and/or continence is not a concern for the owner, bladder marsupialization

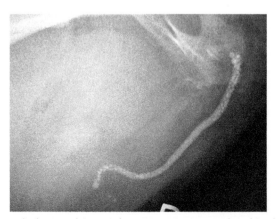

Fig. 3. This radiograph shows calcium carbonate stones accumulated in the urethra.

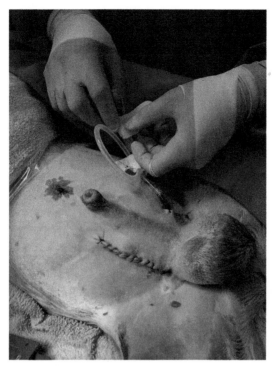

Fig. 4. Postoperative image following a tube cystostomy.

can be performed. Bladder marsupialization is a salvage procedure and owners must be prepared for intensive long-term aftercare associated with lifelong incontinence. Other complications with bladder marsupialization include cystitis, ascending urinary tract infections, and possible stricture of the stoma. With this procedure, the apex of the bladder is sutured to the ventral body wall and skin at a 3 to 5 cm paramedian incision site. A stoma is created between the bladder and the ventral body wall to allow for permanent drainage of urine.[22]

Because of the complications and intensive aftercare associated with bladder marsupialization, vesiculopreputial anastomosis may prove to be a better option.[23] Vesiculopreputial anastomosis is a newer surgical procedure that requires a more skilled surgical technique to be successful. It is not without complications such as dehiscence, fistulas, and infection. However, it offers the benefit of less maintenance, as urine is diverted into the prepuce for evacuation.[24]

The urethral process is the narrowest part of the urethra and is a common location for urinary calculi to lodge. If the stone is lodged in the urethral process, urethral obstruction can be corrected by simply amputating the urethral process of an exteriorized penis. This procedure can be accomplished with the sedated animal sitting up on its rump. The preputial cavity should be disinfected by lavaging with a weak iodine solution. Local analgesia can be achieved by instilling 1% lidocaine into the preputial cavity and held in place by occluding the preputial orifice with index finger and thumb. Epidural anesthesia can also be used. The glans penis is then exteriorized, and the urethral process is amputated close to its attachment to glans at a 60° angle (**Fig. 5**). Cutting the urethra at this angle will create the widest aperture at the opening.

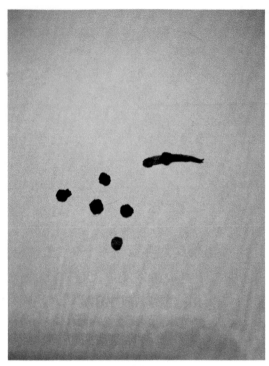

Fig. 5. Amputated urethral process with uroliths.

Unfortunately, the reoccurrence rate of urethral obstruction following urethral process removal is about 50%, as there is frequently more than one urolith present.[25]

Postoperative care is key for successful outcomes. Expression of pain can be particularly difficult to assess accurately in prey species such as small ruminants, which can lead to inadvertently undermedicating an animal in pain. Goats are becoming increasingly common as family pets and the demand for high-quality medical care that exceeds their value as a production animal is becoming more commonplace. A multimodal approach to pain management could include antiinflammatories (meloxicam, flunixin meglumine), opiates (morphine, butorphanol, buprenorphine, fentanyl patches), and acupuncture.[26] Cannabidiol products and intrathecal indwelling catheters could be included, as they become more economically feasible and clinically acceptable practices.

If surgery is not an option and the decision is made to treat medically, phenothiazine tranquilizers are superior to alpha-2 agonists for sedation.[27,28] Fluids (0.9% NaCl) may be necessary to stabilize the patient. If hyperkalemic, dextrose should be added to the fluids (2%–5%). Calcium (23% calcium gluconate) should also be added to the fluids if indicated by the blood work. Urethral catheterization and retropulsion is technically challenging due to the anatomic roadblock of the subischial urethral diverticulum.[29] Complications with this method include urethritis, urethral rupture, and urethral stricture formation. Walpole solution (glacial acetic acid) can be injected intravesicularly into sedated patients via ultrasound-guided cystocentesis to decrease the urine pH to less than 6.5.[30] This treatment is the most successful when treating struvite crystalluria[9]; however, the success rate of this procedure leading to permanent urethral patency is very low.[30] In cases of ruptured bladder or urethra the addition of Walpole solution would be contraindicated. Broad-spectrum antibiotics, nonsteroidal antiinflammatories, and urinary acidifiers may also be indicated. Owners should be aware of the guarded prognosis in cases of urethral or bladder rupture.[3]

ULCERATIVE POSTHITIS

Ulcerative posthitis is an infectious and inflammatory condition of the prepuce and penis of the male small ruminant.[31] It is also known as enzootic balanoposthitis, pizzle rot, and sheath rot.[32] It is more common in castrated males but can also affect bucks and rams.[33] It is a chronic condition, characterized by scabs and ulceration of the skin and mucosa of the prepuce and is caused by overgrowth of the gram-positive organism *Corynebacterium renale*, a normal bacterial inhabitant of the prepuce, due to environmental mucosal changes exacerbated by a high protein diet.[34]

When ruminants are fed a high protein diet, characterized by a dietary protein concentration greater than 16%, they commonly excrete increased urea concentrations in their urine. The increase in urea alkalinizes the urine, which allows for the urease-producing bacteria found in the urinary tract to break down the urea to release excess ammonia. The increase in ammonia results in irritation and ulceration of the prepuce allowing for overgrowth of *C renale*. If the resulting infection is severe, fibrosis, scarring, and stricture of the preputial opening can occur, which can interfere with urination. This may result in the patient becoming uremic and can be fatal if left untreated.[35]

Clinical signs of ulcerative posthitis include pain when urinating, dysuria, urine pooling in the prepuce, and kicking at the abdomen. Intact males may show decreased willingness to breed (libido) due to discomfort associated with lesions contacting the female during intromission. This infection can also be passed to females at breeding resulting in vulvitis.[36]

Presumptive diagnosis is based on physician examination, clinical signs, and dietary history. On physical examination swelling may be noted at the front of the prepuce, and the area is painful on palpation. Definitive diagnosis requires consistent clinical signs of the disease in addition to a positive preputial swab culture to confirm presence of the causative organism.[31] In addition to *C renale,* caprine herpesvirus 1 and *Actinobacillus seminis* have also been reported to cause ulcerative posthitis.[37,38]

Treatment of ulcerative posthitis depends on the severity of the lesions.[1] Focal care consists of clipping the preputial hair and cleaning the area with a nonirritating antiseptic or antibiotic solution. Because of the contagious nature of this disease, clippers and fibers should be dealt with in a manner to prevent spread by cleaning them with a bactericidal spray designed for clippers.[39] If stenosis of the preputial orifice has occurred, measures need to be taken to reestablish the patency of the prepuce. Care needs to be taken when surgically repairing the prepuce due to the risk of additional stricture or the development of adhesions.[40] Once opened, cleaned, and clipped, a topical antibiotic such as Neosporin should be applied to the lesions.[41] Systemic antimicrobial therapy with penicillin or cephalosporin should be considered if there is concern of ascending infection to internal structures.[42] In mild cases, the addition of an acidifying agent, that is, ammonium chloride, to the feed to acidify the alkaline urine may be sufficient.[40]

Prevention is considered superior to treatment of clinical disease. Dietary protein concentration that is less than 16% crude protein is considered ideal.[43] Diets should focus on maximizing hay intake, and consideration should be given to the addition of a urinary acidifier to help control ulcerative posthitis.[40] Any animal diagnosed with ulcerative posthitis should be separated from the herd. Additional biosecurity principles, such as quarantine of new animals for at least 30 days, reducing visitor traffic, and no reuse of needles, should be put in place to prevent spread of the disease.[1]

VULVITIS

There are many different types of vulvitis described in small ruminant. The focus here includes ulcerative, enzootic, and granular vulvitis. Determining which condition is present is the first step to managing their resolution.

Ulcerative vulvitis is inflammation of the vulva characterized by erosion and ulceration of the associated tissues. The cause of ulcerative vulvitis is unclear and numerous organisms (*Mycoplasma spp., Histophilus spp., Trueperella pyogenes*) have been implicated as a cause of infection.[32] Ulcerative vulvitis is relatively common in small ruminants but often includes other surrounding structures such as the vestibule and vagina.[44] When the vagina is involved it is referred to as vulvovaginitis. The anatomy of the small ruminant vulva is fairly simple but susceptible to injury during parturition and coitus. These organisms and poor vulva conformation have been proposed as contributing factors resulting in ulcerative vulvitis.[38,40] Ulcerative vulvitis typically begins as an inflammatory reddening of the vulva and is associated with marked swelling.[45] If left untreated it may progress to development of a yellow exudate with ulceration and scab formation around the vulva, vestibule, and caudal vagina. The glans clitoridis may also be swollen, red, and ulcerated.[46]

Enzootic vulvitis is the female analogue of pizzle rot in the male. It is associated with high protein diets and local infection with *C renale*.[47] Many of the same diagnostics and treatment recommendations for ulcerative posthitis can be implemented with both ulcerative and enzootic vulvitis.

Granular vulvitis is the term used when the infection can be attributed to *Ureaplasma spp*.[48] It is characterized by hyperemia and lymphoid proliferation of the affected tissues. Considered a venereal disease in small ruminants, the male is often implicated as a major distributor of infection.[49] *U spp.* has been identified as a possible causative agent of ovine infertility and abortion.[50] Venereal transmission of the disease has been documented, and several months may pass between exposure of females to infected males and development of vulvitis in the females.[40] The first clinical sign may be the presence of blood on or around the vulva after the start of mating.[32] Production loss results from decreased energy due to pain, incapacitation of breeding animals, loss of breeding soundness, and deformation of external genitalia.[47]

The type of vulvitis encountered will determine the causes that need to be addressed. In the presence of pathogenic microorganisms an ulcerative vulvitis is most likely. A high protein diet can lead to enzootic vulvitis. Postcoital infection often results in a granular vulvitis. However, any predisposing conditions including poor perineal conformation and exuberant perivulvar tissue all can contribute to the inflammatory process seen with vulvitis. Neoplasia, trauma, parasites, and contagious ecthyma should be ruled out before making a diagnosis of vulvitis. Treatment is often unnecessary, especially with milder cases of the disease. When more severe infections are present, topical or systemic antibiotics and antiinflammatories may be indicated. Other recommendations for controlling the disease include changes in diet, careful sire selection, improved hygiene and cleaning practices, and isolation and quarantine of all new stock.[32,38,40]

URINARY TRACT INFECTIONS

Urinary tract infections are an infection of any part of the urinary system, kidneys, ureters, bladder, and urethra. Most infections in small ruminants involve the lower urinary tract including the bladder and the urethra.[1] Females are at greater risk of developing a urinary tract infection than are males. When the infection is limited to the bladder, it can be painful but successfully treated with antibiotics. Left untreated, serious consequences can occur and spread to the kidneys resulting in pyelonephritis.[51] The causes for the infection vary although most infections are acquired from an ascending infection. Postpartum exposure to contaminants during parturition is an ideal time for one of these infections to occur.[52] The most common etiologic organisms are *C renale*, *Escherichia coli*, staphylococci, and streptococci.[51] Clinical signs include stranguria characterized by painful, frequent urination expelled slowly in small amounts. Urinalysis will reveal hematuria or pyuria, with red blood cells, neutrophils, and, in some cases, bacteria visible in microscopic sediment.[1] Treatment should be an appropriate broad-spectrum antibiotic selected based on culture and sensitivity testing and should be excreted through urine. Additional renal involvement should be ruled out with further diagnostics. These can include ultrasonography and bloodwork including a chemistry to evaluate the kidneys.[14,53] Once the infection has been diagnosed, isolation of diseased animals, particularly with *C renale*, is recommended to limit the spread of the organism. Cleaning and disinfecting of contaminated areas and equipment with bleach is advisable.[53,54]

CLINICS CARE POINTS

- When amputating the urethral process, this procedure can be easier with sedation/epidural and with animal sitting on its rump. A scalpel blade and cutting against a surface such as a tongue depressor will allow for a cleaner more precise cut than with scissors.
- During corrective surgery of obstructive urolithiasis the prognosis for a successful outcome increases if the urethra can be flushed normo/retrograde during the procedure.
- Realistic expectations of success and lifetime aftercare expectations need to be discussed with every blocked small ruminant owner so they understand that this is not a quick fix or an easy solution.
- It is crucial to educate owners on the management considerations associated with obstructive urolithiasis in order to prevent it from occurring.
- Postoperative management of obstructive urolithiasis should be focused on pain control as well as acidification of the urine to prevent further stone formation.

DISCLOSURE

The author has nothing to disclose.

REFERENCES

1. Jones M, Miesner MD, Baird A, et al. Diseases of the urinary system. In: Pugh DG, Baird AN, editors. Sheep and goat medicine. Maryland Heights (MO): Elsevier; 2012. p. 325–60.
2. McIntosh GH. Urolithiasis in animals. Aust Vet J 1978;54(6):267–71.
3. Riedi AK, Nathues C, Knubben-Schweizer G, et al. Variables of initial examination and clinical management associated with survival in small ruminants with obstructive urolithiasis. J Vet Intern Med 2018;32(6):2105–14.
4. Chase C, Lutz K, McKenzie E, et al. Blackwell's five-minute veterinary consult: ruminant. Hoboken (NJ): John Wiley & Sons; 2017.

5. Jensen R, Swift BL. Diseases of sheep. Philadelphia: Lea & Febiger; 1982.
6. Ewoldt JM, Anderson DE, Miesner MD, et al. Short- and long-term outcome and factors predicting survival after surgical tube cystostomy for treatment of obstructive urolithiasis in small ruminants. Vet Surg 2006;35(5):417–22.
7. George JW, Hird DW, George LW. Serum biochemical abnormalities in goats with uroliths: 107 cases (1992-2003). J Am Vet Med Assoc 2007;230(1):101–6.
8. Underwood WJ, Blauwiekel R, Delano ML, et al. Biology and diseases of ruminants (sheep, goats, and cattle). In: Fox J, Anderson L, Otto G, et al, editors. Laboratory animal medicine. Amsterdam (the Netherlands): Elsevier; 2015. p. 623–94.
9. Nagy DW. Urolithiasis in small ruminants. In: Proceedings for the Central Veterinary Conference in Kansas City; August 29 - September 1, 2009.
10. Makhdoomi D, Gazi MA. Obstructive urolithiasis in ruminants-A review. Vet World 2013;6(4).
11. Jones ML, Gibbons PM, Roussel AJ, et al. Mineral composition of uroliths obtained from sheep and goats with obstructive urolithiasis. J Vet Intern Med 2017;31(4):1202–8.
12. Navarre CB. Urolithiasis: causes, treatments & prevention. In: Proceedings from the North American Veterinary Conference, Orlando, Florida, January 18–22, 2003. p. 280–2.
13. Rankins DL Jr, Pugh D. Feeding and nutrition. In: Pugh DG, Baird AN, editors. Sheep and goat medicine. Maryland Heights (MO): Elsevier/Saunders; 2012. p. 18–49.
14. Carlson G. Clinical Chemistry Tests. In: Smith BP, editor. Large animal internal medicine. 3rd edition. St Louis (MO): Mosby; 2002. p. 389–412.
15. Van Metre DC, Fubini SL. Ovine and caprine urolithiasis: another piece of the puzzle. Vet Surg 2006;35(5):413–6.
16. Angelos JA. Urolithiasis in small ruminants - Part 1. In: Proceedings of the North American Veterinary Conference, Orlando, Florida, January 18–22, 2014.
17. Angelos JA. Urolithiasis in small ruminants - Part 2. In: Proceedings of the North American Veterinary Conference, Orlando, Florida, January 18–22, 2014.
18. Ewoldt JM, Jones ML, Miesner MD. Surgery of obstructive urolithiasis in ruminants. Vet Clin North Am Food Anim Pract 2008;24(3):455–65.
19. Videla R, van Amstel S. Urolithiasis. Vet Clin North Am Food Anim Pract 2016; 32(3):687–700.
20. Parrah J, Moulvi B, Gazi M, et al. Importance of urinalysis in veterinary practice. Vet World 2013;6(9):640–6.
21. Tamilmahan P, Mohsina A, Karthik K, et al. Tube cystostomy for management of obstructive urolithiasis in ruminants. Vet World 2014;7(4):234–9.
22. May KA, Moll HD, Wallace LM, et al. Urinary bladder marsupialization for treatment of obstructive urolithiasis in male goats. Vet Surg 1998;27(6):583–8.
23. Haven ML, Bowman KF, Engelbert TA, et al. Surgical management of urolithiasis in small ruminants. Cornell Vet 1993;83(1):47–55.
24. Cypher EE, van Amstel SR, Videla R, et al. Vesicopreputial anastomosis for the treatment of obstructive urolithiasis in goats. Vet Surg 2017;46(2):281–8.
25. Anderson DE. Small ruminant tips - Part 1: Urolithiasis. In: Proceedings of the North American Veterinary Conference, Orlando, Florida, January 14–18, 2012.
26. Hamed M, Rizk A, Mosbah E, et al. Evaluation of different anesthetic drugs combination for pain management in goats undergoing tube cystostomy. Global Veterinaria 2015;14(2):251–61.

27. Metre DC. Medical and surgical management of urolithiasis. In: Proceedings of the North American Veterinary Conference, Orlando, Florida, January 14–18, 2012.

28. van Metre DC, House JK, Smith BP, et al. Obstructive urolithiasis in ruminants: medical treatment and urethral surgery. Compend Contin Educ Pract Vet 1996; 18(3):317–27.

29. Hinkle RF, Howard JL, Stowater JL. An anatomic barrier to urethral catheterization in the male goat. J Am Vet Med Assoc 1978;173(12):1584–6.

30. Janke JJ, Osterstock JB, Washburn KE, et al. Use of Walpole's solution for treatment of goats with urolithiasis: 25 cases (2001–2006). J Am Vet Med Assoc 2009; 234(2):249–52.

31. Jones ML. Ulcerative posthitis. Current veterinary therapy 5: food animal practice. St. Louis (MO): Saunders Elsevier; 2008. p. 327.

32. Greig A. Ulcerative balanitis and vulvitis. In: Aitken ID, editor. Diseases of sheep. Ames (IA): Blackwell Publishing; 2007. p. 143–5.

33. Jones M. Ulcerative Posthitis. In: Anderson DE, editor. Current veterinary therapy E-Book: food animal practice. St. Louis (MO): Elsevier Health Sciences; 2009. p. 328–9.

34. Loste A, Ramos JJ, Garcia L, et al. High prevalence of ulcerative posthitis in Rasa Aragonesa rams associated with a legume-rich diet. J Vet Med A Physiol Pathol Clin Med 2005;52(4):176–9.

35. Brook A, Southcott W, Stacy B. Etiology of ovine posthitis: Relationship between urine and a causal organism. Austral Vet J 1966;42(1):9–12.

36. Mickelsen WD, Menon MA. Current therapy in large animal theriogenology. Philadelphia: Saunders; 1997. p. 519–23.

37. Uzal FA, Woods L, Stillian M, et al. Abortion and ulcerative posthitis associated with caprine herpesvirus-1 infection in goats in California. J Vet Diagn Invest 2004;16(5):478–84.

38. Kidanemariam A, Gouws J, van Vuuren M, et al. Ulcerative balanitis and vulvitis of Dorper sheep in South Africa: a study on its aetiology and clinical features. J S Afr Vet Assoc 2005;76(4):197–203.

39. Southcott W. Epidemiology and control of ovine posthitis and vulvitis. Austral Vet J 1965;41(8):225–34.

40. Van Metre D. Ulcerative posthitis and vulvitis. In: Smith BP, editor. Large animal internal medicine. 4th edition. St Louis (MO): Mosby Elsevier; 2009. p. 949–50.

41. Byers SR. Ulcerative posthitis and vulvitis. 5th editionn. St. Louis, MO: Mosby; 2015.

42. Radostits O, Gay C, Hinchcliff K, et al. A textbook of the diseases of cattle, sheep, goats, pigs and horses. Veterinary medicine. 10th edition. London: Bailliere; 2007. p. 1576–80.

43. Petrovic MP, Stanojkovic A, Petrovic VC, et al. Relevant factors affecting the fertility of rams. J Mount Ag Balkans 2017;20(1):77–91.

44. Pritchard GC, Scholes SF, Foster AP, et al. Ulcerative vulvitis and balanitis in sheep flocks. Vet Rec 2008;163(3):86–9.

45. Dent C. Ulcerative vulvitis and posthitis in Australian sheep and cattle. Vet Bulletin 1971;41:719–23.

46. Ihemelandu EC. Ulcerative vulvitis in goats. Vet Rec 1972;91(8):197.

47. Momont H, Checura C. Vulvitis. In: Chase C, Lutz K, McKenzie E, et al, editors. Blackwell's five-minute veterinary consult: ruminant. 2nd edition. Hoboken (NJ): Wiley-Blackwell; 2017. p. 948–9.

48. Ball HJ, McCaughey WJ. Experimental production of vulvitis in ewes with a ureaplasma isolate. Vet Rec 1982;110(25):581.
49. McCaughey W, Ball H, Irwin D. Isolation of ureaplasma from ewes following synchronised mating. Irish Vet J 1981;35:210–3.
50. Livingston CW Jr, Gauer BB, Shelton M. A specific ureaplasmal serotype associated with ovine uterine infections. Am J Vet Res 1978;39(10):1699–701.
51. Higgins RJ, Weaver CR. Corynebacterium renale pyelonephritis and cystitis in a sheep. Vet Rec 1981;109(12):256.
52. Yeruham I, Elad D, Avidar Y, et al. A herd level analysis of urinary tract infection in dairy cattle. Vet J 2006;171(1):172–6.
53. Dominguez BJ. Urinary tract infection. In: Smith BP, editor. Large animal internal medicine. St. Louis (MO): Mosby; 2015. p. 882–4.
54. Al-Dabbagh S, Ali H, Khalil I, et al. A study of some antibiotics; disinfectants and antiseptics efficacy against some species of pathogenic bacteria. Assiut Vet Med J 2015;61(147):210–7.

Management of Reproductive Diseases in Male Small Ruminants

Jamie L. Stewart, DVM, PhD[a],*, Clifford F. Shipley, DVM[b]

KEYWORDS

- Balanitis • Buck • Epididymitis • Genital • Orchitis • Posthitis • Ram • Urolithiasis

KEY POINTS

- Routine breeding soundness examinations in rams and bucks are crucial to identifying reproductive tract lesions that can severely impact breeding success.
- Exteriorization of the penis should be performed with every reproductive examination to ensure the penis and prepuce are free of masses or lesions.
- Early diagnosis of infectious diseases is important because once clinical signs develop (such as epididymitis or orchitis) prognosis begins to worsen.
- Ancillary diagnostics, such as testicular or transrectal ultrasound examination, can aid the practitioner in determining prognosis of reproductive tract diseases.
- Immediate culling should be recommended in males diagnosed with chlamydiosis or brucellosis owing to their infectious and abortifacient potentials.

INTRODUCTION

In 2020, the US Department of Agriculture reported a total of 5.2 million sheep and 2.7 million goats in the United States.[1] This inventory of small ruminants has remained relatively stable over the past 5 years, but most operations still rely on a successful breeding season to ensure profitability. In any situation where conception rates are lower than expected, evaluation of the male should be the first step in diagnosing a cause. In breeding operations, animals can be housed at a ratio of up to 1 male per 50 females. Smaller farms may rely on only 1 or 2 males to cover the entire flock or herd, and development of a reproductive disease in a sire can have disastrous consequences. For this reason, yearly routine breeding soundness examinations of males are recommended to rule out subfertility, identify reproductive tract lesions, and

[a] Department of Large Animal Clinical Sciences, Virginia-Maryland College of Veterinary Medicine, Virginia Polytechnic Institute and State University, 205 Duckpond Drive, Blacksburg, VA 24061, USA; [b] Department of Veterinary Clinical Medicine, College of Veterinary Medicine, University of Illinois, 2001 South Lincoln Avenue, Urbana, IL 61801, USA
* Corresponding author.
E-mail address: jlstewart13@vt.edu

Vet Clin Food Anim 37 (2021) 105–123
https://doi.org/10.1016/j.cvfa.2020.10.005
0749-0720/21/© 2020 Elsevier Inc. All rights reserved.

vetfood.theclinics.com

prevent such negative consequences before the breeding season. In small ruminants, which typically exhibit seasonal changes in reproductive status, this examination should occur early in the fall with enough time for producers to find a replacement sire if necessary.[2] For operations breeding outside the natural reproductive season (spring or summer), males should be reexamined closer to the time of breeding. The effects of season on sperm quality and quantity can vary widely between species, breeds, and even individuals, so males intended for out-of-season breeding should be evaluated closely for physiologic testicular degeneration and decreased semen quality. As a result of these natural changes, bucks and rams should not be failed on a breeding soundness examination performed out of season unless a specific disease process is identified. Rather, males that do not perform well out of season should be reserved for use during in-season breeding provided they pass the examination in the fall.

The routine breeding soundness examination includes an assessment of overall health that includes body condition score, foot and leg evaluation, and FAMACHA scoring. A thorough history with information regarding breeding results in previous seasons, health issues, and vaccine schedule can be beneficial. Depending on the purpose of the examination, serologic testing for specific diseases may be warranted (and may be required if sale or interstate transport is involved). Examination of the reproductive organs (penis/prepuce, scrotal contents, with or without the accessory sex glands) and semen evaluation are also required.[3] The presence of white blood cells in ejaculates ($\geq$10 white blood cells per low power field [magnification of $\times$100]) may be an early sign of disease that warrants subsequent testing for pathogens.[4] Breeding classifications for small ruminants can either be assigned using a point score system[5] or by simply categorizing each male as satisfactory, questionable, or unsatisfactory.[2,3]

Even with the most prepared clients, issues can arise throughout breeding and may require reevaluation if a problem is observed within the herd or flock. This review details some of the most common reproductive diseases found in rams and bucks and provides insight into their diagnosis and management.

UROLITHIASIS

Urolithiasis is a common condition in sheep and goats that often results in complete obstruction of the urethra. Although reported more frequently in castrated males, intact males are also commonly affected with uroliths. Diet is the most important predisposing factor for bucks and rams. High grain diets, such as those used to condition males before the breeding season, increase the secretion of phosphorus into the urine and favor the development of struvite stones.[6] Prevention is always ideal and can be achieved by proper nutritional planning and pulse feeding of ammonium chloride during conditioning periods to acidify the urine and discourage the production of struvite stones. Additionally, appropriate mineral supplementation and fresh water sources should be offered to encourage fluid intake. Owners should be made aware of any signs of urolithiasis (posturing to urinate, straining to urinate, dribbling urine), because it is commonly confused for constipation during the early stages. Early intervention, before complete obstruction, requires a keen eye and significantly improves the prognosis for recovery.

For valuable intact males, the recommended course of treatment is a surgical tube cystotomy.[7] This technique is preferred because it allows the surgeon to clear the bladder of any remaining uroliths to prevent reobstruction. Additionally, a Foley catheter is placed into the bladder to provide an alternate urination route for the male and give the urethra time to heal inflammation while the stones dissolve. A nonsurgical method has been described using a percutaneous approach to insert the Foley catheter into the bladder with subsequent infusion of an acidifying solution (Walpole's solution, commonly).[8] In the authors' experience, this method fails more often than its surgical counterpart owing to the catheter becoming occluded with crystals. However, it might be an ideal low-cost alternative for less valuable intact males when maintaining breeding potential is desired. In cases where urethral rupture is observed, the owner should be informed that preserving breeding ability is no longer an option and that a salvage procedure (such as a perineal urethrostomy or bladder marsupialization) should be considered to allow the animal to go to market.

Medical management can be attempted to treat urolithiasis, but is more effective in the early stages when there is only partial urethral obstruction. Ultrasound-guided cystocentesis and percutaneous infusion of Walpole's solution to acidify the urine relieved urethral obstruction in 80% of goats in 1 case series.[9] However, it is worth nothing that 30% of these goats had to be reexamined for recurrence of the urethral obstruction.[9] In chronic urolithiasis cases, where surgery is preceded by medical management attempts, cavernositis and fibrosis may occur, resulting in erection failure despite correction of the urethral obstruction.[10] Therefore, early surgical intervention should be considered in valuable males to maximize the likelihood of success.

DISEASES OF THE PENIS AND PREPUCE

Infections of the penis (balanitis), prepuce (posthitis), or both (balanoposthitis) can be a significant cause of reproductive failure in the male. Depending on the etiology, these conditions are usually painful, leaving the male unwilling to mate. Certain conditions can also lead to phimosis or paraphimosis, where the male is unable to retract or exteriorize its penis, respectively. Although sometimes difficult, it is always crucial to exteriorize the penis completely when performing a breeding soundness examination to ensure the penis and urethral process seem to be normal. In most males, penis exteriorization can be facilitated by placing the male on its rump and applying pressure to the sigmoid flexure caudal to the scrotum (**Fig. 1**).

One of the most commonly described causes of balanoposthitis in small ruminants is "pizzle rot." This disease is multifactorial, with diet and anatomic defects both contributing to the overgrowth of commensal bacteria, usually *Corynebacterium renale*.[11] Diets high in protein (>16%) tend to favor the production of urea in the urine, which is then broken down into ammonia by urease enzymes produced from *C renale*.[12] When conditioning males before the breeding season, care must be made to ensure that protein concentrations in the diet are not higher than 12% to 14%, because this factor will increase urine pH and contribute to urea production.[6] An outbreak of pizzle rot in up to 95% of rams has been reported in rams with diets consisting of mostly alfalfa and ryegrass.[13] If an outbreak of lesions such as these is observed, careful reevaluation and adjustment of the diet is crucial. Existing infections can be managed with antibiotics and anti-inflammatories, but will continue to be a problem if the diet is not adjusted.

A thorough examination, including complete exteriorization of the penis with ancillary diagnostics may be crucial in determining prognosis and management options for males with balanoposthitis (**Fig. 2**A). Preputial or penile swabs may be obtained and submitted for bacterial culture to rule out infectious agents such as *Mycoplasma* and *Ureaplasma* spp.[14–16] Any noticeable lesions on the penis or prepuce should be biopsied and submitted for histopathology to rule out the presence of neoplasia, such as squamous cell carcinoma (**Fig. 2**B).[17] Papillomavirus can also be diagnosed

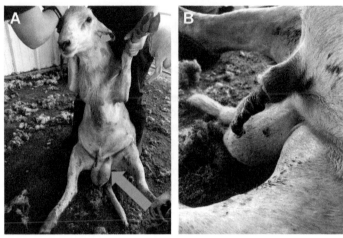

Fig. 1. Exteriorization of the penis in the male small ruminant is an important part of examination that is often overlooked. (*A*) Penis exteriorization can be facilitated by placing the male on his rump and applying pressure to the sigmoid flexure, located caudal to the scrotum (*arrow*). (*B*) Once the penis is exteriorized, it can be examined for abnormalities in mucous membrane color, the presence of any masses or lesions, and integrity of the urethral process (where urethral obstruction commonly occurs).

by performing immunohistochemistry on biopsied tissue.[17] Although papillomavirus on its own tends to be self-limiting, it is infectious and can predispose males to developing neoplastic conditions that carry a grave prognosis.[17] Herpesviruses have also been reported to cause outbreaks of infectious balanoposthitis in rams (*ovine herpesvirus* type 2)[18] and bucks (*caprine herpesvirus* type 1)[19] and can be diagnosed by

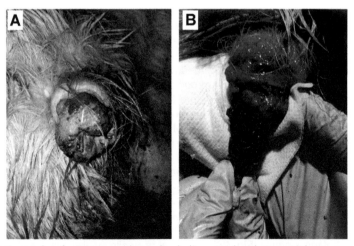

Fig. 2. Photographs of a 4.5-year-old Boer buck diagnosed with preputial squamous cell carcinoma. (*A*) Cranial view of the posthitis at initial presentation. (*B*) Lateral view of the exteriorized penis with numerous squamous cell carcinoma lesions. (*From* Grimmer ED, Canisso IF, Hsiao SH, et al. Squamous cell carcinoma and papilloma virus in the prepuce of a Boer buck. Clin Theriogenology 2017;9(4):595-599; with permission.)

performing virus isolation or polymerase chain reaction on preputial swabs. Because abortions may be linked to these diseases,[19] it is important to separate males from females when lesions are observed. Little is known about the long-term implications of herpesvirus infection in male small ruminants. One report found that lesions developed in a buck 1 day after mating with a *caprine herpesvirus*–infected female.[20] The penis and prepuce of the buck healed by about 15 days after infection, whereas preputial viral shedding continued for up to 24 days after infection.[20] Given that herpesviruses are known to develop latency and recrudesce during periods of stress, recommendations to cull any positive males or females should be made based on the flock or herd status.

Penile and preputial lesions can result from a variety of other common conditions. *Orf virus* can present with pustules or ulcers at the preputial opening or on the penis in rams.[11] Lesions on the preputial orifice, including those from infections (such as *Orf*), fly myiasis, or trauma, can lead to incomplete erections in both bucks and rams.[21] The best way to manage these conditions is to obtain a diagnosis and treat the underlying cause. Rams with suspected or diagnosed *Orf* should be isolated from other animals until all lesions have healed (typically 3 weeks). In some countries, combinations of antiviral drugs (such as cidofovir) and sucralfate have been used topically to treat *Orf* with acceptable results.[22] In addition to being cost prohibitive for many clients, it is also worth noting that these drugs are off label in the United States and require an active veterinarian–client–patient relationship to prescribe; they should only be used if indicated under the Animal Medicinal Drug Use Clarification Act of 1994. Vaccinations against *Orf* should be implemented if infection is endemic within the flock. Common treatments for most diseases of the prepuce should include sexual rest and isolation, fly spray, anti-inflammatories, and/or antimicrobials as determined by the veterinary practitioner based on physical examination findings.

DISEASES OF ACCESSORY SEX GLANDS

Accessory sex gland diseases are rare in small ruminants compared with bulls. In a post mortem analysis of 1000 feral bucks, bulbourethral cysts were reported in 33 (3.3%), vesicular adenitis in 1 (0.1%), and vesicular gland hypertrophy in 1 (0.1%).[23] The clinical relevance of bulbourethral cysts are likely negligible, because they are speculated to be congenital and seemingly have no effect on fertility.[24] Infectious organisms commonly associated with lesions in accessory sex glands are those that are typically associated with orchitis or epididymitis (**Table 1**), such as *Actinobacillus seminis*,[25–28] *Histophilus somni*,[25] *Trueperella pyogenes*,[29] *Chlamydophila abortus*,[30–32] and *Brucella ovis*.[33]

In rams experimentally inoculated with *A seminis*, lesions in the vesicular glands were observed more frequently (40% of inoculated rams; 21/52) than in other accessory sex glands and were associated with both descending infection from the vas deferens or epididymis and ascending infection from the urethra and prepuce.[26,28] Ampulla lesions were observed in 38% of inoculated rams (20/52) and were more frequently associated with descending infection (inoculation of the vas deferens or epididymis).[26,28] Interestingly, the prevalence of ampullitis and vesicular adenitis was found to be higher in rams with concurrent epididymitis (81% and 80%, respectively) than in those without (19% and 20%, respectively).[28] Bulbourethral gland lesions were observed in 23% of inoculated rams (12/52) and more frequently associated with ascending infection (inoculation of the urethra or prepuce).[26,28] Bulbourethral adenitis occurred more frequently in rams without concurrent epididymitis (63%) than those with epididymitis (37%).[28] Lesions in the prostate were not observed

Table 1
Common bacterial causes of lesions in the reproductive tract of rams and bucks

Pathogen	Species	Clinical Effects	Diagnosis
Actinobacillus seminis	Ram	Testicular degeneration,[25,56] epididymitis,[25,26,56] orchitis,[25,56] vesicular adenitis,[25,26,28] ampullitis,[25,26,28] bulbourethral adenitis,[25,26,28] sperm granuloma[56]	Serology (CF, ELISA), Gram stain, culture, or PCR of ejaculate
	Buck	Orchitis,[47,48] epididymitis[47,48]	
Brucella melitensis	Ram and Buck	Orchitis or periorchitis,[50] epididymitis[50]	Serology (CF, AGID, ELISA, FPA); Gram stain, culture, or PCR of ejaculate
Brucella ovis	Ram (more commonly) and Buck	Testicular degeneration,[33] orchitis or periorchitis,[50,51] epididymitis,[33,44,50,51] vesiculitis,[33,51] sperm granuloma[33,51]	Serology (CF, AGID, ELISA, FPA); Gram stain, culture, or PCR of ejaculate
Chlamydophila abortus	Ram and Buck	Orchitis,[32,67,68] epididymitis,[32,68] vesicular adenitis,[30–32] abortions[32,45,68,69]	Serology (CF, FA); culture or PCR of ejaculate
Corynebacterium pseudotuberculosis	Ram and Buck	Orchitis,[42] epididymitis,[42,44] testicular degeneration,[39] abortions[40,41]	Culture of ejaculate or aspirate of lesion
Histophilus somni	Ram	Testicular degeneration,[25] epididymitis,[25] orchitis,[25] vesiculitis,[25] ampullitis,[25] bulbourethritis[25]	Serology (CF); Gram stain, culture, or PCR of ejaculate
Trueperella pyogenes	Ram and Buck	Orchitis or periorchitis,[29,46] epididymitis,[11,29,44,46] vesiculitis[29]	Culture of ejaculate

Abbreviations: AGID, immunodiffusion in agar gel; CF, complement fixation; ELISA, enzyme-linked immunosorbent assay; FA, fluorescent antibody; FPA, fluorescence polarization assay; PCR, polymerase chain reaction.
Data from Refs.[11,25,26,28–33,40–42,44–48,50,51,56,67–69]

frequently, regardless of inoculation site (4% of inoculated rams; 2/52).[28] Accessory sex gland lesions were not observed in rams with intranasal or intraconjunctival routes of *A seminis* infection, suggesting that respiratory secretions are not a major source of transmission of this pathogen.[26,28] Rather, infection of ram lambs with *A seminis* could occur as a sequela to umbilical infection early in life, from trauma to the scrotal contents, through homosexual behavior, or even from in utero transplacental transmission from the dam.[26]

Although not routinely performed, transrectal ultrasound examinations can be performed in small ruminants if an infection in the accessory sex glands is suspected. If a high number of white blood cells are noted in an ejaculate, the most common site of infection in the ram or buck is in the testis or epididymis. However, if both seem to be normal on examination, the practitioner should consider transrectal ultrasound examination of the accessory sex glands as a diagnostic tool.[34] As opposed to bulls, small ruminants contain a disseminate prostate (rather than a distinct body) that should be homogenous in appearance and located along the wall of the pelvic urethra (**Fig. 3A**). The paired vesicular glands can be visualized dorsolateral to the bladder and are also homogenous in appearance (**Fig. 3B**). Distention of these glands with echogenic fluid, change in echogenicity, or obvious asymmetry is consistent with infection (**Fig. 3C**). Gross changes in vesicular gland size were observed post mortem in 30% of rams inoculated intraepididymal with *A seminis* and 0% of rams inoculated with *H somni*.[25] Mild to moderate inflammatory lesions were observed on histopathologic examination of vesicular glands in more than 50% of rams inoculated with either *A seminis* or *H somni*.[25]

As with most reproductive tract diseases, treatment of accessory sex gland lesions tends to be unrewarding, especially once clinical signs have emerged. If there is an outbreak of reproductive tract diseases in a group of young males, metaphylactic treatment with oxytetracycline or macrolide antibiotics may help to decrease the incidence or prevent the progression of clinical disease.[27] In herd situations, affected males with poor prognoses should be euthanized and necropsied. Samples of the accessory sex glands, epididymides, and testes should be collected and submitted for histopathology, culture, and sensitivity testing to facilitate further herd management decisions. If necropsy is not possible, a semen sample can be collected from affected males for cytologic analysis and culture (with or without sensitivity testing). The ejaculate should be collected as cleanly as possible with manual penis exteriorization to prevent contamination by preputial organisms. Any antibiotic therapy indicated by sensitivity testing should adhere to guidelines set by the Food Animal Residue Avoidance Databank and recommended meat withdrawal times should be followed. If no significant pathogens are identified on culture, but an infectious organism is suspected based on cytology, polymerase chain reaction testing should be considered to detect organisms such as *C abortus* or *Brucella* spp. Animals diagnosed with chlamydiosis or brucellosis should be immediately culled owing to their infectious and abortifacient potentials.

DISEASES OF THE SPERMATIC CORD

The neck of the scrotum should be palpated for any swellings or masses that may interact with the structures in the spermatic cord and alter sperm quality. Varicoceles are often associated with testicular degeneration owing to thrombosis of testicular blood supply.[35] This condition is usually spontaneous, especially in older rams, and can be either bilateral or unilateral.[35] Some cases may be secondary to scarring from previous trauma.[36] Idiopathic unilateral varicoceles in rams typically occur on

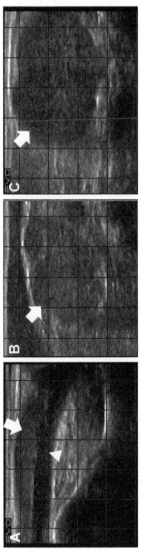

Fig. 3. Transrectal ultrasound examination of accessory sex glands in normal (*A, B*) and abnormal (*C*) Boer bucks. (*A*) Small ruminants possess a disseminate prostate (rather than a distinct body) that is homogenous in appearance (*arrow*) and located along the wall of the pelvic urethra (*arrowhead*). (*B*) The paired vesicular glands (*arrow*) can be visualized dorsolateral to the bladder and are also homogenous in appearance with small anechoic foci. (*C*) An image of a vesicular gland (*arrow*) from a buck with concurrent epididymitis. Note the increase in size and change in echogenicity compared with the normal buck (*B*).

the left side owing to the angle at which the left testicular vein empties into the left renal vein.[36] Unilateral varicoceles can cause subfertility in affected males owing to altered blood flow and thermoregulation of both the ipsilateral and contralateral testes.

Hydrocele is a similar condition where fluid accumulates around either one or both testes and can be idiopathic or associated with inflammation or trauma. In cases of hydrocele, the scrotal circumference may present larger than expected for the animal's age (**Fig. 4**A). Fluid is typically palpable around the testis and can be confirmed with ultrasound examination (**Fig. 4**B). In idiopathic cases with unilateral testicular involvement, semen quality may be initially unaffected. However, as the diseases progresses, the hydrocele fluid can be replaced by fibrous tissue (**Fig. 4**C), resulting in greater testicular asymmetry and pain on palpation. If varicocele or hydrocele conditions are diagnosed before severe testicular changes occur, hemicastration may preserve fertility in valuable males. However, culling is usually the most economical option.

Inguinal or scrotal herniation is another differential for an enlargement of the scrotal neck of small ruminants (**Fig. 5**A). This enlargement should be soft on palpation and may or may not be reducible. Transcrotal ultrasound examination can confirm the presence of herniation by observing intestinal contents (**Fig. 5**B). Herniation is thought to be a heritable and recessive trait so affected young males should be castrated and/ or culled.[37] In unilateral cases where trauma is known or suspected, hemicastrations can be performed to preserve function of the unaffected testis.[38] In cases where hemicastrations are performed to preserve breeding ability, owners should be informed that males should not be bred to as many females as before surgery to maintain acceptable pregnancy rates. This option should be reserved for smaller herds or flocks or those with ample male coverage.

As mentioned elsewhere in this article, ultrasound examination (if available) is a useful tool to assist with the diagnosis and prognosis of scrotal swellings. Intrascrotal

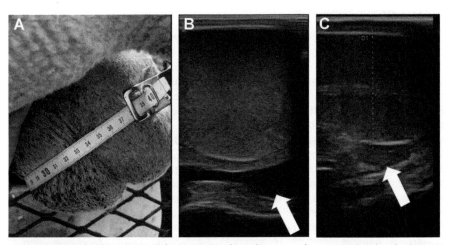

Fig. 4. This ram lamb presented for a routine breeding soundness examination in August. (*A*) The scrotal circumference was large for his age. (*B*) Palpation and ultrasound examination confirmed the presence of anechoic fluid (*arrow*) around the right testis, but semen quality was unaffected. (*C*) Testicular ultrasound examination of the same ram 6 months later. The anechoic fluid is no longer present but fibrous tissue (*arrow*) was in its place. During the examination, the scrotum was enlarged and painful on palpation.

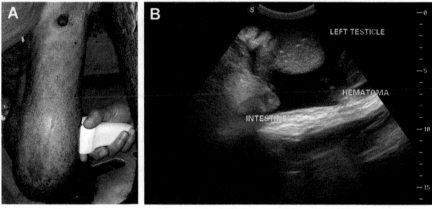

Fig. 5. (A) This ram presented for acute enlargement in the scrotal neck that was suspected to result from trauma. The mass was soft on palpation. (B) Ultrasound examination confirmed the diagnosis of herniation with intestinal involvement so an emergency hemi-castration was performed to preserve breeding ability.

abscesses may palpate as a firm enlargement, but ultrasound examination can be used to determine the involvement of adjacent structures. If there is no underlying involvement, abscesses can be drained and flushed, but males should be isolated from the rest of the flock or herd until the site has completely healed. Culture should be performed either before or after abscess drainage as certain pathogens (*Coryne-bacterium pseudotuberculosis*) can have long-term deleterious effects on ram fertility, are highly infectious, and pose a risk for causing abortions with transmission to the flock.[39–41]

DISEASES OF THE EPIDIDYMIS

Epididymitis is the most common pathology of the reproductive tract of small ruminants. On reproductive examinations, palpation of the scrotal contents should always include distinction of the epididymal cauda (tail), corpus (body), and caput (head). Although a visual examination may suggest testicular asymmetry (**Fig. 6**A), palpation is crucial to distinguish these structures and accurately diagnose epididymitis (**Fig. 6**B).[42] Testes are often concurrently small and palpate soft owing to outflow obstruction and secondary testicular degeneration. Ultrasound examination of the epididymides will reveal echogenic material (**Fig. 6**C). If concurrent with testicular degeneration, the presence of multiple hyperechoic foci (mineralization) may be observed within the testicular parenchyma (see **Fig. 6**C).[43] Culture of the ejaculate can be used to determine the etiology. *C pseudotuberculosis*, the causative agent of caseous lymphadenitis, has been known to cause clinical epididymitis in bucks and rams.[36,44] Other differentials for epididymitis in small ruminants include chlamy-diosis,[44,45] specific pyogenic bacteria (eg, *T pyogenes*[11,29,44,46]), opportunistic bacteria (eg, *A seminis*,[11,44,47,48] *H somni*,[11] *Escherichia coli*,[44] *Moraxella* spp.,[44] *Mannheimia haemolytica*,[11] *Bibersteinia trehalosi*,[11] *Pasteurella multocida*,[11,44] and both *Staphylococcus* and *Streptococcus* spp.[44]), brucellosis (*Brucella mellitensis*[49,50] or *B ovis*[44,50,51]), and viruses (*Sheep* or *Goat Pox Viruses*,[11] lentiviruses,[11] *Bluetongue virus*[11]). The most common bacterial isolates for epididymitis are summarized in **Table 1**.

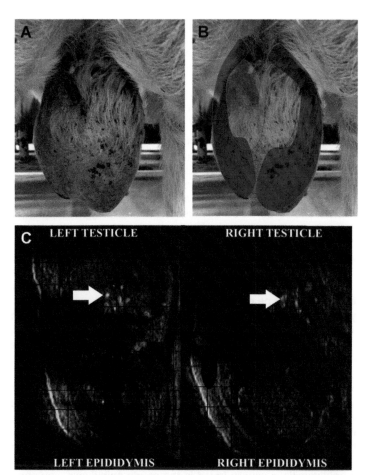

Fig. 6. Gross and ultrasound findings of a buck presented for subfertility and diagnosed with *Corynebacterium pseudotuberculosis*. (*A*) On visual examination (as viewed from the caudal aspect), it appears that the right testis is enlarged compared with the left. (*B*) However, palpation of the scrotal contents revealed that both testes were small and soft (*blue*), and the cauda epididymides were bilaterally enlarged and firm (*red*). (*C*) Ultrasound examination revealed echogenic material within both epididymides. Bilateral testicular degeneration was also evident owing to the presence of multiple hyperechoic foci (mineralization, *arrows*) within the testicular parenchyma. (*From* Stewart JL, Vieson MD, Shipley CF. Corynebacterium pseudotuberculosis as a pathogen of the reproductive tract of male small ruminants: case study and review. Clin Theriogenology. 2018;10(2):107-117; with permission.)

In young rams, *A seminis* and *H somni* are the most common causes of epididymitis and tend to occur during puberty.[11] As described for accessory sex gland lesions elsewhere in this article, respiratory secretions do not seem to be a major source of transmission for *A seminis*.[26] Rather, it is more likely that the organisms are transmitted to ram lambs either in utero or after birth (through umbilical infection or scrotal trauma). These infections remain latent until puberty, when hormone changes trigger their colonization of the reproductive tract (the epididymis, most commonly).[11,26] Homosexual behavior between males can allow for quick dissemination of this pathogen throughout the flock. Other opportunistic bacteria likely have similar mechanisms of action, highlighting the need to ensure a clean environment during the prepartum, peripartum, and postpartum periods of small ruminants.[52] Ram lambs born from ewes infected with chlamydial organisms may also develop epididymitis, orchitis, or vesicular adenitis and shed the organism in semen later in life.[32] Although not a major cause of lesions in males, asymptomatic shedding of chlamydial organisms in the semen can cause infertility, metritis, and abortions in females, so affected males should be culled.[32]

Any ram with clinical epididymitis must be tested for *B ovis*. In some cases, the presence of abscesses may cause an outflow obstruction and culture or polymerase chain reaction of an ejaculate may be negative. In these situations, serologic testing is indicated. Whenever *B ovis* is diagnosed, all rams within the flock should undergo serologic testing regardless if clinical signs are present. In the United States, any *B ovis*–positive ram should be culled because there is currently no approved vaccine or treatment available. *Brucella melitensis* is not currently known to be in the United States and should be reported if found. In other countries where brucellosis is endemic, vaccination alone has been found to appropriately control outbreaks within sheep and goat operations.[53] When feasible, test and slaughter-based programs (with or without concurrent vaccinations in countries where it is available) can help to eradicate brucellosis, but may be cost prohibitive.[53]

Cytology and culture of the ejaculate will usually allow for isolation of the causative pathogen in epididymitis cases and should be performed cleanly as described for accessory sex gland lesions elsewhere in this article. Ultrasound examination can be used to help with determining prognosis for recovery. In a herd outbreak situation, necropsy of an affected male may help to better define the pathogenicity of the specific organism and ensure an accurate diagnosis. Treatment decisions should be made at the discretion of the veterinarian based on examination and diagnostic findings. Broad spectrum antibiotics, such as oxytetracyclines and macrolides, may be useful against opportunistic pathogens if caught early before extensive damage to the epididymides and testes occur. However, in more advanced cases (such as observed in **Fig. 6**), treatment is generally unrewarding and culling is recommended.

Although epididymitis is usually found in the cauda epididymis, any abnormalities palpated within the corpus or caput epididymis should also be critically examined. Sperm granulomas typically present as a swelling in the caput epididymis. Bilateral sperm granulomas are a common congenital manifestation of polled intersex goats caused by partial or complete blockage of the efferent ducts draining the epididymis.[54] These ducts eventually become distended and may rupture, resulting in testicular degeneration.[54] Affected polled intersex males should be culled, even if only one testis is involved, because the condition tends to form in the contralateral testis over time. Unilateral epididymal aplasia has also been implicated as a congenital cause of spermiostasis and sperm granuloma formation in rams and bucks.[24,55] Sperm granulomas have also been associated with epididymitis, likely secondary to occlusion of ducts with purulent material.[33,51,56] Regardless of the cause, the prognosis for fertility is poor when sperm granulomas are present and culling is recommended.

DISEASES OF THE TESTIS

Orchitis may occur in small ruminants as a result of trauma, infection, or neoplasia. Differentials for suppurative orchitis in small ruminants include the same pathogens described previously for epididymitis and accessory sex glands (see **Table 1**). Although rare, *B melitensis* has been reported as a cause of orchitis in a buck as determined by serology and testicular culture.[57] Although *B ovis* commonly causes epididymitis in rams, experimental infection has led to the development of titers and excretion of bacteria in the semen of goats.[51] As with epididymitis, brucellosis should always be ruled out in cases of orchitis owing to its severity, and affected males should be culled.

Rams experimentally inoculated with *T pyogenes* all developed clinical signs of orchitis with subsequent adverse effects on sperm quality.[58] Ultrasound changes were observed by day 30, before any gross abnormalities were appreciable, and included a wider appearance of the mediastinum testis, presence of hyperechogenic foci, and increased echogenicity of the scrotum and tunics.[58] Interestingly, the infection seemed to be self-limiting, and by day 71 no organisms and minimal white blood cells were detected in the ejaculates.[58] Consistently, all adverse effects observed on sperm morphology, motility, and concentration were resolved by day 85.[58] It is worth noting that even though lesions were unilateral, semen quality of the rams seemed to be of subfertile quality for up to 2 months after initial infection.[58] Consequently, sexual rest for 2 months should be the minimum recommendation made to owners if *T pyogenes* is diagnosed as a cause of orchitis in bucks or rams. It is also important to remember that the prognosis for recovery can vary between animals owing to differences in virulence among *T pyogenes* strains.[59] The decision to implement sexual rest versus cull should largely depend on the reproductive value of the particular animal involved. Subsequent ultrasound examination, ejaculate cultures, and semen analyses should be performed to monitor progression and ensure recovery is made before allowing males to breed.

Testicular ultrasound examination can be used to confirm diagnosis and determine prognosis in males with orchitis (**Fig. 7**).[60] If semen culture does not provide a diagnosis, culture and/or cytologic analysis from a fine needle aspirate of any lesions observed via ultrasound examination should be performed.[42] In contrast with the findings with *T pyogenes*,[58] the presence of abscesses from *C pseudotuberculosis* throughout the testicular parenchyma and inability to culture the organism in semen should present concerns about the integrity of the efferent ducts.[42] Findings such as these indicate a grave prognosis for recovery of breeding potential, and affected males should be culled.

Neoplasia, although rare, can also be included as a differential for testicular enlargement and can be diagnosed either by cytologic analysis of a fine needle aspirate or histologic analysis of a biopsy sample. Seminoma,[61,62] leiomyoma,[63] and adenocarcinoma[64] have all been reported in descended testes of rams and bucks. If only 1 testis seems to be involved, a hemicastration can be performed to preserve breeding potential in valuable males. However, histopathology of the affected testis is strongly recommended to determine if there is any venous or lymphatic involvement or metastatic potential. Leydig[65] and Sertoli[66] cell tumors have all been associated with abdominal testes of goats with the polled intersex condition. Bucks or rams with undescended cryptorchid testes have an increased risk for the development of testicular neoplasia in the retained testis, and castration should be recommended.

Cryptorchidism is failure of either one or both testes to descend from the abdominal cavity into the scrotum. Frequently, an owner may obtain a male thought to be castrated, only for it to start acting and smelling like an intact male. In these cases, the right testis is most often retained, owing to its anatomic positioning within the abdomen. A definitive diagnosis can be made by testing a blood sample for the presence of testosterone. However, the development of behavioral changes and smell around the time of puberty are almost pathognomonic for the presence of a functional gonad. Ultrasound examination can be used to help identify the position of the

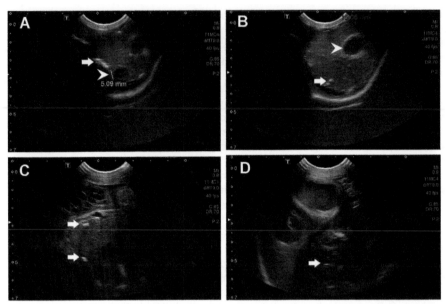

Fig. 7. Ultrasound images of the right (*A*, *B*) and left (*C*, *D*) testis associated with *Corynebacterium pseudotuberculosis* orchitis in a Boer buck. Large 5- and 15-mm abscesses can be visualized in the right testis (*arrowheads*). Multiple hyperechoic foci (*arrows*) are consistent with mineralization and testicular degeneration bilaterally. (*From* Stewart JL, Vieson MD, Shipley CF. Corynebacterium pseudotuberculosis as a pathogen of the reproductive tract of male small ruminants: case study and review. Clin Theriogenology 2018;10(2):107-117; with permission.)

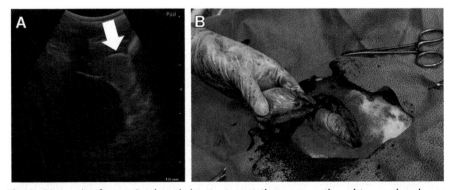

Fig. 8. Diagnosis of a retained testis in a pet goat that owners thought was already castrated. The male goat had begun developing male-like scent and behavior. (*A*) Ultrasound image of a testis (*arrow*) that was identified on the right side of the abdomen, in close proximity to the bladder. (*B*) A paramedian surgical approach was made over the site identified on ultrasound examination, and the retained testis was easily found and surgically removed.

retained testis within the abdomen to determine the best surgical approach (**Fig. 8**). Animals that are intended to be kept long term (ie, pets) should undergo surgery to remove the retained testis owing to its increased risk for neoplasia and undesirable development of male behavior and smell. Surgery may be cost prohibitive with males intended for slaughter, but recommendations should be made to separate these males from females because many are still able to produce viable spermatozoa. Breeding these males is contraindicated owing to the heritable nature of this condition, so hemicastrations to preserve breeding potential should be discouraged.

SUMMARY

Reproductive tract diseases are a common cause of subfertility and infertility in male small ruminants. Clinical lesions of the reproductive tract can usually be identified during routine breeding soundness examinations and include balanoposthitis, epididymitis, or orchitis. Serologic screening and isolation of incoming males is critical for preventing introduction of diseases into a herd or flock. Subclinical manifestations of infectious diseases may be initially identified through the presence of white blood cells in the ejaculate, and follow-up diagnostics (such as ultrasound examination and culture) may be warranted. If significant bacterial isolates are identified in the subclinical stage, treatment may be beneficial. The development of clinical signs usually indicates that damage within the reproductive tract has occurred and the prognosis worsens. The decision to cull versus treat should be made at the discretion of the veterinarian after a thorough examination, diagnostics, and discussion of prognosis with the owner. Many reproductive tract disorders (infectious or noninfectious) can be prevented through proper herd or flock management. Factors such as diet, biosecurity protocols, and environment should be evaluated closely if an outbreak of any reproductive disorder occurs.

CLINICS CARE POINTS

- Breeding soundness examinations should be performed routinely in rams and bucks for early identification of reproductive tract lesions that can adversely impact breeding success.
- Early diagnosis of most reproductive tract diseases in male small ruminants will improve the likelihood of treatment success and minimize long-term deleterious effects on fertility.
- Laboratory testing, such as serologic screening of incoming males or semen bacterial culture of clinically affected males, should be performed in all herds or flocks to prevent and manage outbreaks.
- Bacterial agents that cause reproductive tract infections in young bucks and rams may be transmitted transplacentally or through umbilical infection early in life; therefore, ensuring a clean environment during parturition and the subsequent neonatal period is critical.
- Rams and bucks with clinical signs of infectious diseases, such as with epididymitis or orchitis, do not respond well to treatment and should be culled.
- Ultrasound examination of the scrotal contents can aid the practitioner in determining prognosis of reproductive tract diseases.

DISCLOSURE

The authors have nothing to disclose.

REFERENCES

1. National Agricultural Statistics Service (NASS). Sheep and Goats. 2020. Available at: https://downloads.usda.library.cornell.edu/usda-esmis/files/000000018/n296xf83n/m900pb410/shep0120.pdf. Accessed April 1, 2020.
2. Shipley CF. Breeding soundness examination of the male ovine, caprine and cervidae species. Clin Ther 2016;8(4):445–8.
3. Ott RS, Memon MA. Breeding soundness examinations of rams and bucks, a review. Theriogenology 1980;13(2):155–64.
4. Kimberling CV, Arnold KS, Schweitzer DJ, et al. Correlation of the presence of seminal white blood cells and the prevalence of separated spermatozoal heads with subclinical Brucella ovis infection in rams. J Am Vet Med Assoc 1986;189(1):73–6.
5. Ley WB, Sprecher DJ, Thatcher CD, et al. Use of the point-score system for breeding soundness examination in yearling Dorset, Hampshire and Suffolk rams. Theriogenology 1990;34(4):721–33.
6. Gurung NK, Rush J, Pugh DG. Feeding and Nutrition. In: Pugh DG, Baird AN, Edmondson M, et al, editors. Sheep, goat, and cervid medicine. 3rd edition. Philadelphia: Elsevier; 2021. p. 15–44.
7. Ewoldt JM, Jones ML, Miesner MD. Surgery of obstructive urolithiasis in ruminants. Vet Clin North Am Food Anim Pract 2008;24(3):455–65.
8. Streeter RN, Washburn KE, McCauley CT. Percutaneous tube cystostomy and vesicular irrigation for treatment of obstructive urolithiasis in a goat. J Am Vet Med Assoc 2002;221(4):546–9.
9. Janke JJ, Osterstock JB, Washburn KE, et al. Use of Walpole's solution for treatment of goats with urolithiasis: 25 cases (2001-2006). J Am Vet Med Assoc 2009;234(2):249–52.
10. Todhunter P, Baird AN, Wolfe DF. Erection failure as a sequela to obstructive urolithiasis in a male goat. J Am Vet Med Assoc 1996;209(3):650–2.
11. Gouletsou PG, Fthenakis GC. Microbial diseases of the genital system of rams or bucks. Vet Microbiol 2015;181(1–2):130–5.
12. Brook AH, Southcott WH, Stacy BD. Etiology of ovine posthitis: relationship between urine and a causal organism. Aust Vet J 1966;42:9–12.
13. Loste A, Ramos JJ, García L, et al. High prevalence of ulcerative posthitis in rasa aragonesa rams associated with a legume-rich diet. J Vet Med A Physiol Pathol Clin Med 2005;52(4):176–9.
14. Kidanemariam A, Gouws J, van Vuuren M, et al. Ulcerative balanitis and vulvitis of Dorper sheep in South Africa: a study on its aetiology and clinical features. J S Afr Vet Assoc 2005;76(4):197–203.
15. Göçmen H, Alçay S, Rosales RS, et al. Characterisation of genital Mycoplasma species from preputial swabs of bucks and rams. Kafkas Univ Vet Fak Derg 2020;26(2):305–8.
16. Gregory L, Rizzo H, Gaeta NC, et al. Interference of Mycoplasma spp. or Ureaplasma spp. in ovine semen quality. J Microbiol Res 2012;2(5):118–22.
17. Grimmer ED, Canisso IF, Hsiao SH, et al. Squamous cell carcinoma and papilloma virus in the prepuce of a Boer buck. Clin Ther 2017;9(4):595–9.
18. Pritchard GC, Scholes SFE, Foster AP, et al. Ulcerative vulvitis and balanitis in sheep flocks. Vet Rec 2008;163(3):86–9.
19. Uzal FA, Woods L, Stillian M, et al. Abortion and ulcerative posthitis associated with caprine herpesvirus-1 infection in goats in California. J Vet Diagn Invest 2004;16:478–84.

20. Camero M, Larocca V, Lovero A, et al. Caprine herpesvirus type 1 infection in goat: not just a problem for females. Small Rumin Res 2015;128:59–62.
21. Fthenakis GC, Karagiannidis A, Alexopoulos C, et al. Clinical and epidemiological findings during ram examination in 47 flocks in southern Greece. Prev Vet Med 2001;52:43–52.
22. Spyrou V, Valiakos G. Orf virus infection in sheep or goats. Vet Microbiol 2015;18: 178–82.
23. Tarigan S, Ladds P, Foster R. Genital pathology of feral male goats. Aust Vet J 1990;67(8):286–90.
24. Ladds PW. Congenital abnormalities of the genitalia of cattle, sheep, goats, and pigs. Vet Clin North Am Food Anim Pract 1993;9(1):127–44.
25. Moustacas VS, Silva TMA, Costa LF, et al. Clinical and pathological changes in rams experimentally infected with Actinobacillus seminis and Histophilus somni. ScientificWorldJournal 2014;1–10. https://doi.org/10.1155/2014/241452.
26. Al-Katib WA, Dennis SM. Experimental transmission of *Actinobacillus seminis* infection to rams. Vet Rec 2005;157:143–7.
27. Al-Katib WA, Dennis SM. Ovine genital actinobacillosis: a review. N Z Vet J 2009; 57(6):352–8.
28. Al-Katib WA, Dennis SM. Pathological changes in accessory sex organs of rams following experimental infection with Actinobacillus seminis. N Z Vet J 2008;56(6): 319–25.
29. Ribeiro MG, Risseti RM, Bolaños CAD, et al. Trueperella pyogenes multispecies infections in domestic animals: a retrospective study of 144 cases (2002 to 2012). Vet Q 2012;35(2):82–7.
30. Nietfeld JC. Chlamydial infections in small ruminants. Vet Clin North Am Food Anim Pract 2001;17(2):301–14.
31. Storz J, Carroll E, Stephenson E, et al. Urogenital infection and seminal excretion after inoculation of bulls and rams with chlamydiae. Am J Vet Res 1976;37(5): 517–20.
32. Rodolakis A, Laroucau K. Chlamydiaceae and chlamydial infections in sheep or goats. Vet Microbiol 2015;181:107–18.
33. Carvalho Júnior CA, Moustacas VS, Xavier MN, et al. Andrological, pathologic, morphometric, and ultrasonographic findings in rams experimentally infected with Brucella ovis. Small Rumin Res 2012;102:213–22.
34. Gonzalez-Bulnes A, Pallares P, Vazquez MI. Ultrasonographic imaging in small ruminant reproduction. Reprod Domest Anim 2010;45(Suppl 2):9–20.
35. Ezzi A, Ladds PW, Hoffmann D, et al. Pathology of varicocele in the ram. Aust Vet J 1988;65(1):11–5.
36. Foster RA. Pathology of male reproductive organs. Clin Ther 2010;2(4):531–44.
37. Roberts SJ. Scrotal hernia in rams. A case report. Cornell Vet 1988;78(4):351–2.
38. Braun WF, Cole WJ. Unilateral scrotal hernia repair in a ram lamb. J Am Vet Med Assoc 1985;187(5):500.
39. Mahmood ZK, Jin ZAM, Jesse FF, et al. Relationship between the Corynebacterium pseudotuberculosis, phospholipase D inoculation and the fertility characteristics of crossbred Boer bucks. Livest Sci 2016;191:12–21.
40. Dennis SM, Bamford VW. The role of corynebacteria in perinatal lamb mortality. Vet Rec 1966;79:105–8.
41. Alonso JL, Simon MC, Girones O, et al. The effect of experimental infection with Corynebacterium pseudotuberculosis on reproduction in adult ewes. Res Vet Sci 1992;52(3):267–72.

42. Stewart JL, Vieson MD, Shipley CF. Corynebacterium pseudotuberculosis as a pathogen of the reproductive tract of male small ruminants: case study and review. Clin Ther 2018;10(2):107–17.

43. Ahmad N, Noakes DE, Middleton DJ. Use of ultrasound to diagnose testicular degeneration in a goat. Vet Rec 1993;132:436–9.

44. Lozano EA. Etiologic significance of bacterial isolates from rams with palpable epididymitis. Am J Vet Res 1986;47(5):1153–6.

45. Appleyard WT, Aitken ID, Anderson IE. Attempted venereal transmission of Chlamydia psittaci in sheep. Vet Rec 1985;116(20):535–8.

46. Gouletsou PG, Fthenakis GC. Ovine orchitis, with special reference to orchitis associated with Arcanobacterium pyogenes. Small Rumin Res 2006;62:71–4.

47. dos Santos FA, de Azevedo EO, de Azevedo SS, et al. Isolation of Actinobacillus seminis from a goat with clinical epididymo-orchitis in Brazil. Braz J Microbiol 2014;45(1):205–9.

48. Santos FA, Figueiredo Da Costa D, Ferreira Da Silva A, et al. Microbiological, molecular, and histopathological findings in goats experimentally infected with Actinobacillus seminis. Microb Pathog 2019;133. https://doi.org/10.1016/j.micpath.2019.103555.

49. Nasruddin NS, Mazlan M, Saad MZ, et al. Histopathology and immunohistochemistry assessments of acute experimental infection by Brucella melitensis in bucks. Open J Pathol 2014;04(02):54–63.

50. Ali A, Derar DR, Osman SA, et al. Scrotal enlargement in rams and bucks in Qassim region, central of Saudi Arabia: clinical and ultrasonographic findings and seroprevalence of brucellosis. Trop Anim Health Prod 2019;51:2109–14.

51. Burgess GW, Spencer TL, Norris MJ. Experimental infection of goats with Brucella ovis. Aust Vet J 1985;62(8):262–4.

52. Walker RL, LeaMaster BR. Prevalence of Histophilus ovis and Actinobacillus seminis in the genital tract of sheep. Am J Vet Res 1986;47(9):1928–30.

53. Blasco JM, Molina-Flores B. Control and eradication of Brucella melitensis infection in sheep and goats. Vet Clin North Am Food Anim Pract 2011;27:95–104.

54. Söller M, Padeh B, Ysoki MW, et al. Cytogenetics of Saanen goats showing abnormal development of the reproductive tract associated with the dominant gene for polledness. Cytogenetics 1969;8:51–67.

55. Ladds PW, Briggs GD, Foster RA. Epididymal aplasia in two rams. Aust Vet J 1990;67(12):457–8.

56. Al-Katib WA, Dennis SM. Early sequential findings in the genitalia of rams experimentally infected with Actinobacillus seminis. N Z Vet J 2008;56(2):50–4.

57. Ahmad R, Niaz B. Orchitis due to brucellosis in a buck. Pak Vet J 1998;18(2):108–9.

58. Gouletsou PG, Fthenakis GC, Cripps PJ, et al. Experimentally induced orchitis associated with Arcanobacterium pyogenes: clinical, ultrasonographic, seminological and pathological features. Theriogenology 2004;62:1307–28.

59. Risseti RM, Zastempowska E, Twarużek M, et al. Virulence markers associated with Trueperella pyogenes infections in livestock and companion animals. Lett Appl Microbiol 2017;65(2):125–32.

60. Scott PR. Applications of diagnostic ultrasonography in small ruminant reproductive management. Anim Reprod Sci 2012;130:184–6.

61. Shortridge EH, Cordes DO. Seminomas in sheep. J Comp Pathol 1969;79(2):229–32.

62. Oliveira Cosentino I, Felipe Alvarez Balaro M, Beatriz A, et al. Metastatic seminoma in a male alpine goat: clinical and histopathological approach. Acta Sci Vet 2019;47(Suppl 1):405.
63. Foster RA, Ladds PW, Hoffmann D. Testicular leiomyoma in a ram. Vet Pathol 1989;26:184–5.
64. Searson JE. Testicular adenocarcinoma in a ram. Vet Pathol 1980;17:391–3.
65. Monteagudo LV, Arruga MV, Bonafonte JI, et al. Bilateral Leydig cell tumor in a six-year-old intersex goat affected by Polled Intersex Syndrome. Vet Pathol 2008;45(1):42–5.
66. Canisso I, Coffee L, Ortved K, et al. Bilateral Sertoli and interstitial cell tumours in abdominal testes of a goat with polled intersex syndrome (PIS). Reprod Domest Anim 2014;49(6):e64–9.
67. Aitken ID, Longbottom D. Chlamydial abortion. In: Aitken ID, editor. Diseases of sheep. Oxford (United Kingdom): Blackwell Publishing Ltd; 2008. p. 105–12. https://doi.org/10.1002/9780470753316.ch16.
68. Rodolakis A, Salinas J, Papp J. Recent advances on ovine chlamydial abortion. Vet Res 1998;29(304):275–88. Available at: https://hal.archives-ouvertes.fr/hal-00902529. Accessed April 3, 2020.
69. Appleyard WT, Aitken ID, Anderson I. Outbreak of chlamydial abortion in goats. Vet Rec 1983;113(3):63.

Estrus Synchronization in the Sheep and Goat

Hayder Mohammed Hassan Habeeb, PhD[a],*, Michelle Anne Kutzler, MBA, DVM, PhD[b]

KEYWORDS

- Breeding season • Gonadotropin • Male sex pheromone • Out-of-season
- Ovulation • Progestogen

KEY POINTS

- Sheep and goats are seasonally polyestrous animals, which means they exhibit spontaneous estrus and ovulation during periods of short daylight but not during periods of long daylight.
- Estrus synchronization and manipulation have been used by producers to provide uniform lamb and kid meat production and dairy sheep and goat milk production, to concentrate work and labor cost, and to plan for the lambing and kidding time.
- Estrus synchronization can be accomplished during the breeding season and out of season using hormonal and nonhormonal methods.

INTRODUCTION

Sheep and goat are seasonally polyestrous animals, which means they exhibit spontaneous estrus and ovulation during periods of short daylight (breeding season) but not during periods of long daylight (out of season). Because their gestation length is 5 months long, ewes and does can only have one lamb or kid crop each year without intervention. This factor limits the individual productivity and profitability of each animal. The number of lamb and kid crops per individual can be increased to 3 every 2 years or 5 every 3 years if females become pregnant outside of the breeding season.[1] This will also provide an out-of-season supply of lamb and kid meat and sheep and goat milk for consumers. To stimulate the ewes and does to exhibit estrus and ovulation outside of their breeding season, breeders can use estrus synchronization.[1,2] However, both the ovulation rate and pregnancy rate decrease out of season.[3,4]

To increase the ovulation rate with out-of-season estrus induction, a variety of methods have been used (eg, progesterone, gonadotropins, male sex pheromone).

[a] Department of Animal Production, College of Agriculture, Al-Qasim Green University, Babylon, Hella 51013, Iraq; [b] Animal and Rangeland Science, Oregon State University, 112 Withycombe Hall, Corvallis, OR 97331, USA
* Corresponding author. ,
E-mail addresses: Hayder75r@yahoo.com; Hayder.habeeb@agre.uoqasim.edu.iq

Vet Clin Food Anim 37 (2021) 125–137
https://doi.org/10.1016/j.cvfa.2020.10.007
0749-0720/21/© 2020 Elsevier Inc. All rights reserved.
vetfood.theclinics.com

PG-600 is a gonadotropin hormone used off label by US sheep and goat producers to induce ovulation in ewes outside of the breeding season.[5–9] However, the most commonly used dose of PG-600 (3–5 mL per ewe)[6,7,9,10] overstimulates the ovaries, resulting in increased follicle size and estradiol-17β concentration.[6,10,11] Consequently, fertilization rates are decreased.[6,10,12,13] To better understand breeding management during the breeding season and out of season, seasonality and cyclicity as well as hormonal and nonhormonal methods for estrous cycle manipulation and estrus induction are discussed.

SEASONALITY

Sheep and goat are seasonally polyestrous animals, meaning that regular spontaneous estrous cycles occur during periods of decreasing or short daylight (early fall to late winter).[14,15] Sheep and goats go into anestrus during periods of increasing or long daylight (early spring to late summer).[16] A decreased secretory pattern of melatonin secretion occurs as daylight increases, which results in increased release of dopamine from A15 dopamine neurons in the retrochiasmatic area of the hypothalamus.[17,18] Increasing dopamine secretion inhibits kisspeptin from the arcuate nucleus in the hypothalamus, resulting in inhibition of gonadotropin-releasing hormone (GnRH) secretion.[18,19] Decreasing GnRH secretion results in lower luteinizing hormone (LH) and follicle-stimulating hormone (FSH) secretion and ovarian follicular activity gradually becomes static. During this period of static ovarian activity, estradiol-17β concentrations remain low, which activates the estradiol-17β responsive inhibitory neural system in the brain and inhibits GnRH and LH pulse frequency.[20,21]

With decreasing daylight, less ultraviolet light is transmitted through the retina to the suprachiasmatic nucleus and superior cervical ganglion, which results in increased melatonin secretion from the pineal gland.[2,14] Melatonin inhibits the hypothalamic inhibitory A15 dopamine neurons, which results in a decrease in hypothalamic sensitivity to estradiol-17β. Decreased hypothalamic sensitivity to estradiol-17β stimulates kisspeptin release in the hypothalamic arcuate and preoptic nuclei, stimulating GnRH, LH, and FSH secretion.[22,23] FSH secretion stimulates follicular development and increases estradiol-17β secretion. As the estradiol-17β concentration increases, hypothalamic sensitivity to estradiol-17β decreases, which in turn increases GnRH and LH pulse frequency culminating in the LH surge.[24,25]

The first ovulation of the breeding season occurs after the LH surge, but resultant corpus luteal formation and diestrus is represented by a significantly shortened luteal phase[26,27] with minimal progesterone production.[28–31] This process is the result of down-regulation of genes involved in progesterone synthesis (eg, steroidogenic acute regulatory protein, 3β-hydroxysteroid dehydrogenase, and vascular endothelial growth factor).[26,31–33] The second ovulation of the breeding season is characterized by a normal length luteal phase, but estrous behavior around the time of ovulation is lacking (silent) owing to insufficient progesterone priming. As a result, natural mating with subsequent pregnancy cannot occur until the third estrous cycle of the season unless progesterone supplementation is used.[29,32] Unlike the out-of-season period, the inhibitor of GnRH and LH pulse frequency during the breeding season is progesterone. At the end of diestrus when progesterone concentrations with luteolysis, GnRH and LH secretion increases, which triggers the next LH surge and ovulation.

CYCLICITY

In sheep and goats, the length of the estrous cycle ranges from 14 to 19 days (average, 17 days) and 18 to 24 days (average, 21 days), respectively.[34] The estrous cycle is divided into 4 stages: proestrus, estrus, metestrus, and diestrus. As mentioned else-where in this article, ovarian estradiol-17β and progesterone provide positive and negative feedback to the hypothalamus and pituitary gland, respectively. The inhibi-tory effect of progesterone is mediated by increasing the inhibitory effect of the neuro-transmitter, dynorphin. Dynorphin acts on the hypothalamus to inhibit the GnRH pulse frequency, which inhibits LH pulse frequency.[23] When progesterone decreases at the end of the luteal phase, GnRH pulse frequency increases, which results in FSH-mediated follicle development and estradiol-17β secretion.[32,35]

Estradiol-17β is a product of 2 ovarian cell types (granulosa cells and theca cells) and 2 gonadotropins (LH and FSH). In response to LH, follicle theca cells produce testosterone,[36] which diffuses into adjacent granulosa cells and is aromatized to estradiol-17β. The expression of the enzyme aromatase in granulosa cells is regulated by FSH.[37] Estradiol then acts on its receptor in the hypothalamic arcuate nucleus to stimulate the release of kisspeptin, which increases GnRH and LH pulse frequency.[38] This increase in the LH pulse frequency then increases estradiol-17β, which is respon-sible for the estrous behavior exhibited by ewes and does.[39,40] Increasing concentra-tions of estradiol-17β will also stimulate additional LH secretion, culminating in an LH surge and ovulation.[38,41] Ovulation occurs 24 to 27 hours from the onset of behavioral estrus.[42,43]

NOVEL MALE SEX PHEROMONE

Introducing a novel male ram or buck ("ram or buck effect") to cycling ewes and does can trigger an ovulatory LH surge through a series of neuroendocrine events within the hypothalamus and pituitary gland.[44] Sex pheromones produced by the ram or buck sudoriferous gland act on receptors within the ewe or doe olfactory bulb, stimulating neurons in the ventromedial and arcuate nuclei in the hypothalamus, leading to an in-crease in kisspeptin secretion and the onset of estrus.[18,40,45-48] The ewe or doe response to a novel male's sex pheromones can even overcome the inhibitory effect of progesterone except in the midluteal phase.[49] However, estrous behavior and ovulation responses to a novel male's sex pheromones can vary between ewes.[50]

The introduction of sex pheromones from a novel male to anestrous ewes or does can also trigger an LH surge[40,51,52] that induces ovulation in 46% to 50% of ewes and 10% to 16% of does without any other treatment.[45,53-57] Even though estrus induction from male sex pheromone in anestrous ewes and does is effective, similar to the first ovulation of the breeding season, estrous behavior is silent and ovulation is followed by a shortened luteal phase in ewes and does.[31,32,58-60] It is important to note that the stage of anestrus may affect the female response to male sex pheromones, such that the estrus induction rate is lower in early anestrus compared with late anestrus.[58,61] However, other investigators have reported no relationship between the length of anestrus and the estrus induction response to novel male sex pheromones.[30] This dif-ference may be a result of breed difference; breeds that express greater seasonality (eg, Suffolk sheep) only responded to novel male sex pheromone in late anestrus, whereas breeds that express less seasonality (eg, Polypay) responded to novel males at any time during anestrus.[38]

In ruminants, prior exposure to a progestogen is necessary for both expressions of normal estrous behavior and normal luteal function after ovulation.[32,62,63] Knights and coworkers[64] found that the percentage of out-of-season ewes exhibiting estrous behavior was higher after progestogen treatment with novel male sex pheromone exposure (77%) compared with just ram exposure (20%). Administering progestogens before exposing out-of-season ewes to a novel male not only increases induction of normal estrous behavior and ovulation, but also results in pregnancy in about 50% of females mated.[65] As a result, it is common to use progestogens in combination with novel male sex pheromone to improve out-of-season reproductive performance.[58,62,63,66]

Progestogen priming is not the only way to enhance the effect of novel male sex pheromones. Administration of FSH with progestogens increases the estrus induction response in out-of-season ewes (79%) compared with the out-of-season ewes only exposed to novel rams (12%).[67] In does during the breeding season, administration of FSH with a norgestomet implant (6 mg for 11 days) was more likely to result in estrus (90%) compared with does treated with norgestomet alone (70%).[68] Prepuberal Boar goat, treated with norgestomet (2 mg) in combination with buck introduction and pregnant mare serum gonadotropin (PMSG) (300 IU) had a significantly higher estrus response rate (91%) compared with prepuberal does exposed to novel buck alone (16%).[55] With or without progestogens, the use of gonadotropins with novel male sex pheromones can increase the estrus induction response in out-of-season ewes and does.

ESTRUS INDUCTION AND SYNCHRONIZATION DURING THE BREEDING SEASON
Progestogens

Treatment with progestogens (natural or synthetic forms of progesterone) is a common method for estrus synchronization in small ruminants. Progesterone administration for 10 to 14 days results in a return to estrus in 2 days after progesterone withdrawal.[69] Ewes treated with intravaginal progesterone (300 mg controlled internal drug release [CIDR] or 500 mg intravaginal sponge) for 12 days in combination with ram introduction demonstrated 100% and 94% estrous behavior, respectively.[70] Decreasing the amount of progesterone (eg, using a 40 mg or 20 mg intravaginal sponge) or decreasing the treatment duration from 12 days to 6 days did not negatively affect follicular development and ovulation during the breeding season.[71] However, daily progesterone injections for 17 days result in lower fertilization rates compared with no treatment as a control group (28.0% and 66.7%, respectively).[72] In dairy goats, treatment with norgestomet (6 mg for 11 days) in combination with a single injection of PMSG (750 IU) at the time of implant removal was more likely to result in estrus (90%) compared with the control group (70%).[68] But, change the type of progesterone and gonadotropin did not enhance significantly the estrous response in does treated with 5 days CIDR (300 mg) in combination with prostaglandin F2α (PGF2α) and equine chorionic gonadotropin (eCG) (250 IU) compared with a control group (85% and 87%, respectively) during the breeding season.[73] However, treatment with medroxyprogesterone acetate (MPA) (60 mg per doe for 17 days) in combination with an intramuscular injection of GnRH (125 mg) at progestogen removal was less likely to result in estrus (12%) compared with does treated with MPA in combination with PMSG injection (400 IU) at progestogen removal (57%).[74]

Prostaglandin F2α

PGF2α is produced from endometrial glands in response to oxytocin to cause luteolysis at the end of the luteal phase when there is no pregnancy. In ewes and does, this process occurs on day 11 to 12 and around day 13 after estrus, respectively.[75,76] Intramuscular administration of PGF2α or a synthetic analog will induce premature lysis of the corpora lutea during diestrus and accelerate the onset of estrus and ovulation.[69] PGF2α is ineffective at estrus synchronization when administered during a stage of the estrous cycle when corpora lutea are unresponsive to PGF2α (eg, metestrus, proestrus, estrus).[77–79] However, a second PGF2α (15 mg. im) treatment 9 to 10 days after the initial treatment results in estrus induction in 72% of cycling ewes.[70] This is still lower than the estrus induction response rate (94%) in ewes following treatment with a CIDR for 12 days.[70] Also, it is important to mention that lambing rate is decreased following administration of 2 PGF2α (D-Cloprostenol; 0.15 mg) injections.[80]

In goats, Boer does treated with 2 intermuscular injections of PGF2α (125 μg in does 11 days apart) resulted in low estrus response (33%) compared with does treated with a double intermuscular injection of PGF2α in combination with eCG (300 IU) (100%).[81] In the same experiment, using the same protocol but with 5 mg, FSH injection did not enhance estrus response (33%).

ESTRUS INDUCTION AND SYNCHRONIZATION OUT OF SEASON
Progesterone

As mentioned elsewhere in this article, the introduction of a novel male alone can induce ovulation in anestrous ewes and does. However, the male introduction alone is not sufficient to result in estrous behavior with a subsequent normal luteal phase.[1,26,32] Prior progestogen treatment can overcome this problem. Anestrous ewes treated with melengestrol acetate before ram introduction had a significantly higher estrus induction rate (90%) compared with anestrous ewes exposed to novel male sex pheromones alone (4%).[1] The estrus induction rate was increased to 100% when anestrous ewes were treated with zeranol in addition to melengestrol acetate (MGA) and ram introduction. In goat, injection of progesterone just before buck introduction had a significant higher estrus induction compare to buck effect only during out of season.[82] Prepuberal Boar goat, treated with norgestomet (2 mg) in combination with buck introduction and PMSG (300 IU) had a significantly higher estrus response rate (91%) compared with prepuberal does exposed to a novel buck alone (16%).[55]

Adding FSH or eCG (a gonadotropin with FSH-like activity) to the estrus induction protocol increases out-of-season response rates. Ram exposure did not affect ovulation rate when anestrous ewes were treated with intravaginal progesterone and eCG (500 mg) 1 day before progesterone withdrawal.[83] Oral administration of MPA (60 mg MPA per ewe per day for 20 days) in combination with eCG (30 mg per ewe per day for 16 days) to anestrous ewes increased fertility after estrus induction compared with treatment with eCG alone.[84] However, the duration of progestogen treatment with FSH can affect fertility because induction of estrous behavior and ovulation rates in anestrous ewes was highest following a 5-day CIDR treatment compared with a 12-day treatment (79% and 3.3 ± 0.6 ovulations vs 66% and 2.2 ± 0.4 ovulations, respectively).[64] In goats, anestrus does treated with progesterone impregnant sponges (40 mg per doe for 10 days) with a single injection of eCG (500 IU), 2 days before sponge withdrawal resulted in high estrus response (100%) compared with progesterone alone (0%).[85]

Prostaglandin F2α

Estrus induction will not occur with PGF2α alone during anestrus because there is no luteal tissue.[86] However, using 2 PGF2α injections (D-Cloprostenol; 0.15 mg 10 days apart) in combination with GnRH (4.2 μg [buserelin]) before the first PGF2α injection resulted in a higher lambing rate in out-of-season ewes.[80] In Boar goats, using 2 injections of PGF2α (11 days apart) resulted in low (20%) estrus response compared with PGF2α (62.5 μg cloprostenol at sponge removal) injection in combination with progestogen (60 mg MAP; 8 days) (86%) during out-of-season does.[87]

Gonadotropins

Follicle-stimulating hormone

Using gonadotropins with progesterone and ram introduction is necessary to maximize the pregnancy rate in out-of-season ewes. FSH is a gonadotropic hormone produced by the anterior pituitary that acts on receptors within ovarian granulosa cells. When administered during the breeding season, FSH induces superovulation. Administration of FSH (200 mg) to ewes during the breeding season resulted in a higher ovulation rate with a greater number of the transferable embryos.[88] However, at a higher dosage, FSH can impair fertility in cycling ewes by decreasing embryo survival.[8]

During the management of out-of-season breeding, a single injection of FSH (Folltropin 68 mg) 12 hours before progesterone withdrawal (0.3 g progesterone [CIDR-G]) and introduction of ram resulted in only a small increase in the ovulation rate compared with a single injection of FSH 36 hours before progesterone and introduction of ram in out-of-seaon ewes.[3] However, the treatment of anestrous ewes with a single injection of FSH (55 mg) 24 hours before CIDR withdrawal results in a pregnancy rate of 52% compared with 0% in anestrous ewes not receiving any treatment.[64]

Equine chorionic gonadotropin

Equine CG is a gonadotropic hormone produced by the endometrial cups in pregnant mares from 45 to 100 days of gestation.[89] Similar to FSH, eCG acts on receptors within ovarian granulosa cells to induce estrus in sheep and goats. Varying dosages of eCG have been used in sheep. Administration of eCG (500 IU) to Dorper ewes during out of season after progestogen treatment removal (65 mg MPA; 12 days) and ram exposure increased pregnancy rates (60%) compared with ram exposure alone (40%).[90] When eCG was administered to haired sheep, under tropical conditions, 24 hours before progestogen (fluorogestone acetate sponge; 5 days) removal, 400 IU eCG enhanced fertility rates compared with 100 IU, but did not differ from 200 IU (100 IU, 45.4%; 200 IU, 61%; 400 IU, 81.8%).[91] In addition, litter sizes were higher with 400 IU eCG (400 IU, 177.2%; 200 IU, 113%; 100 IU, 68.2%) during out of season.[91] In goat, administration of different dosage of eCG (300, 500 IU) to Morocco goat during out of season 2 days before flurogestone acetate (FGA) treatment removal (20 mg for 11 days) and with or without PGF2α did not differ in estrus response (100%, 87%, 100%, and 100%).[92] Treatment of eCG (300 IU) to Boer does during out of season after progestogen treatment implant removal (65 mg FGA; 14 days) and PGF2α increased estrus response (100%) compared with 2 PGF2α (33%).[81]

PG-600

PG-600 is a product labeled for estrus induction in pigs that contains both eCG (80 IU/mL) and human chorionic gonadotropin (40 IU/mL). Sheep and goat producers have used PG-600 for out-of-season estrus induction for many years. The dosage most commonly reported in the literature (5 mL per ewe) has been found to overstimulate the ovary,[10] resulting in abnormally large follicles with increased estradiol-17β concentrations at the time of ovulation.[11] As a result, out-of-season fertilization rates are decreased by 42% when PG-600 is used compared with fertilization rates of ewes bred during the breeding season.[12,13] In addition, out-of-season treatment with PG-600 in combination with progestogens and ram exposure resulted in a lower fertilization rate compared with anestrous ewes treated with only progestogens and ram exposure.[8] However, out-of-season treatment with PG-600 in combination with progestogens and ram exposure did not decrease the pregnancy or fecundity rate compared with ewes treated with progestogens and ram exposure alone.[93]

Administration of PG-600 (2.0–3.5 mL per ewe) 1 day before progestogen withdrawal improved reproductive performance in out-of-season ewes.[9,94] Our laboratory investigated the effect of different dosages of PG-600 on ovulation and pregnancy rate after CIDR removal (300 mg, 9 days) during the breeding season and out of season.[10,93] A high ovulation rate was associated with 5 mL PG-600 during the breeding season, but the pregnancy rate decreased with 5 mL PG-600 in both seasons.

In goat, the administration of PG-600 for estrus induction is poorly reported. In dairy goats, during the transition period, treatment with PG-600 (300 IU) 36 hours before norgestomet implantation (3 mg, 9–12 days) and PGF2α (125 μg [Estrumate]) at the time of implant removal increased the pregnancy rate (90%) compared with does treated with PMSG (300 IU) 36 hours before norgestomet implant removal (76%).[94,95] However, in the same report, the estrus and litter size did not differ among groups. Also, Spanish does treated with different dosages of PG-600 (0, 0.2, 0.45, 0.8, 1.6, and 3.2 mL) after norgestomet implant removal (3 mg, 12 days) resulted in no effect on estrus induction during the breeding and out of season.[6] In addition, the dose level of PG-600 greater than 0.45 mL resulted in an increased ovulation rate in both seasons. It is important to mention that the dose level (3.2 mL) of PG-600 has a potential superovulation effect but lower than that might be sufficient for estrus synchronization in goat.[6]

SUMMARY

Estrus induction and synchronization are methods producers can use to provide uniform lamb and kid meat production and sheep and goat milk production, to concentrate work and labor cost, and to plan for the lambing and kidding time. To stimulate the ewes and does to exhibit estrus and become pregnant outside of the natural breeding season, producers can use a combination of methods. It is this author's opinion that for estrus synchronization during the breeding season, male sex pheromones in combination with progestogen (CIDR) and PGF2α in ewes and does should be used. For out-of-season estrus induction, male effect in combination with progesterone and gonadotropin (PG-600; 2–3.5 mL in sheep, <3.2 mL in goat) should be used for best reproductive outcomes.

CLINICS CARE POINTS

- Sheep and goats are seasonality polyestrus.
- Both extrinsic (eg, light, pheromones) and intrinsic (eg, pituitary and gonadal hormones) regulate sheep and goat seasonality.
- Estrus induction and synchronization are tools that are used by sheep and goat producers to provide for year-round meat and milk production.
- Estrus induction and synchronization protocols used in sheep and goats used a combination of methods including the male effect, progestogens, and gonadotropins.

DISCLOSURE

The author has nothing to disclose.

REFERENCES

1. Powell MR, Kaps M, Lamberson WR, et al. Use of melengestrol acetate-based treatments to induce and synchronize estrus in seasonally anestrous ewes. J Anim Sci 1996;74:2292–302.

2. Dawson LJ. Estrus synchronization in goats. Clin Ther 2013;5:270–9.
3. Knights M, Baptiste QS, Dixon AB, et al. Effects of dosage of FSH, vehicle and time of treatment on ovulation rate and prolificacy in ewes during the anestrous season. Small Rumin Res 2003;50:1–9.
4. deNicolo G, Morris ST, Kenyon PR, et al. Effect of weaning pre- or post-mating on performance of spring-mated ewes and their lambs in New Zealand. N Z J Agric Res 2006;49:255–60.
5. Jabbar G, Umberger SH, Lewis GS. Melengestrol acetate and norgestomet for the induction of synchronized estrus in seasonally anovular ewes. J Anim Sci 1994;72:3049–54.
6. Wildeus S. Estrus and ovarian response in norgestomet synchronized Spanish does to graded doses of PMSG/HCG. J Anim Sci 1997;75(16). Abstract.
7. Cline MA, Ralston JN, Seals RC, et al. Intervals from norgestomet withdrawal and injection of equine chorionic gonadotropin or P.G. 600 to estrus and ovulation in ewes. J Anim Sci 2001;79:589–94.
8. Windorski EJ, Schauer CS, Wurst AK, et al. Effects of melengestrol acetate and P.G. 600 on fertility in Rambouillet ewes outside the natural breeding season. Theriogenology 2008;70:227–32.
9. D'Souza KN, Rastle-Simpson SL, Redhead AK, et al. Gonadotropin stimulation using P.G. 600?? on reproductive success of non-lactating anestrous ewes. Anim Reprod Sci 2014;148:115–20.
10. Habeeb HMH, Hazzard T, Stormshak F, et al. Effect of different dosages of PG-600 on ovulation and pregnancy rates in ewes during the breeding season. Transl Anim Sci 2019;3:429–32.
11. Safranski TJ, Lamberson WR, Keisler DH. Use of melengestrol acetate and gonadotropins to induce fertile estrus in seasonally anestrous ewes. J Anim Sci 1992;70:2935–41.
12. Lunstra DD, Christenson RK. Fertilization and embryonic survival in ewes synchronized with exogenous hormones during the anestrous and estrous seasons. J Anim Sci 1981;53:458–66.
13. Ryan JP, Hunton JR, Maxwell WMC. Increased production of sheep embryos following superovulation of merino ewes with a combination of pregnant mare serum gonadotrophin and follicle stimulating hormone. Reprod Fertil Dev 1991; 3:551–60.
14. Rawlings NC, Bartlewski PM. Clinical reproductive physiology of ewes. In: Youngquist RS, Threlfall WR, editors. Current therapy in large animal theriogenology. 2nd edition. St. Louis (MO): Saunders; 2007. p. 642–9.
15. Fatet A, Pellicer-Rubio MT, Leboeuf B. Reproductive cycle of goats. Anim Reprod Sci 2011;124:211–9.
16. Downey BR. Regulation of the estrous cycle in domestic animals– a review. Can Vet J 1980;21:301–6.
17. Thiéry JC, Gayrard V, Le Corre S, et al. Dopaminergic control of LH secretion by the A15 nucleus in anoestrous ewes. J Reprod Fertil Suppl 1995;49:285–96.
18. Wakabayashi Y, Nakada T, Murata K, et al. Neurokinin B and dynorphin A in kiss-peptin neurons of the arcuate nucleus participate in generation of periodic oscillation of neural activity driving pulsatile gonadotropin-releasing hormone secretion in the goat. J Neurosci 2010;30:3124–32.
19. Weems P, Smith J, Clarke IJ, et al. Effects of season and estradiol on KNDY neuron peptides, colocalization with D2 dopamine receptors, and dopaminergic inputs in the ewe. Endocrinology 2017;158:831–41.

20. Barrell GK, Moenter SM, Caraty A, et al. Seasonal changes of gonadotropin-releasing hormone secretion in the ewe. Biol Reprod 1992;46:1130–5.
21. Tanaka T, Mori Y, Hoshino K. Hypothalamic GnRH pulse generator activity during the estradiol-induced LH surge in ovariectomized goats. Neuroendocrinology 1992;56:641–5.
22. Clarke IJ, Caraty A. Kisspeptin and seasonality of reproduction. New York: Springer; 2013. p. 411–30.
23. Nestor CC, Bedenbaugh MN, Hileman SM, et al. Regulation of GnRH pulsatility in ewes. Reproduction 2018;156:83–99.
24. Robinson JE, Max Radford H, Karsch FJ. Seasonal changes in pulsatile luteinizing hormone (lh) secretion in the ewe: relationship of frequency of LH pulses to day length and response to estradiol negative feedback. Biol Reprod 1985;33:324–34.
25. Clarke IJ. The preovulatory LH surge. A case of a neuroendocrine switch. Trends Endocrinol Metab 1995;6:241–7.
26. Chemineau P. Possibilities for using bucks to stimulate ovarian and oestrous cycles in anovulatory goats - a review. Livest Prod Sci 1987;17:135–47.
27. Rodríguez Iglesias RM, Ciccioli NH, Ferrería J, et al. Short-lived corpora lutea syndrome in anoestrous ewes following 17β-oestradiol or MAP treatments applied before an allogenic sexual stimulation with rams and oestrous ewes. Anim Reprod Sci 2013;136:268–79.
28. Oldham CM, Martin GB, Knight TW. Stimulation of seasonally anovular merino ewes by rams. I. Time from introduction of the rams to the preovulatory LH surge and ovulation. Anim Reprod Sci 1979;1:283–90.
29. Legan SJ, I'anson H, Fitzgerald BP, et al. Importance of short luteal phases in the endocrine mechanism controlling initiation of estrous cycles in anestrous ewes. Endocrinology 1985;117:1530–6.
30. Chanvallon A, Sagot L, Pottier E, et al. New insights into the influence of breed and time of the year on the response of ewes to the "ram effect. Animal 2011; 5:1594–604.
31. Brown HM, Fabre Nys C, Cognié J, et al. Short oestrous cycles in sheep during anoestrus involve defects in progesterone biosynthesis and luteal neovascularisation. Reproduction 2014;147:357–67.
32. Chemineau P, Pellicer-Rubio MT, Lassoued N, et al. Male-induced short oestrous and ovarian cycles in sheep and goats: a working hypothesis. Reprod Nutr Dev 2006;46:417–29.
33. Adib A, Freret S, Touze JL, et al. Progesterone improves the maturation of male-induced preovulatory follicles in anoestrous ewes. Reproduction 2014;148:403–16.
34. Underwood WJ, Blauwiekel R, Delano ML, et al. Biology and Diseases of Ruminants (Sheep, Goats, and Cattle). In: Fox JG, editor. Laboratory animal medicine. 3rd edition. Elsevier Inc; 2015. p. 623–94.
35. Caraty A, Skinner DC. Progesterone priming is essential for the full expression of the positive feedback effect of estradiol in inducing the preovulatory gonadotropin-releasing hormone surge in the ewe. Endocrinology 1999;140: 165–70.
36. Hillier SG, Whitelaw PF, Smyth CD. Follicular oestrogen synthesis: the "two-cell, two-gonadotrophin" model revisited. Mol Cell Endocrinol 1994;100:51–4.
37. Monniaux D. Short-term effects of FSH in vitro on granulosa cells of individual sheep follicles. Reproduction 1987;79:505–15.
38. Martin GB, Oldham CM, Cognié Y, et al. The physiological responses of anovulatory ewes to the introduction of rams - A review. Livest Prod Sci 1986;15:219–47.

39. Imwalle DB, Lehrer AR, Katz LS. Intravaginal impedance and sexual behavior of ovariectomized goats given estrogen alone or in combination with progesterone. J Anim Sci 2007;85:1908–13.

40. Hawken PAR, Martin GB. Sociosexual stimuli and gonadotropin-releasing hormone/luteinizing hormone secretion in sheep and goats. Domest Anim Endocrinol 2012;43:85–94.

41. Lindsay DR, Cognie Y, Pelletier J, et al. Influence of the presence of rams on the timing of ovulation and discharge of LH in ewes. Physiol Behav 1975;15:423–6.

42. Dávila FS, Bosque-González AS del B, Barragán HB. Reproduction in Goats. In: Kukovics S, editor. Goat science. Herceghalom (Hungary): IntechOpen; 2017. p. 87–105. Available at: https://www.intechopen.com/books/goat-science/reproduction-in-goats. Accessed March 12, 2020.

43. Robertson HA. The endogenous control of estrus and ovulation in sheep, cattle, and swine. Vitam Horm 1969;27:91–130.

44. Martin GB, Oldham CM, Lindsay DR. Increased plasma LH levels in seasonally anovular merino ewes following the introduction of rams. Anim Reprod Sci 1980;3:125–32.

45. Oldham CM, Martin GB. Stimulation of seasonally anovular merino ewes by rams. II. Premature regression of ram-induced corpora lutea. Anim Reprod Sci 1979;1: 291–5.

46. Romano J, Christians C, Crabo B. Continuous presence of rams hastens the onset of estrus in ewes synchronized during the breeding season. Appl Anim Behav Sci 2000;66:65–70.

47. Ergül Ekiz E, Ekiz B, Koçak Ö. Effects of ram presence during synchronization period and previous experience on certain estrus parameters and sexual behaviors in Kivircik ewes. Turkish J Vet Anim Sci 2013;37:189–93.

48. Fabre-Nys C, Cognié J, Dufourny L, et al. The Two populations of kisspeptin neurons are involved in the ram-induced LH pulsatile secretion and LH surge in anestrous ewes. Endocrinology 2017;158:3914–28.

49. Hawken PAR, Beard AP, Esmaili T, et al. The introduction of rams induces an increase in pulsatile LH secretion in cyclic ewes during the breeding season. Theriogenology 2007;68:56–66.

50. Evans ACO, Duffy P, Crosby TF, et al. Effect of ram exposure at the end of progestagen treatment on estrus synchronisation and fertility during the breeding season in ewes. Anim Reprod Sci 2004;84:349–58.

51. Martin GB, Cognié Y, Schirar A, et al. Diurnal variation in the response of anoestrous ewes to the ram effect. J Reprod Fertil 1985;75:275–84.

52. Martin GB, Scaramuzzi RJ, Lindsay DR. Effect of the introduction of rams during the anoestrous season on the pulsatile secretion of LH in ovariectomized ewes. J Reprod Fertil 1983;67:47–55.

53. Minton JE, Coppinger TR, Spaeth CW, et al. Poor reproductive response of anestrous Suffolk ewes to ram exposure is not due to failure to secrete luteinizing hormone acutely. J Anim Sci 1991;69:3314–20.

54. Flores JA, Véliz FG, Pérez-Villanueva JA, et al. Male Reproductive Condition Is the Limiting Factor of Efficiency in the Male Effect During Seasonal Anestrus in Female Goats. Biol Reprod 2000;62(5):1409–14.

55. Mellado M, Olivas R, Ruiz F. Effect of buck stimulus on mature and pre-pubertal norgestomet-treated goats. Small Rumin Res 2000;36(3):269–74.

56. Delgadillo JA, Fitz-Rodríguez G, Duarte G, et al. Management of photoperiod to control caprine reproduction in the subtropics. Reprod Fertil Dev 2004;16: 471–81.

57. Vielma J, Hernandez H, Veliz FG, et al. Buck vocalisations stimulate estrous behaviour in seasonally anovulatory female goats. Reprod Domest Anim 2005; 40:360–8.

58. Chemineau P. Effect on oestrus and ovulation of exposing creole goats to the male at three times of the year. J Reprod Fertil 1983;67:65–72.

59. Ungerfeld R, Forsberg M, Rubianes E. Overview of the response of anoestrous ewes to the ram effect. Reprod Fertil Dev 2004;16:479–90.

60. Fabre-Nys C, Chanvallon A, Dupont J, et al. The "ram effect": a "non-classical" mechanism for inducing LH surges in sheep. PLoS One 2016;11:1–22.

61. Lindsay DR, Signoret JP. Influence of behaviour on reproduction. In: Proceedings of the 9th International Congress on Animal Reproduction and Artificial Insemination. Editorial Garsi 1980;1:83-92.

62. Chemineau P. Effects of a progestagen on buck-induced short ovarian cycles in the creole meat goat. Anim Reprod Sci 1985;9:87–94.

63. Wheaton JE, Windels HF, Johnston LJ. Accelerated lambing using exogenous progesterone and the ram effect. J Anim Sci 1992;70:2628–35.

64. Knights M, Maze TD, Bridges PJ, et al. Short-term treatment with a Controlled Internal Drug Releasing (CIDR) device and FSH to induce fertile estrus and increase prolificacy in anestrous ewes. Theriogenology 2001;55:1181–91.

65. Knights M, Hoehn T, Marsh D, et al. Reproductive management in the ewe flock by induction or synchronization of estrus. Morgantown, WV: West Virginia Agricultural and Forestry Experiment Station. 2003, pp. 1-21.

66. Ungerfeld R. Combination of the ram effect with PGF2α estrous synchronization treatments in ewes during the breeding season. Anim Reprod Sci 2011;124:65–8.

67. Knights M, Hoehn T, Lewis PE, et al. Effectiveness of intravaginal progesterone inserts and FSH for inducing synchronized estrus and increasing lambing rate in anestrous ewes. J Anim Sci 2001;79:1120–31.

68. Pendleton RJ, Youngs CR, Rorie RW, et al. Follicle stimulating hormone versus pregnant mare serum gonadotropin for superovulation of dairy goats. Small Rumin Res 1992;8:217–24.

69. Dutt RH, Casida LE. Alteration of the estrual cycle in sheep by use of progesterone and its effect upon subsequent ovulation and fertility. Endocrinology 1948;43: 208–17.

70. Godfrey RW, Collins JR, Hensley EL, et al. Estrus synchronization and artificial insemination of hair sheep ewes in the tropics. Theriogenology 1999;51:985–97.

71. Letelier CA, Contreras-Solis I, García-Fernández RA, et al. Ovarian follicular dynamics and plasma steroid concentrations are not significantly different in ewes given intravaginal sponges containing either 20 or 40 mg of fluorogestone acetate. Theriogenology 2009;71:676–82.

72. Foote WC, Waite AB. Some effects of progesterone on estrous behavior and fertility in the ewe. J Anim Sci 1965;24:151–5.

73. Menchaca A, Miller V, Salveraglio V, et al. Endocrine, luteal and follicular responses after the use of the Short-Term Protocol to synchronize ovulation in goats. Anim Reprod Sci 2007;102(1–2):76–87.

74. Robin N, Laforest J, Lussier J, et al. Induction of estrus with intramuscular injections of GnRH or PMSG in lactating goats (Capra hircus) primed with a progestagen during seasonal anestrus. Theriogenology 1994;42:107–16.

75. McCracken JA, Carlson JC, Glew ME, et al. Prostaglandin F2α identified as a luteolytic hormone in sheep. Nat New Biol 1972;238:129–34.

76. Homeida AM, Khalafalla AE. Effects of oxytocin-antagonist injections on luteal regression in the goat. Br J Pharmacol 1987;90:281–4.

77. Rubianes E, Menchaca A, Carbajal B. Response of the 1–5 day-aged ovine corpus luteum to prostaglandin F2α. Anim Reprod Sci 2003;78:47–55.
78. Acritopoulou S, Haresign W. Response of ewes to a single injection of an analogue of PGF-2 alpha given at different stages of the oestrous cycle. J Reprod Fertil 1980;58:219–21.
79. Deaver DR, Stilley NJ, Dailey RA, et al. Concentrations of ovarian and pituitary hormones following prostaglandin F2 alpha-induced luteal regression in ewes varies with day of the estrous cycle at treatment. J Anim Sci 1986;62:422–7.
80. Mirzaei A, Mohebbi-Fani M, Omidi A, et al. Progesterone concentration and lambing rate of Karakul ewes treated with prostaglandin and GnRH combined with the ram effect during breeding and non-breeding seasons. Theriogenology 2017;100:120–5.
81. Bukar MM, Yusoff R, Haron AW, et al. Estrus response and follicular development in Boer does synchronized with flugestone acetate and PGF2α or their combination with eCG or FSH. Trop Anim Health Prod 2012;44:1505–11.
82. Lassoued N, Khaldi G, Cognié Y, et al. Effect of progesterone on ovulation length and duration of the ovarian cycle induced by the male effect in the Barbarine ewe and the local Tunisian goat. Reprod Nutr Dev 1995;35:415–26.
83. Iida K, Kibayashi N, Kohno H, et al. Comparative study of induction of estrus and ovulation by three different intravaginal devices in ewes during the non-breeding season. J Reprod Dev 2004;50:63–9.
84. Brunner MA, Hansel W, Hogue DE. Use of 6-Methyl-17-Acetoxyprogesterone and pregnant mare serum to induce and synchronize estrus in ewes. J Anim Sci 1964;23:32–6.
85. Lu MC, Takayama K, Nakanishi Y, et al. Luteal lifespan and fertility after estrus synchronization in goats. J Vet Sci 2008;9:95–101.
86. Miguel-Cruz EE, Mejía-Villanueva O, Zarco L. Induction of fertile estrus without the use of steroid hormones in seasonally anestrous Suffolk ewes. Asian-Australas J Anim Sci 2019;23:1673–85.
87. Greyling JPC, Van Niekerk CH. Different synchronization techniques in Boer goat does outside the normal breeding season. Small Rumin Res 1991;5:233–43.
88. García-Salas A, Cortez-Romero C, Salazar-Ortiz J, et al. Administration of exogenous hormones in ovulatory and embryonic response in Pelibuey sheep. Reprod Domest Anim 2017;52:446–51.
89. Hoppen HO. The equine placenta and equine chorionic gonadotrophin — an overview. Exp Clin Endocrinol Diabetes 1994;102:235–43.
90. Martinez-Tinajero JJ, Ruiz-Herluver I, Montanez-Valdez OD, et al. Reproductive performance in dorper ewes synchronized at estrus during non breeding season in tropical conditions. J Anim Vet Adv 2013;10:221–3.
91. Quintero-Elisea JA, Macías-Cruz U, Álvarez-Valenzuela FD, et al. The effects of time and dose of pregnant mare serum gonadotropin (PMSG) on reproductive efficiency in hair sheep ewes. Trop Anim Health Prod 2011;43:1567–73.
92. El Kadili S, Raes M, Bister J, et al. Effect of doses of eCG and cloprostenol on oestrus and ovulation induction in North Moroccan goats during the anoestrus season: Innovation for Sustainability in Sheep and Goats. R. Ruiz, A. López-Francos, L. López Marco (eds). Zaragoza: CIHEAM/NEIKER 2019. (Options Méditerranéennes, Series A: Mediterranean Seminars, No. 123):229–234.

93. Habeeb HMH, Hazzard T, Stormshak F, et al. Ovulation, pregnancy, and lambing rates during nonbreeding season with or without exogenous gonadotropin stimulation. Clin Ther 2020;12:23–8.

94. Cross LJ, Cross RM, Stormshak F. Optimal dose of PG600 when given to progestogen-synchronized ewes during anestrus as affected by day of the year and temperature. Transl Anim Sci 2019;3:433–42.

95. Rowe JD, East NE. Comparison of two sources of gonadotropin for estrus synchronization in does. Theriogenology 1996;45:1569–75.

Use of Hysteroscopy for Diagnosing Causes of Infertility in Camelids

Michelle Anne Kutzler, MBA, DVM, PhD[a],*, Michelle Ing, DVM[b]

KEYWORDS

- Alpaca • Endometritis • Endoscopy • Infertility • Llama • Uterus • Vaginoscopy

KEY POINTS

- Hysteroscopy allows the veterinarian to observe abnormalities on the surface or within the endometrium that cannot be observed using other methods (eg, transrectal ultrasonography).
- It is important to introduce the endoscope completely down to the tips of both uterine horns until the uterine papilla are visualized.
- Three endometrial biopsies (one for culture, cytology, and histopathology) of normal endometrium should be collected during hysteroscopy. Additional biopsies should be collected from abnormal-appearing endometrium.
- Even when no abnormalities are found during the hysteroscopic procedure, previously infertile females tend to become pregnant and maintain their pregnancies following hysteroscopy.

 Video content accompanies this article at http://www.vetfood.theclinics.com.

INTRODUCTION

Endometritis is a common cause of infertility in alpacas and llamas, resulting in 30% to 50% embryo loss in the first 90 days of gestation.[1,2] Endometritis is most commonly the result of overbreeding but can also occur following a dystocia. Endometrial cytology and culture are typically used to confirm a diagnosis of endometritis. In addition, endometrial biopsy can be used to diagnose endometritis as well as determine its chronicity as defined by fibrotic changes within the endometrium.[3]

Imaging the uterine lumen and endometrium using an endoscope (hysteroscopy) for the purposes of diagnosing causes of infertility has been used in horses, cattle, and dogs.[4–12] Vaginoscopy is commonly performed during fertility examinations in

[a] Department of Animal and Rangeland Sciences, Oregon State University, 112 Withycombe Hall, Corvallis, OR 97331, USA; [b] Granite Bay Alpacas, PO Box 2073, Granite Bay, CA 95746, USA
* Corresponding author.
E-mail address: michelle.kutzler@oregonstate.edu

Vet Clin Food Anim 37 (2021) 139–147
https://doi.org/10.1016/j.cvfa.2020.12.004
0749-0720/21/© 2020 Elsevier Inc. All rights reserved.

camelids,[13,14] and this method is quite useful for diagnosing abnormalities within the vagina and cervix (**Fig. 1**). However, there are few reports of using hysteroscopy in llamas and alpacas during a breeding soundness examination. Hysteroscopy allows the veterinarian to observe abnormalities on the surface or within the endometrium that cannot be observed using other methods (eg, transrectal ultrasonography). For example, focal, multifocal, and diffuse endometritis can be visualized using hysteroscopy (**Fig. 2**). Endometritis with endometrial ulceration from repeated penile endometrial abrasion during mating can also be visualized (**Fig. 3**). In addition, mural adhesions, scarring over the uterine papilla (opening of the uterine tube opening), and endometrial cysts can be visualized (**Fig. 4**, Video 1).

PROCEDURE

Before performing a hysteroscopy, a reproductive history should be collected. The breeding history and the female's return to receptivity should be included (**Box 1**). A complete physical examination and reproductive examination should be performed. If there is *ANY* possibility that the female could be pregnant, she should be examined using transrectal B-mode ultrasound scanner with a 7.5 MHz linear array probe to confirm a nonpregnant status. Hysteroscopy would terminate a pregnancy. In addition, it is easier to perform hysteroscopy when the female does not have a corpus

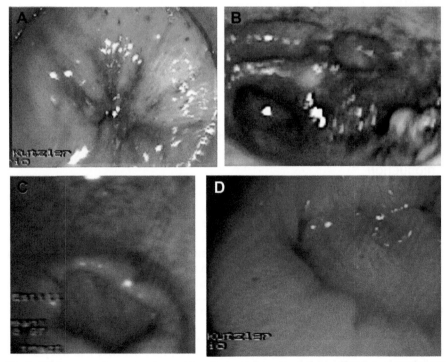

Fig. 1. Vaginoscopy is commonly used for diagnosing cervical abnormalities in camelids. (*A*) The external cervical os in this image is inflamed, and cloudy mucus is visible passing through the cervix into the vagina. (*B*) Extensive cervical damage occurred in this female alpaca during correction of a dystocia. (*C*) Same alpaca as shown in **Fig. 2**B but 8 weeks after the dystocia. The cervical mucosa has healed but the integrity of the cervical os has been lost. (*D*) A normal external cervical os is shown here for reference.

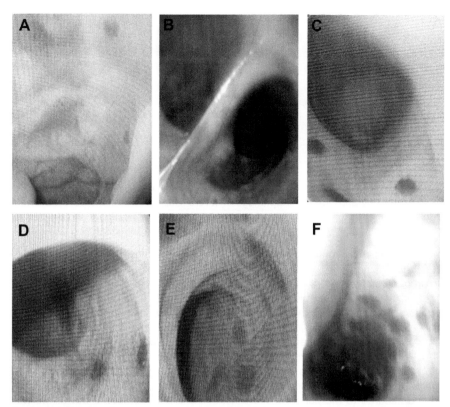

Fig. 2. Multifocal endometritis is common in camelids. (*A*) Uterine body. (*B*) Bifurcation of the uterine horns. (*C*) Base of the left uterine horn. (*D*) Midway along the length of the left uterine horn. (*E*) Base of the left uterine horn. (*F*) Midway along the length of the left uterine horn.

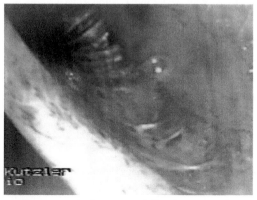

Fig. 3. Linear endometrial mucosal ulcerations following natural mating. During copulation, the male's penis repeatedly abrades the endometrium, which can result in ulceration and endometritis.

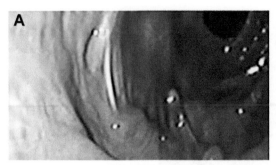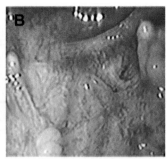

Fig. 4. Several cysts visible on the endometrial surface at the base of the left uterine horn in an alpaca with a history of infertility. (*A*) Image taken from the perspective of the bifurcation of the uterine horn. (*B*) Close-up image of several clusters of endometrial cysts within the base of the left uterine horn.

luteum, which can be confirmed by a serum progesterone concentration below 0.5 ng/mL.[15]

In preparation for the hysteroscopy, the female can be treated with 0.5 to 2.5 mg of estradiol benzoate or estradiol cypionate intramuscularly 12 to 48 hours before the procedure.[2,16] Pretreatment with estrogen will relax the cervix, facilitating passage of the endoscope as well as increase the innate immune function within the endometrium.[17–19] Females are restrained within a camelid chute and administered butorphanol (0.1–0.2 mg/kg) intramuscularly to provide mild sedation and general analgesia during the procedure. It has been the authors' experience that most patients will remain standing for the procedure with administration of butorphanol. The tail is wrapped and secured to the fleece or the neck of the animal to keep it out of the way (**Fig. 5**).

Fecal contents are removed from the rectum, the perineum is cleaned with a disinfectant soap, and a glass speculum is passed into the vagina (**Fig. 6**). A chemically disinfected video-endoscope (0.9 cm diameter) with a working length of 1.5 m is passed

---

Box 1
Examples of questions to ask while collecting a reproductive history

- Was this female a twin?
- At what age was this female first bred?
- How many times has the female been bred?
- How often has the female been bred?
- How long did each of the breedings last?
- How long did the female reject the male following breeding becoming receptive again?
- Has this female been confirmed pregnant via ultrasound, and if so, how many times?
- Has this female ever aborted?
- Has this female had a cria and if so, how many times?
- Has this female ever had a dystocia?
- Has this female exhibited abnormal reproductive behaviors (eg, mounting other females, orgling)?

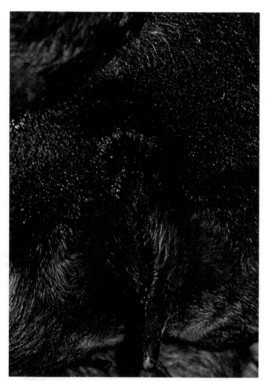

Fig. 5. Before performing a hysteroscopic examination, the tail is the wrapped and secured to the fleece or the neck of the animal to keep it out of the way during the procedure.

through a vaginal speculum. The external os of the cervix is visualized and the endoscope is gently passed through the cervix (**Fig. 7**). Once through the cervix, the uterus is insufflated with filtered-room air to visualize the endometrium (**Fig. 8**). It is important to introduce the endoscope completely down to the tips of both uterine horns to access the integrity of uterine papilla (opening of the uterine tubes) (Video 2).[2] Any abnormalities should be noted and photographed.

At least 3 endometrial biopsies should be collected using the biopsy instrument for the endoscope. The first biopsy should be submitted for aerobic and anaerobic bacterial culture as well as *Ureaplasma*, *Mycoplasma*, and fungal culture. The next biopsy should be used to make impression smears on a glass microscope slide for an

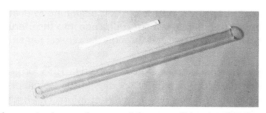

Fig. 6. Example of a vaginal speculum used for camelid reproductive examinations. This vaginal speculum is made of tempered (shatter-resistant) glass and is 2 cm in diameter by 25 cm long.

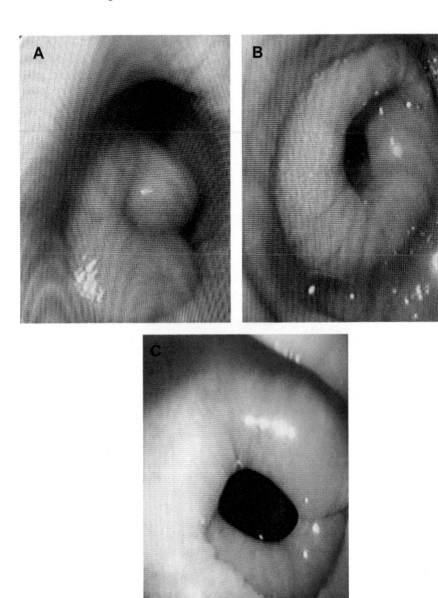

Fig. 7. Visualization of the external cervical os at the beginning of the hysteroscopy proced-ure. (*A*) The cervix is not yet dilated. (*B*) The cervix is beginning to dilate with insufflation. (*C*) The cervix is dilated sufficiently to pass the endoscope into the uterus. Note the bifurca-tion of the uterine horns can be visualized through the cervical lumen.

endometrial cytology. The last biopsy should be fixed in 10% formalin or Bouin's fixa-tive solution for histopathology. Like other species, endometrial biopsies in camelids are useful for determining the underlying cause of infertility.[3] If abnormalities in the endometrium are visualized, additional site-directed biopsies should be collected from these areas. It is important to collect biopsies from both normal-appearing and abnormal-appearing endometrium.

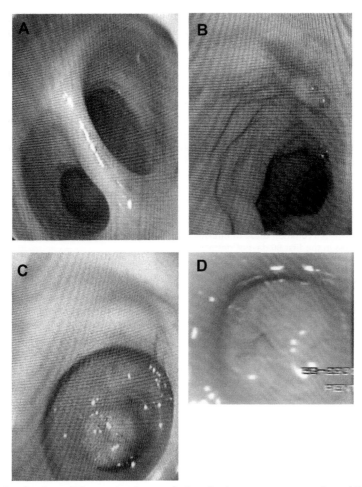

Fig. 8. Visualization of the uterine lumen during the hysteroscopy procedure. (*A*) Bifurcation of the uterine horns as viewed from the uterine body. (*B*) Lumen of one of the uterine horns. (*C*) Lumen of the tip of one of the uterine horns. Note the presence of the uterine papilla (opening of the uterine tube) at the end of the uterine horn. (*D*) Closer view of the uterine papilla. Careful examination of the surface of the uterine papilla is necessary to rule-out the presence of scar tissue covering the opening of the uterine tube.

POSTPROCEDURE CARE AND CONSIDERATIONS

Following the hysteroscopic examination, the uterine lumen is lavaged. This can be accomplished a single time through the endoscope or daily using an indwelling intrauterine catheter. With an indwelling intrauterine catheter, camelid owners can continue to administer the uterine lavage through the indwelling catheter for a total of 5 daily treatments before removing the catheter. Choice of lavage solutions varies but, in most instances, involves the use of sterile lactated ringers' solution (LRS) or 0.9% saline with or without the addition of antibiotics. It is one of the author's (MK) preferences to add 10 g of gentamycin per milliliter of LRS before lavaging the uterus. Lavage fluid volumes vary from 200 to 500 mL total for each lavage.

The authors have performed more than 100 hysteroscopic procedures in camelids and have not had any complications. However, complications such as endometritis, hemorrhage, uterine perforation, vaginitis, vaginal tears, and venous air emboli have been reported in dogs and humans following hysteroscopy.[8,10,20,21]

It has been the authors' clinical experience that even when no abnormalities are found during the hysteroscopic procedure, previously infertile females tend to become pregnant and maintain their pregnancies following hysteroscopy. This possible therapeutic effect may be a response to prehysteroscopy estrogen treatment, dilation of the uterine horns during hysteroscopy, and/or posttreatment uterine lavages. Research is needed with sham-treated controls to determine if the therapeutic benefit of hysteroscopy is real or just perceived.

CLINICS CARE POINTS

- Endometritis is a common cause of infertility in alpacas and llamas, resulting in 30% to 50% embryo loss in the first 90 days of gestation.
- Imaging the uterine lumen and endometrium using an endoscope (hysteroscopy) for the purposes of diagnosing causes of infertility has been used in horses, cattle, and dogs.
- Hysteroscopy allows for site-directed biopsies of abnormal endometrium; however, it is important to collect biopsies from both normal-appearing and abnormal-appearing endometrium for histopathology.
- Although complications have not been reported in camelids, complications reported in dogs and humans following hysteroscopy include endometritis, hemorrhage, uterine perforation, vaginitis, vaginal tears, and venous air emboli.

DISCLOSURE

The authors have nothing to disclose.

SUPPLEMENTARY DATA

Supplementary data to this article can be found online at https://doi.org/10.1016/j.cvfa.2020.12.004.

REFERENCES

1. Pearson LK, Rodriguez JS, Tibary A. Disorders and diseases of pregnancy. In: Cebra CE, Anderson DE, Tibary A, et al, editors. Llama and alpaca care. St Louis (MO): Elsevier; 2014. p. 256–73.
2. Tibary A. Breeding soundness evaluation and subfertility in female llamas and alpacas. In: Youngquist RS, Threlfall WR, editors. Current therapy in large animal theriogenology. 2nd edition. Philadelphia: WB Saunders; 2007. p. 878–83.
3. Powers BE, Johnson LW, Linton LB, et al. Endometrial biopsy technique and uterine pathologic findings in llamas. J Am Vet Med Assoc 1990;197(9):1157–62.
4. Schneeweiss W, Krump L, Metcalfe L, et al. Endoscopic-assisted resection of a pedunculated uterine leiomyoma with maximal tissue preservation in a cow and a mare. Vet Surg 2015;44(2):200–5.
5. Madoz LV, De la Sota RL, Suzuki K, et al. Use of hysteroscopy for the diagnosis of postpartum clinical endometritis in dairy cows. Vet Rec 2010;167(4):142–3.

6. Rambags BP, Stout TA. Transcervical endoscope-guided emptying of a transmural uterine cyst in a mare. Vet Rec 2005;156(21):679–82.
7. Janicek JC, Rodgerson DH, Boone BL. Use of a hand-assisted laparoscopic technique for removal of a uterine leiomyoma in a standing mare. J Am Vet Med Assoc 2004;225(6):911–4, 880.
8. Gerber D, Nöthling JO. Hysteroscopy in bitches. J Reprod Fertil Suppl 2001;57: 415–7.
9. Watts JR, Wright PJ, Lee CS, et al. New techniques using transcervical uterine cannulation for the diagnosis of uterine disorders in bitches. J Reprod Fertil Suppl 1997;51:283–93.
10. Watts JR, Wright PJ. Investigating uterine disease in the bitch: uterine cannulation for cytology, microbiology and hysteroscopy. J Small Anim Pract 1995;36(5): 201–6.
11. Bracher V, Allen WR. Videoendoscopic evaluation of the mare's uterus: I. Findings in normal fertile mares. Equine Vet J 1992;24(4):274–8.
12. Devine DA, Lindsay FE. Hysteroscopy in the cow using a flexible fibrescope. Vet Rec 1984;115(24):627–8.
13. Tan RH, Dascanio JJ. Infertility associated with persistent hymen in an alpaca and a llama. Can Vet J 2008;49(11):1113–7.
14. Belknap EB, Schmidt AR, Carleton CL. Double cervices in two llamas. J Am Vet Med Assoc 1990;197(8):1049–50.
15. Leon JB, Smith BB, Timm KI, et al. Endocrine changes during pregnancy, parturition and the early post-partum period in the llama (Lama glama). J Reprod Fertil 1990;88(2):503–11.
16. Cavilla MV, Bianchi CP, Aba MA. Oestradiol-17beta plasma concentrations after intramuscular injection of oestradiol benzoate or oestradiol cypionate in llamas (Lama glama). Acta Vet Scand 2010;52(1):13.
17. Bianchi C, Sahlin L, Meikle A, et al. Endometrial population of oestrogen receptors alpha and beta and progesterone receptors A and B during the different phases of the follicular wave of llamas (Lama glama). Reprod Domest Anim 2010;45(5):872–80.
18. Fahey JV, Wright JA, Shen L, et al. Estradiol selectively regulates innate immune function by polarized human uterine epithelial cells in culture. Mucosal Immunol 2008;1(4):317–25.
19. Powell SA, Smith BB, Tim KI, et al. Expression of estrogen receptors alpha and beta in the corpus luteum and the uterus from nonpregnant and pregnant llamas. Mol Reprod Dev 2007;74(8):1043–52.
20. Stoloff DR, Isenberg RA, Brill A. Venous air and gas emboli in operative hysteroscopy. J Am Assoc Gynecol Laparosc 2001;8(2):181–92.
21. Brundin J, Thomasson K. Cardiac gas embolism during carbon dioxide hysteroscopy: risk and management. Eur J Obstet Gynecol Reprod Biol 1989;33(3): 241–5.

Udder Health for Dairy Goats

Paula Menzies, DVM, MPVM*

KEYWORDS

- Goat • Mastitis • Somatic cell counts • CMT • Staphylococcus aureus
- Udder health

KEY POINTS

- *Staphylococcus aureus* is the most important cause of clinical mastitis in goats and non-aureus staphylococci (NAS) are the most common isolates from subclinical mastitis; pathogenicity varies between species of NAS.
- Poor udder hygiene practices, and dirty, wet environment and milking equipment are associated with streptococcal mastitis.
- Somatic cell counts and CMT can be used as screening tests for mastitis and as an indicator of poor udder health. However, normal values are higher than with cattle and sheep. Use logarithmic transformation (e.g. somatic cell scores) to better interpret values.
- High bacterial counts in the milk are common in many goat dairies reflecting poor milk quality; mastitis may contribute as a cause.
- Proper udder preparation, milking procedure and post-milking management are key factors in mastitis control.

 Video content accompanies this article at http://www.vetequine.theclinics. com/

INTRODUCTION

Mastitis is defined as inflammation of the udder with change to the physiology and/or anatomy of the udder as evidenced by swelling, heat, changes in the appearance of milk, and possible systemic illness. The inflammation may be caused by trauma, infusion of an irritating substance, or an infectious microorganism, such as bacteria, viruses, and mycotic agents. Infection of the udder is termed, *intramammary infection (IMI)*. Udder health is comprised of those measures to control mastitis, including IMI. The ultimate goals are to keep the goat and its udder healthy and to optimize production of quality milk.

Milk quality is measured by several parameters, that is, bacterial counts, somatic cell counts (SCCs), freezing point, presence of inhibitors, and odor, appearance,

Department of Population Medicine, Ontario Veterinary College, University of Guelph, Guelph Ontario N1G 2W1, Canada
* 690 Colquhoun Street, Fergus, Ontario N1M 1S3, Canada.
E-mail address: pmenzies@uoguelph.ca

Vet Clin Food Anim 37 (2021) 149–174
https://doi.org/10.1016/j.cvfa.2020.12.002
vetfood.theclinics.com

and taste. These measures often are used to regulate to the production of healthy milk that is to be consumed by the public. Each jurisdiction has its own regulatory levels. Mastitis is one of the important factors affecting milk quality.

When developing an udder health program, have a discussion with the client regarding the costs associated with mastitis versus the costs of an udder health program (**Table 1**). Benefits can be identified as improved milk production and quality and reduction in costs associated with the effects of mastitis.

IMPORTANT DIFFERENCES IN MILK PRODUCTION OF GOATS VERSUS CATTLE
Anatomy and Physiology

The udder of the goat is very different from that of the dairy cow, much more than having only 2 glands rather than 4. Some of these issues relate directly to managing udder health.

Gland cistern capacity
Gland cistern capacity is the volume of the gland cistern of the udder, which can hold greater than 40% to 80% of milk volume as opposed to 30% for dairy cattle.[1] This is

---

Table 1
Costs associated with mastitis and an udder health program

Costs Associated with Mastitis	Costs of an Udder Health Program
<ul><li>Lower milk production<ul><li>Lower volume of milk</li><li>Lower level of components</li><li>Higher feed costs for milk produced</li></ul></li><li>Loss of bonus for high-quality milk</li><li>Penalties/rejection of low-quality milk</li><li>Higher turnover due to involuntary removals (culled/died)<ul><li>Replacement costs = cost of doe raised or purchased to replace minus slaughter value of culled doe/value of dead doe</li><li>Lower milk production of doelings</li><li>Lost opportunity sales of replacements</li><li>Increased cost of dead stock management</li></ul></li><li>Treatment costs<ul><li>Drugs, equipment, labor, laboratory investigation, veterinary visits</li><li>Discarded milk from treatments</li><li>Increased risk of rejection/penalties due to inhibitors</li></ul></li><li>Increased management costs<ul><li>Record keeping needs and potential errors</li><li>Segregation of goats with contagious mastitis</li></ul></li><li>Welfare costs<ul><li>Kid illness and death</li><li>Doe illness and death</li></ul></li><li>Public health costs<ul><li>Higher risk of zoonotic pathogens in the milk, particularly important for raw milk markets</li></ul></li></ul>	<ul><li>Improvements in housing, for example, lower stocking densities, better ventilation, cleanliness of bedding</li><li>Improvements in milking equipment and its maintenance</li><li>Increased labor at milking to assure proper milking practices</li><li>Products to improve hygiene at milking, for example, gloves, udder wash/teat dips, paper towels</li><li>Detection/monitoring for subclinical mastitis, for example, SCC/CMT and culturing milk from suspect cases</li><li>Therapies to control the incidence of mastitis, for example, dry period intramammary products, vaccines</li><li>Veterinary costs for implementation and review of the udder health program, including goal setting</li></ul>

important because poor stimulation of milk let-down, that is, poor level of oxytocin release and thus milk ejection, still may see milk being removed by the machine but without the alveolar milk component, which contains most of the fat. Additionally, incomplete milk-out due to poor udder conformation and teat placement can leave as much as 20% of the milk in the gland cistern after milking. Improper stimulation, therefore, may lead to incomplete milk-out and overmilking, and, along with poor udder conformation, may lead to excessive machine stripping, all of which are risk factors for teat damage and mastitis.

Ectopic mammary tissue

Occasionally, mammary tissue may be present in places other than in the mammary gland and is not evident until the doe lactates for the first time. A common site is at the annular ring of the teat between the teat and gland cisterns. Another is around the vulva. With the former, there is a risk of mastitis and scarring in these tissues as well as in the gland.

Apocrine secretion of milk

In cattle, milk is produced by merocrine secretion but in sheep and goats, the secretion is apocrine; milk globules are pinched off the cell, surrounded by the cell membrane, and may contain cytoplasmic particles containing mitochondrial DNA as well as milk components (**Fig. 1**). This has implications on how SCC machines are calibrated and the accuracy of counting.

Goat Milk Production Practices

There are many common practices used in commercial goat dairies that differ from cattle and many of these have a direct impact on udder health.

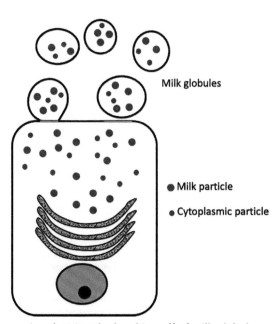

Fig. 1. Apocrine secretion showing the breaking off of milk globules containing milk and fat particles as well as cytoplasmic particles.

Seasonal milk production

Goats are short-day seasonal breeders, with most freshenings (kiddings) occurring in the spring and peak milk occurring in the early summer months. The normal dry period is in the winter months. Although producers may attempt to have does freshen off-season in an attempt to produce year-round milk, there still is more milk shipped in the spring-summer than in the autumn-winter from most commercial goat dairies. Goats that freshen in the autumn (ie, short days) tend to have lower milk production unless the photoperiod is manipulated to mimic spring/summer (ie, long days).[2,3] This may have the effect that at times of the year, SCC values may rise to very high levels—possibly reflecting a herd mostly in late lactation rather than an udder health issue.

Length of dry period

There is little research on the appropriate length of the dry period in goats, but there is evidence that a dry period of less than 28 days is associated with lower milk yield in the following lactation.[4] It is a common practice in many commercial dairies, however, to omit the dry period and milk through kidding. This practice is said to lower the incidence of pregnancy toxemia; however, more research is needed to fully understand the effects on udder health.

Extended lactations

Many goat dairies practice extended lactations with does often milked for 2 years or more before kidding again. Although it has been shown to be associated with increased incidence of pseudopregnancy,[5] it often is done because the producer has difficulty in drying the doe at the traditional time, that is, after 10 months of lactation. It appears that goats with extended lactations (2 years) produce a similar amount of lifetime milk as does with traditional lactation lengths,[6] but of course give birth to fewer kids. Koop and colleagues[7] did not find higher bulk tank SCC in goat herds with a higher proportion of goats with extended lactations, but there is a trend for individual SCCs to increase throughout lactation with animals with lactations longer than 10 months having SCCs that continue to rise through the second and third years of lactation (Gerit Koop, personal communication, 2020). The effect on udder health has not yet been well studied.

MASTITIS—THE DISEASE
Clinical Mastitis

Clinical mastitis presents with visible signs of infection including with abnormal including and may or may not be associated with systemic signs, depending on the severity of the infection.

Severe clinical mastitis

In cases of severe clinical mastitis, the doe is clinically ill with fever and off-feed. Additionally, there are marked changes to the udder and milk. The disease can be acute severe with a sudden onset or more chronic in nature. Signs include high fever, usually 40.5°C (105°F) or higher (normal, approximately 39.5°C or 103°F); depression; partial or complete lack of appetite; moderate to severe dehydration; and grinding teeth from pain. The gland is swollen, hot, and painful to touch and usually has an inflamed appearance. The doe may appear lame because of a reluctance to have the leg touch the udder. The milk may be watery in appearance or red-tinged from blood or appear like reddish serum—with or without clots of milk present. In some cases, the udder becomes abscessed (**Fig. 2**); these abscesses may break and drain and are a risk for

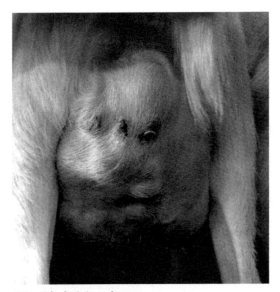

Fig. 2. Chronic mastitis with draining abscesses.

environmental contamination. Does with abscessed udders may be chronically ill or show few systemic effects.

Acute necrotizing gangrenous mastitis

About 8 to 10% of clinical mastitis cases develop necrotizing gangrene, usually due to Staphylococcus aureus and less commonly *Mannheimia haemolytica* or *Pseudomonas aeruginosa* infection and often secondarily infected with clostridial bacteria. The skin is cool to the touch and usually blueish in color, indicating damage to blood vessels from bacterial toxins. The blood-tinged serum milked from the teat also may contain gas (**Fig. 3**). Does are extremely ill and if they survive with supportive treatment (intravenous fluids, antibiotics, nonsteroidal anti-inflammatory drugs, and stripping),

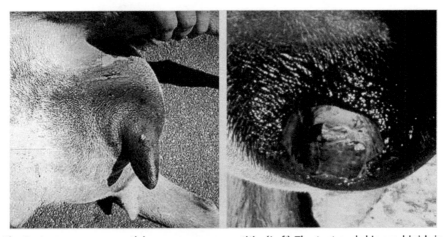

Fig. 3. Acute severe necrotizing gangrenous mastitis. (*Left*) The teat and skin are bluish in color. (*Right*) Teat removed, demonstrating the udder tissue is necrotic.

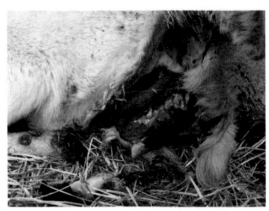

Fig. 4. Necrotic gland has sloughed leaving a large infected wound. (*Courtesy of* G. Zobel, PhD, Hamilton, New Zealand.)

the gland, and other affected tissues slough over the ensuing weeks (**Fig. 4**). During this phase, animals are unsuitable for milking. The decaying tissue is at risk for fly-strike and contaminate the environment. Affected goats should be euthanized, or with appropriate nursing care and, once drug withdrawal periods are met and healing is complete, they can be sold to slaughter. They should not be retained for milking.

Moderate clinical mastitis
This condition may be acute or chronic in nature. The doe is not systemically ill but the udder may be uneven, swollen, and inflamed (**Fig. 5**). The milk also is abnormal in appearance with clots and/or discoloration of the milk.

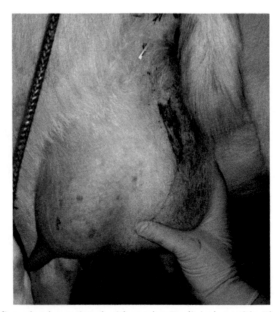

Fig. 5. Swollen, firm gland associated with moderate clinical mastitis. Blue color likely due to livestock spray indicating treatment.

Mild clinical mastitis

This condition may not be noted clinically until the milk is examined. It may be acute or chronic in nature.

Subclinical Mastitis

Subclinical mastitis by far is the most common presentation of mastitis. There are no clinical changes to the doe and the milk has a normal appearance. Mastitis may be present, however, and be causing an increase in somatic cells and a decrease in milk production. Subclinical mastitis must be detected either using tests that detect the somatic cells or by culturing the milk. Because most mastitis in does is subclinical, it is economically critical to detect and control.

Agalactia

If no milk can be expressed from the gland or udder, consider the following:

- The milk-producing tissue of the glands may be destroyed by an infection.
- The teats may have a blockage—either congenital or acquired from trauma—or scarring secondary to mastitis.
- The doe may not be producing milk either because she is ill, nutritionally starved, or at the end of her lactation.
- Apparent agalactia may occur if the milk let-down mechanism is not working (eg, stress or improper udder preparation) or the kids have nursed out all of her milk.

IMPORTANT MASTITIS PATHOGENS IN GOATS

There have been many surveys of mastitis pathogens in goats, with good agreement between findings in different countries with a few exceptions. **Table 2** summarizes the different pathogens and disease caused in dairy goats.

Contagious Goat-to-Goat or Fomite-to-Goat

These are organisms that most likely are transmitted from another infected goat, not necessarily from the milk or udder, or from a fomite (eg, milk cup or hands) contaminated with that organism. In some cases, the bacteria have colonized the person milking the goats (nasal/skin colonization).

Staphylococcus aureus

S aureus is the most commonly identified cause of clinical mastitis in dairy goats. It is estimated that close to 50% of goat herds are infected with this organism.[9] Incidence of acute, severe mastitis is lower, with most herds experiencing fewer than 3% of animals affected annually. A higher incidence likely means the prevalence of *S aureus* subclinical mastitis is high in that herd. There appears to be no host specificity between bacterial lineages,[10] although there are differences in virulence-associated genes between species; this may account for differences in clinical disease in goats and cattle.[11] In goats, the same lineages are found in cases of clinical mastitis as in subclinical mastitis so that identification of subclinical infections with *S aureus* is important to controlling this pathogen in a dairy goat herd.[12] As in other species, important antimicrobial resistance (AMR) genes are found in isolates of *S aureus* from caprine mastitis cases as well as other staphylococcal isolates. It is known that some of these genes may be transferred between bacterial species, meaning that AMR gene in *S epidermidis* may be transferred to *S aureus* and vice versa.[13]

Table 2
Characteristics of important udder pathogens of goats

Name of Organism	Class	Clinical Type	Prevalence	Comments
Primarily contagious goat-to-goat or fomite-to-goat				
S aureus	B	ASCI; ANG; MCI; SCI	Most common cause of clinical mastitis	Associated with very high SCC >10^6 cells/mL milk; difficult to cure; AMR strains identified internationally. Contagious from milkers (hands and nasal carriage) as well as from goat udders and skin.
M haemolytica	B	ASCI; ANG	Uncommon in dairy herds	Shared biotypes with isolates from nasopharynx of nursing kids. In sheep requires teat damage to cause mastitis
NAS (*S caprae, S chromogenes, S epidermidis, S simulans, S. xylosus*)	B	MCI; MiCI; SCI	Most common isolate	Many species involved and pathogenicity varies between species. Self-cure and reinfection common. Can be associated with mild to marked elevation in SCC. Contagious from milker's hands as well as goats
Streptococcus agalactiae	B	unknown	Rare in goats	Theoretically could be transmitted from cattle but not identified on surveys.
Mycoplasma agalactiae	B	MCI; MiCI; SCI	Not reported in Canada. One report in the United States	Termed, *contagious agalactia*. This disease occurs in regions of the Mediterranean in dairy sheep and goats. There is no successful treatment. Some vaccines are used to control.
Mycoplasma mycoides subsp *capri*	B	ASCI; SCI	Reported in the United States, Canada, and internationally	Also causes septicemia, septic arthritis, meningitis, and pleuropneumonia in goat kids consuming infected colostrum/milk.
CAEV	V	MCI; SCI	Common internationally	Infections often are clinically inapparent; however, histologically there often is inflammation and damage resulting in production losses.

(continued on next page)

Table 2 (continued)				
Name of Organism	Class	Clinical Type	Prevalence	Comments
Primarily environmental				
Streptococcus dysgalactiae, Streptococcus uberis, and *Enterococcus* spp	B	MCl; SCl	Lower prevalence within herd (3%–15%); 20%–50% of herds infected	Associated with dirty environment (wet, dirty bedding) and contamination of teats, udder, and teat cups. May be associated with high milk bacterial counts.
Coliforms (*E coli, Klebsiella* sp)	B	ASCl–SCl	Low prevalence in herds	Associated with dirty environment.
Pseudomonas aeruginosa	B	ASCl–SCl	Outbreaks are not uncommon	Associated with dirty water or contaminated water products. Also may be contagious. Rarely susceptible to antimicrobial therapy.
Listeria monocytogenes	B	ASCl; SCl	Disease rare but infection not uncommon	Associated with contaminated feed, bedding. May shed in subclinical cases. Zoonotic risk.
Candida albicans and *Cryptococcus* spp	Y	ASCl–SCl	Outbreaks are not uncommon	Usually associated with poor hygiene at milking, overtreatment with intramammary antibiotics or contamination of infusion tubes.

Abbreviations: Class of organism: B, bacteria; M, mycoplasma; V, virus; Y, yeast. Rype of mastitis caused: ANG, acute, necrotizing gangrenous; ASCl, acute, severe clinical; MCl, mModerate clinical; MiCl, mild clinical; SCl, subclinical.

Mannheimia haemolytica

The bacterium *M haemolytica* rarely is isolated from dairy goats, although the disease can be very severe, that is, acute severe necrotizing gangrenous mastitis. In dairy sheep, it has been demonstrated that the strains isolated from the pharynx of lambs are identical to the strains isolated from mastitis, and teat damage increases the likelihood of infection from this source.[14] This is important to understand when the dairy goat herd allows nursing of kids.

Non-aureus staphylococci species

NAS is a large group of bacteria with many species associated with mastitis in ruminants. Because there are other sources of NAS bacteria than the milk (eg, skin), assuring that the isolates are not contaminants is important. If 2 or more colony types are identified on culture, or fewer than 100 colony-forming units (CFUs)/mL milk are grown, then there is a risk that the sample was contaminated.[15] NAS infections are associated with elevated SCC compared with no-infection.[16] Species that have been identified as associated with higher SCCs include *S caprae, S epidermidis, S simulans, S xylosus,* and possibly *S chromogenes*.[15,16] Approximately half of NAS infections are eliminated during the dry period, with those glands with higher SCC prior to drying being less likely to clear.[17] It has been shown that if S caprae was cultured from the teat ends prepartum, those goats were more likely to have an IMI prior to 10 days in milk.[18] Infections detected later in lactation (>10 DIM) were more likely to be eliminated, and uninfected glands were more likely to become infected if the contralateral gland was infected. S caprae and S xylosus are more likely to persist.[19] Effect on milk production is mixed depending on species with small or no differences found.[16,19] More work needs to be done on this aspect by species rather than only typing as NAS.

Mycoplasma species

In the Mediterranean region of Europe, *Mycoplasma agalactiae* (contagious agalactia) is a common infection but it appears to be uncommon or absent from North American dairy goats, although veterinarians should always be alert for its potential presence.[20] *Mycoplasma mycoides* subsp *capri* has been reported in the United States as well as in many other countries. It can cause severe to subclinical mastitis, but also septicemia, meningitis, and arthritis in goat kids that consume infected milk and pleuropneumonia in all ages.[21] There is suggestion that *Mycoplasma bovis* can infect goats but no evidence yet it is a cause of mastitis in that species.

Caprine arthritis encephalitis virus

It is well-known that caprine arthritis encephalitis virus (CAEV) infects the alveolar epithelium of the udder and causes interstitial lymphocytic inflammation leading to chronic damage; this leads to reduced milk production and a moderate elevation of SCC. The effect of being seropositive on milk production appears to be putative although results vary between studies. Leitner and colleagues[22] found that only first lactation does had significantly lower milk production, with a nonsignificant trend in second lactation; Martínez-Navalón and colleagues[23] found a 10% reduction overall. CAEV seropositivity has been shown to be associated with higher SCC and should be taken into account when investigating bacterial causes of mastitis using SCC.[15,23] The association with increased risk of bacterial IMI is either weak or nonexistent, however. But the positive effect overall on udder health of eliminating CAEV infection from dairy goat herds is significant. Norwegian dairy goat herds monitored for SCC before and after herd-level CAEV eradication have significantly lower SCC values at all stages of lactation and parity (Olav Østerås, personal communication, 2020).

Environmental

The environmental group of organisms is present in the environment of the goat, for example, bedding and water—although, in some cases, the infection can be acquired from a goat.

Streptococcus dysgalactiae, Streptococcus uberis, and Enterococcus species

Mastitis tends to be moderately clinical to subclinical. The bacteria, *Streptococcus dysgalactiae*, *Streptococcus uberis*, and *Enterococcus* spp, are acquired from the environment when dirty and / or wet, as well as contaminated fomites such as teat cups[24]; These bacteria may also be considered contagious, so it important to identify all infected goats and isolate and either treat or cull. The Chatzopoulos and colleagues speculate that the teat cups may have been contaminated from dirty teats and udder from bedding. As well as maintaining clean bedding, it is important that the teats and udder be prepped properly prior to milking. This may help to reduce infections. Of note is the possibility of shedding of high numbers of bacteria—at least soon after infection—which may influence milk bacterial counts[25] (Phillip Wilman, personal communication, 2015).

Coliforms

The coliform organisms, usually *Escherichia coli* or *Klebsiella pneumonia*, sometimes are cultured from cases of mastitis in goats from severe clinical to subclinical mastitis but appear much less common than other mastitis pathogens. As with dairy cattle, investigate environmental cleanliness. Because these infections are extremely sudden and severe, antibiotic treatment of the IMI may not be effective; however, the treatment of the systemic signs of pain and dehydration is essential to lessening the adverse effects on the doe. Salmonella bacteria are an uncommon infection in goats and pose most risk because the bacteria can be transmitted through consumption of unpasteurized milk and cheeses.

Pseudomonas aeruginosa

Outbreaks of pseudomonas mastitis in dairy goats most often are associated with exposure to contaminated water but may be contagious as well. Most cases are acute, severe clinical with dehydration and high fever but some goats may be inapparent carriers. Investigate possible sources of exposure to contaminated water, for example, wet areas in pens or yards, teat dips, and udder washes, as well as equipment used to perform those tasks, milk meters, drinking troughs, and so forth.[26] As with environmental streptococcus infections, it also is important to identify potential carriers and cull, because treatment is unlikely to be successful.[27]

Listeria monocytogenes

The bacterium *Listeria monocytogenes* is not commonly associated with severe mastitis although it has been reported. Shedding in the milk with subclinical mastitis, however, is not rare, so there is a zoonotic concern, particularly when raw milk products are consumed or there is a risk of post-pasteurization contamination.[28] Listeria are able to grow at is refrigerator temperatures (5°C [40°F]).

Candida albicans and Cryptococcus species (yeast)

Yeasts are environmental organisms and frequently are found in water sources. They have an increased potential for causing an IMI during milking if the teats are wet when the milking unit is put on. Overtreatment with antibiotics or poor hygiene when inserting mastitis ointment tubes commonly is associated with outbreaks of yeast mastitis. Yeast infections present as acute clinical infections, with fever. Yeast mastitis does not respond to standard antibiotic therapy and antibiotics should not be used to treat infections. The symptoms of these infections could be addressed, however, with the use of pain management therapies and frequent stripping of the affected glands. Candida infections are more likely to cure than Cryptococcus. Nonresponders should be culled.

RISK FACTORS FOR MASTITIS

Table 3 lists many of the risk factors associated with mastitis in dairy goats that should be considered in an udder health program.

DETECTION OF MASTITIS
Clinical examination

Clinical examination should be performed; this includes examination of the udder (size, heat, and firmness), teats, and teat ends (calluses and sores) as well as milk.

Table 3
Risk factors associated with mastitis in dairy goats

Factor	Risk
Kidding time	Weakened immune system; number of kids born; difficult kidding
Stage of lactation	The prevalence of infection increases in late lactation
Nursing kids	The risk increases if kids are allowed to nurse: • Orf (sore mouth) infections can increase risk of S aureus mastitis. • Teat biting causes scarring of the teat, slower milk-out, and secondary bacterial infections. • Cross-sucking or self-sucking after drinking mastitic milk may infect the gland of the kid; this may only be evident when it freshens for the first time as an adult.
Dry-off	Should be done when milk production has dropped sufficiently. Milking once/d reduces milk production. Removal of milk a few days after milk cessation, however, removes the keratin plug and allow entrance of bacteria.
Lactation number	Older does tend to be more at risk of mastitis and are more likely to carry infections (eg, S aureus).
Viral infections	CAE virus—increased risk of bacterial IMI is low; orf virus infections of teat ends
Udder shape and size	Poor shape interferes with milk-out; poor size reduces milk production; poor teat placement and teat size interfere with milk-out. Worn-out suspensory ligaments cause the teats to be low and susceptible to damage. Casu and colleagues[8] found a relationship between udder morphology and SCC in dairy sheep indicating it may be useful also in dairy goats (**Fig. 6**).
Teats	Teat end damage (calluses, sores, or scarring [**Fig. 7**]) from overmilking, excessive vacuum pressures at the teat end, collapsing worn-out liners, irritating chemicals, pointed teat ends, and long milk-out times. Proper placement of the teat cups, for example, falling off, sucking air, is influenced by teat size and diameter, warts, extra teats.
Environment	High stocking densities; poor ventilation; wet and cold floor and dirty bedding; air temperature too hot or cold; high humidity; inclement weather; relocating and mixing does
Milking technique and equipment	• Poor udder preparation and postmilking management, for example, clipping long hair, cleanliness of teats and udder, proper stimulation of milk let-down; method and products for postmilking teat dipping, etc. • Cleanliness of hands, use of gloves • Set-up and maintenance of milking equipment, for example, cracked and worn teat liners; high vacuum levels; inadequate vacuum reserve; incorrect pulsation rate and ratio; overmilking • Milking time, for example, overmilking, number of units per milker, etc., noise in the parlor
Genetics	Resistance to mastitis
Nutrition	Low energy; selenium and vitamin E

Foremilk should be discarded and then the milk examined carefully using a dark sur-faced strip cup. This allows detection of of clots and abnormal color. Yellow-colored milk may be transitional milk or milk still containing colostrum or may indicate mastitis. Strawberry-colored milk may indicate breakage of small blood vessels in the udder leaking blood. Usually this resolves in a few days.

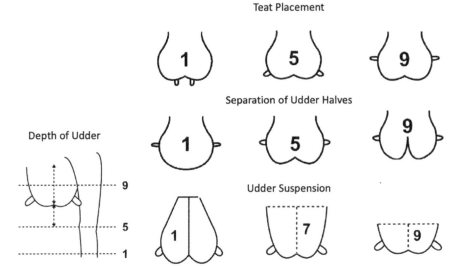

Fig. 6. Scoring system to assist for selection of superior udder morphology. (*Adapted from* Casu S, Pernazza I, Carta A. Feasibility of a linear scoring method of udder morphology for the selection scheme of Sardinian sheep. J Dairy Sci. 2006 89(6):2200-2209; with permission.)

Somatic cell counts

Goats are different than cattle in that the somatic cells are more prevalently neutrophils (30%–70% of cells) even when IMI is absent. Numbers overall tend to be higher than cattle and can be very high at the end of lactation. Additionally, because of apocrine secretion in the goat, the counting technique needs to be calibrated so that cytoplasmic particles, which do not contain DNA, are not counted. For this

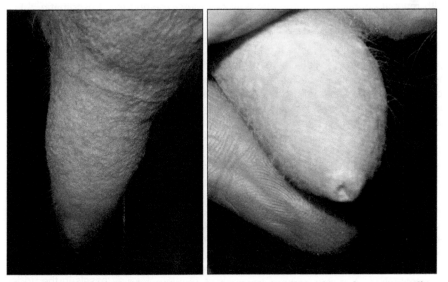

Fig. 7. Teat lesions. (*Left*) Teat end is hyperemic and edematous, likely from poor milking technique. (*Right*) Teat end is callused.

CMT Score	CMT Interpretation	Visual Characteristics of the milk	SCC Range (cells/mL milk)	Suggested Interpreta-tion	Somatic Cell Score	
					Score	Mid-point SCC (cells/mL milk)
N	Negative	The mixture does not change, and remains the same liquid consistency of milk with bluish/purple tinges.	0– 200,000		0	12,500
					1	25,000
					2	50,000
					3	100,000
					4	200,000
T	Trace	The mixture will thicken slightly like very thin porridge; however, it can revert back to its original state when moving the paddle.	150,000 – 500,000		4	200,000
					5	400,000
1	Weak, but positive	There is slight thickening of the milk like thin porridge; no gel forms; when swirled, the mixture will climb the walls of the well; and when poured out, the mixture flows a steady pace.	400,000 – 1,500,000		5	400,000
					6	800,000
					7	1,600,000
2	Distinctly positive	Gel is beginning to form; when swirled, the gel tends to clump in the middle of the well; when poured out, the gel will pour out first; leaving some liquid is remaining in the well.	800,000 – 5,000,000		6	800,000
					7	1,600,000
					8	3,200,000
3	Strongly positive	The entire mixture is gelled; when swirled it clumps in the middle; and when poured out of the paddle, no liquid remains in the well.	> 5,000,000		9	6,400,000

▇ = healthy   ▢ = suspect   ■ = likely mastitis

Fig. 8. Interpretation of California mastitis test scores, somatic cell count range, and somatic cell Score. (*Data from* Schalm OW& Noorlander DO. Experiments and observations leading to development ofthe California mastitis test. J Am Vet Med Assoc. 1957;130(5):199-207; and Shook GE and Ali AKA. An optimum transformation for somatic cell concentration in milk. J Dairy Sci. 1980;63(3):487-490.)

reason, methods must be used that only counts cells containing DNA. This requires that cells are stained firstly before counting, eg, use of pyronin y-methyl green dye with manual counting, or automatic flow cytometry method (eg, Fossomatic™ FC, Foss, Denmark).

It is difficult to indicate a single SCC range as normal for a goat because of the non-IMI factors influencing counts. It appears that a range of 400×10^3 cells/mL milk to 600×10^3 cells/mL milk is achievable in dairy goat herds with superior udder health,[29–32] but that number appears quite variable. When calculating mean values for a herd, it is better to report geometric means or somatic cell scores (SCSs) than arithmetic means to lower the influence of outlier values; distribution in a herd is considered lognormal, that is, the SCC needs to be log transformed to achieve normality. SCSs are calculated using the following formula: SCS = ln (SCC/100)/0.6931 + 3[15]; these scores are reflective of milk production losses in dairy cattle due to increasing SCC but similar research in dairy goats has not been published. **Fig. 8** includes SCS and midpoint SCC values.

There are many factors affecting SCCs other than presence of an IMI and there can be considerable daily variation in a goats. Stage of lactation and length of lactation and parity are both very important.[15] Primiparous does may have low counts throughout lactation, less than 300×10^3/mL milk. Infection in 1 gland may elevate SCC in the un-infected contralateral gland. Season is influential, possibly tied to stage of lactation because most does are in early lactation during the summer and late lactation during the early winter, but also perhaps because of environmental conditions. In Norway, peak SCCs occur during the summer when goats are grazing mountain pastures, but the opposite is true in Canada and the Netherlands, where summer has the lowest SCC values in confinement reared situations. Goats in estrus tend to have higher SCC values, followed by a drop postestrus. This is most marked in does synchronized using exogenous progesterone products.[33] There also is an association with breed type and genetic selection. External stressors of various types may cause a temporary increase on SCC, for example, hoof trimming, mixing and moving, and vaccination—particularly if not done with care.

California mastitis test

The California mastitis test (CMT) is an efficient goat-side test that is easy for producers to use to screen goats.[34,35] Proper technique must be done using equal amounts of milk and CMT solution (detergent-bromocresol purple solution), ideally not more than 5 mL or 1 teaspoon each of milk and solution swirled together in a CMT paddle and interpreted within 15 seconds of mixing. **Fig. 8** outlines the expected reactions and likely SCC associated with that reaction. A video produced by the author, showing the reaction and how to perform a CMT properly, can be found in Video 1. A suggested cutpoint for selecting goats for bacterial culture, but not necessarily treatment, is greater than or equal to CMT 1.

Bacterial culture

It is important to encourage clients to take individual milk samples (gland or composite) when investigating clinical mastitis or elevation of SCC. Sterile vials should be labeled first with animal ID and affected gland. Have your clients record everything and teach them sterile techniques, including teat and udder preparation, wearing gloves, discarding foremilk, teat disinfection, and proper filling of the culture vial without contamination of the milk or lid. Milk should be chilled immediately and transported to the laboratory for culture (or use an on-farm culturing system or frozen for later submission). Work with a local diagnostic laboratory to understand the routine tests being performed. It is preferable to speciate NAS. Antimicrobial sensitivity may be requested depending on how the results are intended to be used. An excellent resource for understanding laboratory testing can be found in the handbook, *Mastitis in Small Ruminants*,[36] which can be downloaded at https://www.izs-sardegna.it/quaderni/Mastitis%20in%20small%20ruminant.pdf. Review the results with clients to determine the importance of the culture results (refer to previous descriptions of the pathogens). Bulk tank samples (or bucket samples for small dairies) can be submitted as a way to possibly screen for pathogens, such as *S aureus*; however, results also may reflect milk quality issues due to biofilms present on milking equipment.

MILKING MANAGEMENT AND MILKING EQUIPMENT

These bullet points should be reviewed with clients. More in-depth information is available in the *A Guide to Udder Health for Dairy Goats*, written by the author and available for download at https://www.iga-goatworld.com/repository.html.

- Milking preparation—this includes hygiene of teats and udders as well as stimulation for proper milk let-down.
  - The udder should be clipped if long hair is present.
  - Wash and sanitize hands or wear gloves (eg, blue nitrile).
  - Strip foremilk and then a sample into a teat cup to examine for abnormal milk. Perform a CMT if any abnormalities seen on clinical examination of udder, teats, or milk.

○ Clean teats and udder using a suitable product starting with the teats and teat ends and wiping up the udder away from the teats; dry prepping alone does not remove dirt and bacteria. This is not done commonly by many dairy goat producers because are mistakenly are believed to be clean if the dirt is not visible and they believe it takes too long. This is a mistake.

○ Single-use paper towels or reusable clothes if washed with bleach at 70°C (approximately 160°F) (bacteria survive in a cold wash).

○ Make sure udder is dry before applying teat cups.

○ If predip is used to lower risk of environmental pathogens, use only approved products and wipe and dry teats after use.

- Milking procedure
  ○ Apply milking units within 1 minute (not longer than 2 minutes) of initial stimulation for optimal milk let-down.
  ○ Attach properly to minimize air admitted into line.
  ○ If milking a single gland, use a clean inflation plug in unused teat cup.
  ○ Avoid overmilking. Peak milk usually is 30 seconds after unit attachment, keeping in mind a large portion of milk is in the gland cistern. Milk-out usually is completed within 1 minute to 3 minutes; overmilking leads to teat end damage.
  ○ Avoid excessive machine stripping. This may be caused by improper stimulation of milk let-down or poor udder conformation and can lead to overmilking and teat damage.
  ○ Make sure the vacuum is broken before removing the teat cups.
  ○ If automatic take-offs are used, make sure the units are lifted up away from the goat to prevent dirt from contaminating the inside of the liner.
  ○ Postmilking, the teats should be immediately disinfected with a suitable product. There should be full coverage of the teat end and sides. Use a nonrecovery teat dip cup and keep dip container free of organic material. If a spray is use, assure that coverage of the teat is adequate.
  ○ Keep the goat standing for at least 30 minutes in a clean environment to allow the teat sphincter to close.
  ○ Flies can transmit some mastitis pathogens; ensure fly control is used in livestock housing areas as well as the milking parlor and pens.

- Milking order and communication of udder health status
  ○ Milk doelings first, followed by healthy multiparous and then goats infected with contagious pathogens (eg, *S aureus*).
  ○ Use a permanent, removable method to identify animals with mastitis, that is visible to the person milking the goats (eg, leg band). Livestock marker or paint may disappear before milk withdrawal period is complete or may persist too long.
  ○ Make sure there is an effective way to communicate treatments to the milkers in the parlor, for example, a white board.

- Equipment set-up and maintenance. There are many valuable resources with in-depth information on this topic. An example is at http://www.omafra.gov.on.ca/english/livestock/goat/goatdairy.html.
  ○ The parlor should be easy for goats to enter and leave without need to force animals. It should be cleaned of organic material between milkings to assure the equipment and udder remain clean.
  ○ Recommendations for pulsation and vacuum levels are found in **Table 4**. Caria and colleagues[37] found that a vacuum level of 35 kPa versus 44 kPa, had excellent milk out and superior milk yield and the units did not drop off. High vacuum levels are associated with teat end damage and increased SCC.

Table 4	
Standard values for milking equipment in dairy goat parlors	
Equipment Parameter	**Standard Value**
Pulsation speed	60–120 cycles/min—90 cycles/min most commonly recommended
Pulsation ratio	50%–60%
Vacuum at peak flow	At the teat: 35–39 kPa (10–11.5 in Hg) Low line system: 35.5 kPa (10.5 in Hg) High line system: 39 kPa (11.5 in Hg) 1 kPa = 0.295 in Hg

Data from Billon P, Fernandez Martinez N, Ronningen O, et al. Quantitative recommendations for milking machine installations for small ruminants. Bulletin of the International Dairy Federation, 370/2002.

- Investigate squawks and liner slips because these may mean liners are worn and need replacement.
- Check liners for cracks and biofilms.
- Review the cleaning system and assure chemicals in the proper concentrations and water temperature is sufficiently hot. Include buckets and pails if used.
- Check for presence of milk residues, stone, and biofilms in equipment.
- Make sure that the client has the equipment serviced and parts replaced as necessary.

MILK QUALITY

Not only does poor milk quality affect the clients due to lost markets but also the milk is unhealthy for consumers. As the herd veterinarian, work with the regulatory inspectors if a client has a sudden or persistent issue with milk quality to help troubleshoot where the issue may be arising. It not always is due to mastitis, but problems with milk quality often mean problems with milk production overall.

Somatic cell counts

SCCs are one of the measures of milk quality; in some jurisdictions, the level is regulated, with bulk tank levels greater than 1.5×10^6 cells/mL of milk being in violation. Many herds struggle to keep below this level, particularly in late autumn-winter when goats are in late lactation. Even in these herds, however, it is recommended to investigate mastitis as contributing to these higher levels. As well as animal health concerns, high SCC values affect the ability to make suitable cheese, affecting processors' ability to use this product.

Bacterial counts

Bacterial counts usually are measured as standard plate counts (number of CFUs) of live aerobic bacteria grown per milliliter of milk). In some jurisdictions, herds with levels greater than 50,000 CFUs/mL milk are in violation. Also, in some jurisdictions, coliform counts are calculated separately as are post-pasteurization bacterial counts. Bacto-Scan™ FC+ (Foss, Demark) is an automated system frequently used in the dairy industry that additionally measures dead bacteria, anaerobic bacteria, and prototheca.

It is used by the Ontario government to assess goat milk quality with values greater than 321,00 individual bacteria cells being in violation. Although high bacterial counts may not be related to mastitis but rather poor milking equipment maintenance and cleaning, in some cases mastitis pathogens have been associated with high bacterial counts, in particular environmental streptococci.

Other criteria include being free of inhibitors, freezing point, and the milk being of normal color and odor.

TREATMENT AND CONTROL OF MASTITIS IN DAIRY GOATS

In many jurisdictions, there are few to no drugs approved for goats being milked for human consumption. This puts additional responsibility on veterinarians that, when using drugs in an extralabel manner, they are certain the drug is safe and efficacious for the purpose prescribed and a sufficient milk withhold is met to assure the milk is unadulterated. Using resources, Food Animal Residue Avoidance Databank (FARAD) in the United States, and global FARAD in other countries such as Canada (eg, CgFARAD), may assist in being provided with a proper dosage and milk withdrawal. In some countries, with some drugs, there is no established maximum residue limit for goats; this means that if a product is detected by regulatory testing, even if at a level lower than the maximum residue limit established for dairy cattle, for example, that level is in violation and the shipment may be rejected. In worst-case situations, a client may be fined.

For these reasons, it is important to review any treatment protocols with a client to assure treated animals are identified and the milk is withheld from the tank for the proper length of time. There are kits that can be used on-farm or in the veterinary practice to detect inhibitors (antimicrobials) in milk. These can be used to screen individual goats or bulk tank samples, although it is important first to make sure that the test (1) is labeled for use in goats (not all are suitable) and (2) is testing for the antibiotic of concern. Also, make sure that the test detects the antibiotic at or below the detection limit used by the regulatory laboratory. There can be false-positive results (as well as false-negative results); submission of a sample directly to the regulatory laboratory may help to sort these issues.

Goats that should be tested are those that receive a drug not licensed for that species, indication or so forth; purchased lactating does; those that were dry-treated but gave birth early; those that have lost their identification, jumped a pen or otherwise their treatment history is uncertain or unknown; and goats that have been treated with the wrong medication or more than one medication of any kind. Encourage your clients to join a food safety program, to keep excellent records and to practice responsible management of livestock medicines, including labeling, storage, and so forth.

Treatment during lactation

There is little information on the efficacy of treatment of lactating does for mastitis, but some research shows some benefit.[34,38] Before deciding to treat, it is important to know the pathogen and, in most cases, the antimicrobial sensitivity pattern because AMR is not uncommon in some common pathogens, such as S aureus, some NAS, and P aeruginosa. Intramammary products in lactating does probably are minimally effective. If a goat is systemically ill, use systemic antibiotics.

Intramammary treatments

Intramammary treatments (ie, mastitis tubes) should not be split between glands; the contents of the entire tube should be inserted into the teat end but the cannula should

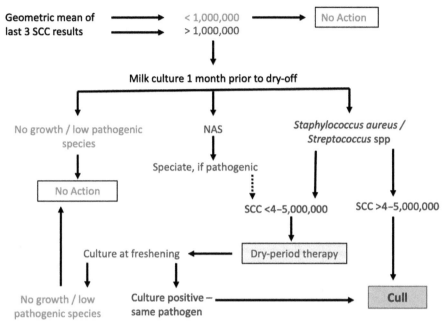

Fig. 9. Algorithm for dry-period mastitis therapy. (*Courtesy of* O. Østerås, PhD, Oslo, Norway.)

not be inserted beyond the sphincter. Outbreaks of mastitis and yeast infections have occurred in dairy sheep and goats when tubes are split. Instruct your clients on proper administration, including proper restraint of the goat (They will kick!), effective cleaning and disinfection of the teat end, and avoidance of contamination of the teat cannula prior to insertion by improper handling. Hands must be clean and dry; gloves are preferred.

Dry period mastitis treatment

Dry period mastitis treatment is not done routinely but may be advantageous in some herds. Little is published specifically on its use in dairy goats, but those results show that treated goats had fewer infections at freshening that untreated goats.[39] Unfortunately, many of the published studies used antimicrobials of high importance to humans, which should not be used in goats. Blanket treatment has been discouraged in dairy cows because of the risk of AMR; rather, SCC is used to prescreen cattle at dry-off for treatment. This is more problematic in dairy goats because many at dry-off have SCC values in excess of 800×10^3 mL milk with no IMI. Culturing all goats prior to dry-off also is not likely practical. More work needs to be done to develop a proper algorithm for selecting goats for treatment. One such algorithm, adapted from one proposed for Norwegian goat dairies, is presented in **Fig. 9** (Olav Østerås, personal communication, 2020). This can be modified to fit the dairies that are worked with. There is no published information on the use of teat sealants in goats; they may be helpful in reducing new infections in the dry period.

Control of Staphylococcus aureus mastitis

As the most common pathogenic species in dairy goats, *S aureus* deserves special attention. As with dairy cattle, the recommendation is to remove infected goats

Table 5
Assessment of udder health in dairy goats

Date of Assessment	Milking System	Farm Name	Herd Veterinarian
Average number of does milked in previous 12 mo		Avg. number of days post-kidding does put into milk-line	Avg. length of lactation (milked)

Measurement of Performance	Previous Level	Goal for Herd[a]	Current Level	Action Needed?	Additional Assessment
Assessment of Clinical Mastitis					
Annual incidence of clinical mastitis[b] (%) Calculate: (number of does with 1 or more cases of clinical mastitis[c] in last 12 mo/average number of does milked in last 12 mo) X 100		< 5%		YES NO	• Investigate stage of lactation, season, parity of animals with clinical mastitis • Culture cases before treating to determine if contagious or environmental organisms • Review milking management, milking equipment
Annual incidence of repeat cases of clinical mastitis (%) Calculate: (Total number of cases of clinical mastitis in last 12 mol average number of does milked in last 12 mo) X 100		<1.5 X above		YES NO	• Culture cases to determine organism. • Investigate reasons for failure to manage clinical cases (eg, treatment protocols)
Prevalence of does with a blind gland (%) Calculate: (number of glands that did not produce milk in the last 12 months/total number of does milked in last 12 mo) X 100		< 5%		YES NO	• Examine history of does with blind glands to determine reason. for example, mastitis, teat damage. • Review culling policy.
Assessment of Sub-Clinical Mastitis					

Measure	Target		Action
Proportion of does with SCC level > 800,000^d (linear score 6) each test (%) *Calculate: (number of does with SCC > 800,000 at last milk test/ number of does tested) X 100*	< 20%	YES NO	• Investigate stage of lactation, season, parity etc. of animals with subclinical mastitis • Review milking hygiene and maintenance of milking equipment
Incidence of new infections during lactation (%) *Calculate: (number of does with SCC > 800,000 at last milk test and ≤ 800,000 at previous milk test/number of does ≤ 800,000 at previous milk test) X 100*	< 5%	YES NO	• Review management of does with contagious mastitis • Review hygiene of environment • Determine prevalence of teat end lesions and their cause (eg, over-milking, high vacuum) • Review biosecurity protocol when purchasing animals • Investigate risk from nursing kids of teat damage
Prevalence of chronic infections (%) *Calculate: (number of does with SCC > 800,000 at 3 or more tests this lactation/total number of lactations assessed) X 100*	< 5%	YES NO	• Determine period of onset of chronic mastitis cases with respect to stage of lactation, parity, season • Culture to determine pathogen type • Investigate status of CAE infection in the herd
Prevalence of infections at first test post-kidding (%) *Calculate: (number of does with SCC > 400,000 at first test post-kidding/total number of first tests) X 100*	< 10%	YES NO	• Determine parity of affected animals • Investigate whether due to damage from nursing kids prior to placing in milk line • Review dry-period mastitis treatment protocols and hygiene at treatment • Investigate dry-off management • Review environment of dry does

Animal Loss Due to Mastitis

(continued on next page)

Table 5
(continued)

Measurement of Performance	Previous Level	Goal for Herd[a]	Current Level	Action Needed?	Additional Assessment
Turnover rate due to mastitis (%) *Calculate: (number of does culled and died due to mastitis/average number of milked in last 12 mo) X 100*		**< 5%**		YES NO	• Review treatment protocols, including methods of detection of does with clinical mastitis • Investigate causative agents causing death (eg, Staphylococcus aureus) • Investigate and review as outlined above under clinical and subclinical mastitis • Review culling policies as well as areas above
Incidence of does dying of mastitis annually (%) *Calculate: (number of does dying of mastitis/avg. number of milked in last 12 mo) x 100*		**< 0.5%**		YES NO	
Proportion of does culled due to mastitis (%) *Calculate: (number of does culled due to mastitis/avg. number of milked in last 12 mo) X 100*		**< 5%**		YES NO	
Proportion of does culled, that were culled due to mastitis (%) *Calculate: (number of does culled due to mastitis/total number of does culled[e] in last 12 mo)*		**< 20%**		YES NO	

[a] *Goal for Herd:* Suggested goal in box, enter goal agreed to by client and veterinarian as achievable within a suitable time period.

[b] A case of clinical mastitis is one in which there is a change to the udder and/or milk of one or more glands as detected by visual inspection.

[c] Count does with multiple cases of clinical mastitis only once.

[d] This cutpoint may be lowered as udder health improves and average herd SCC drops.

[e] Do not include does that were sold for dairy, that is, into another herd to be milked, but only those does sent to slaughter.

From International Goat Association. A Guide to Udder Health for Dairy Goats. Version 1.6. 2016; with permission. Available at https://www.iga-goatworld.com/repository.html.

from the milking string and milk last to prevent transmission to other goats through the milking procedure. When possible, these goats should be dried-off and treated or be culled. Another option is herd vaccination, which might be recommended in herds with a high prevalence of S aureus infections. One such vaccine, VIMCO (HIPRA, Canada, Ottawa Ontario), is licensed for use in dairy goats in several countries, including Canada, and is composed of an inactivated culture of S aureus—a high biofilm producing strain. It appears to reduce the clinical signs associated with infection and SCCs (sheep) and reduce the number of treatments with antibiotics and/or nonsteroidal anti-inflammatory drugs. It does this by inhibiting the ability of the staphylococci bacteria to produce biofilms.[40] Goats are to be vaccinated twice, 5 weeks and 3 weeks prior to freshening. This same protocol is repeated annually when the doe is dry.

Culling

Review with your clients how to decide that a goat should be culled for mastitis. Certainly, those with contagious, pathogenic infections should be considered for removal (eg, S aureus and P aeruginosa) because not only are they rarely superior milking animals but also they are a risk to others in the herd. Goats with 1 gland, severe teat damage, or abscesses in the udder also should be culled from the herd. If CAEV is present in the herd, encourage the client to enroll in a CAE herd status program, if available, or develop a test and remove program. Serologic testing and removal from the herd is more effective than removing kids at birth because most transmission occurs between adults when housed together. Assist clients in making the right decisions.

MONITORING AND ASSESSING UDDER HEALTH

It is important for clients to gather basic information on udder health in their goats. This can include SCC reports on individual goats as well as bulk tank milk, milk culture results, response to treatments (lactating and dry), incidents of clinical mastitis, and culling events due to mastitis as well as milk quality issues. Gathering data on milk-out time and teat end scoring may be helpful as well. One of the most important parts of this exercise is for the client with a veterinarian's help, to set reasonable and achievable goals.

Table 5 allow veterinarians to work with their client to calculate important parameters and set goals. If action is needed, it provides some example areas to investigate.

SUMMARY

Udder health in dairy goats is a challenging undertaking because it requires not only knowledge of the physiology of milking and a good understanding of the common pathogens and their diseases with some important differences from dairy cattle but also understanding the milking process and the equipment used. Work with an expert in this field, particularly one with knowledge on set-up, maintenance, and cleaning of milking equipment. Monitoring udder health through the use of SCCs can be done but has challenges in comparison to dairy cattle and sheep. Treatment is another challenge, not only because there are few to no drugs approved for use in dairy goats but also because there is little peer-reviewed information on safety and efficacy. In this regard, veterinarians must balance caution with knowledge and the need to provide effective treatment and control measures to their clients' herds. On a positive note, new information is being developed around the world to assist veterinarians in developing a sound approach to managing and promoting udder health in dairy goats.

CLINICS CARE POINTS

- There are few to no approved medications for dairy goats producing food for human consumption and very little information on efficacy of treatment. Make sure when using any medication in an extralabel manner to (1) test the milk for antimicrobial residues and/or (2) used FARAD to obtain the best guidance on appropriate milk withdrawals, particularly when using nonantimicrobial medicines.

- Selecting goats for dry-period mastitis treatment must use different criteria than dairy cattle. SCCs can be used to screen goats and high SCC goats (>1,000,000 cells/mL milk) should be cultured and treated if warranted.

- Always strip the foremilk before evaluating the milk for mastitis or before culturing the milk.

DISCLOSURE

The contents of this article were written my me and appropriately referenced.

SUPPLEMENTARY DATA

Supplementary data related to this article can be found online at https://doi.org/10.1016/j.cvfa.2020.12.002.

REFERENCES

1. Marnet PG, McKusick BC. Regulation of milk ejection and milkability in small ruminants. Livest Prod Sci 2001;70:125–33.
2. Logan KJ, Leury BJ, Russo VM, et al. An extended photoperiod increases milk yield and decreases ovulatory activity in dairy goats. Animals 2020;10:1879–89.
3. Zamuner F, DiGiacomo K, Cameron AWN, et al. Effects of month of kidding, parity number, and litter size on milk yield of commercial dairy goats in Australia. J Dairy Sci 2020;103:954–64.
4. Caja G, Salama AAK, Such X. Omitting the dry-off period negatively affects colostrum and milk yield in dairy goats. J Dairy Sci 2006;89:4220–8.
5. Van den Brom R, Klerx R, Vellema P, et al. Incidence, possible risk factors and therapies for pseudopregnancy on Dutch dairy goat farms: a cross-sectional study. Vet Rec 2019;184:770.
6. Douhard F, Friggens NC, Tessier J, et al. Characterization of a changing relationship between milk production and liveweight for dairy goats undergoing extended lactation. J Dairy Sci 2013;96:5698–711.
7. Koop G, Nielen M, van Werven T. Bulk milk somatic cell counts are related to bulk milk total bacterial counts and several herd-level risk factors in dairy goats. J Dairy Sci 2009;92:3455–4364.
8. Casu S, Sechi S, Salaris SL, et al. Phenotypic and genetic relationships between udder morphology and udder health in dairy ewes. Small Rumin Res 2010;88:77–83.
9. Dore S, Liciardi M, Amastiste S, et al. Short communication: Survey on small ruminant bacterial mastitis in Italy, 2013-2014. Small Rumin Res 2016;141:91–3.
10. Mørk T, Tollersrud T, Kvitle B, et al. Comparison of Staphylococcus aureus genotypes recovered from cases of bovine, ovine and caprine mastitis. J Clin Microbiol 2005;43:3979–84.

11. Vautor E, Magnone V, Rios G, et al. Genetic differences among Staphylococcus aureus isolates from dairy small ruminant species: a single-dye DNA microarray approach. Vet Microbiol 2009;133:105–14.

12. Hoekstra J, Rutten VPMG, van den Hout M, et al. Short communication: differences between Staphylococcus aureus lineages isolated from ovine and caprine mastitis but not between isolates from clinical or subclinical mastitis. J Dairy Sci 2019;102:5430–7.

13. Coimbra-e-Souza V, Rossi CC, Jesus-de Frietas LJ, et al. Short communication: diversity of species and transmission of antimicrobial resistance among Staphylococcus spp. isolated from goat milk. J Dairy Sci 2019;102:5518–24.

14. Fragkou IA, Gougoulis DA, Billinis C, et al. Transmission of Mannheimia haemolytica from the tonsils of lambs to the teat of ewes during sucking. Vet Microbiol 2011;148:66–74.

15. Bernier Gosselin V, Dufour S, Middleton JR. Association between species-specific staphylococcal intramammary infections and milk somatic cell score over time in dairy goats. Prev Vet Med 2020;174:104815.

16. Koop G, van Werven T, Schuiling HJ, et al. The effect of subclinical mastitis on milk yield in dairy goats. J Dairy Sci 2010;93:5809–17.

17. Bernier Gosselin V, Dufour S, Calcutt MJ, et al. Staphylococcal intramammary infection dynamics and the relationship with milk quality parameters in dairy goats over the dry period. J Dairy Sci 2019a;102. 4332-4320.

18. Bernier Gosselin V, Dufour S, Adkins PRF, et al. Longitudinal microbiological evaluation of subclinical non-aureus staphylococcal intramammary infections in a lentivirus-infected dairy goat herd. Vet Microbiol 2019b;230:156–63.

19. Koop G, De Vliegher S, De Visscher A, et al. Differences between coagulase-negative Staphylococcus species in persistence and in effect on somatic cell count and milk yield in dairy goats. J Dairy Sci 2012;95:5075–84.

20. Loria GR, Puleio R, Filioussis G, et al. Contagious agalactia: costs and control revisited. Rev Sci Tech 2019;38:695–702.

21. Johnson GC, Fales WH, Shoemake BM, et al. An outbreak of Mycoplasma mycoides subspecies capri arthritis in young goats: a case study. J Vet Diagn Invest 2019;31:453–7.

22. Leitner G, Krifucks O, Weisblit L, et al. The effect of caprine arthritis encephalitis virus infection on production in goats. Vet J 2010;183:328–31.

23. Martínez-Navalón B, Peris C, Gómez EA, et al. Quantitative estimation of the impact of caprine arthritis encephalitis virus on infection on milk production by dairy goats. Vet J 2013;197:311–7.

24. Chatzopoulos DC, Lianou DT, Michael CK, et al. Streptococcus spp from bulk tank milk and milking machine teatcups on small ruminant farms, and factors potentially associated with their isolation. J Dairy Res 2020;87:277–81.

25. Lasagno MC, Vissio C, Reinoso EB, et al. Development of an experimentally induced Streptococcus uberis subclinical mastitis in goats. Vet Microbiol 2012;154:376–83.

26. Kelly EJ, Wilson DJ. Pseudomonas aeruginosa mastitis in two goats associated with an essential oil-based teat dip. J vet Diagn Invest 2016;28:760–2.

27. Yeruham I, Schwimmer A, Friedman S, et al. Investigation and control of mastitis outbreaks caused by Pseudomonas aeruginosa in a sheep flock and a goat herd. Berl Munch Tierarztl Wochenschr 2005;118:220–3.

28. Addis MF, Cubeddu T, Pilicchi Y, et al. Chronic intramammary infection by Listeria monocytogenes in a clinically healthy goat - a case report. BMC Vet Res 2019;15:229–38.

29. Paape MJ, Wiggans GR, Bannerman DD, et al. Monitoring goat and sheep milk somatic cell counts. Small Rumin Res 2007;68(Issues 1–2):114–25.
30. Raynal-Ljutovac K, Pirisi A, de Crémoux R, et al. Somatic cells of goat and sheep milk: Analytical, sanitary, productive and technological aspects. Small Rumin Res 2007;68:126–44.
31. Ruegg P, Reinemann D. Milk quality and mastitis tests. Bov Pract 2002;36:1–33.
32. Souza FN, Blagitz MG, Penna CF, et al. Somatic cell count in small ruminants: friend or foe? Small Rumin Res 2012;107(2–3):65–75.
33. Mehdid A, Diaz JR, Marti A, et al. Effect of oestrus synchronization on daily somatic cell variation in goats according to lactation number and udder health status. J Dairy Sci 2013;96:4368–74.
34. McDougall S, Supré K, De Vliegher S, et al. Diagnosis and treatment of subclinical mastitis in early lactation in dairy goats. J Dairy Sci 2010;93:4710–21.
35. Persson Y, Olofsson I. Direct and indirect measurement of somatic cell count as indicator of intramammary infection in dairy goats. Acta Vet Scand 2011;53:15.
36. Cannas EA, Dore S, Lollai S, et al. Mastitis in small ruminants. Istituto Zooprofilattico Sperimentale della Saardegna and Centro di Referenza Nazionale per le Mastropatie degli Ovini e dei Caprini. 2019. Available at: https://www.izs-sardegna.it/quaderni/Mastitis%20in%20small%20ruminant.pdf. Accessed January 8, 2021.
37. Caria M, Boselli C, Murgia L, et al. Influence of low vacuum levels on milking characteristics of sheep, goat and buffalo. J Ag Eng 2013;XLIV(s2):e43.
38. Doğruer G, Saribay MK, Ergün Y, et al. Treatment of subclinical mastitis in Damascus goats during lactation. Small Rumin Res 2010;90:153–5.
39. Poutrel B, de Cremoux R, Ducelliez M, et al. Control of intramammary infections in goats: impact on somatic cell counts. J Anim Sci 1997;75:566–70.
40. Vasileiou NGC, Chatzopoulos DC, Cripps PJ, et al. Evaluation of efficacy of a biofilm-embedded bacteria-based vaccine against staphylococcal mastitis in sheep - a randomized, placebo-controlled field study. J Dairy Sci 2019;102:9328–44.

Resuscitation Compression for Newborn Sheep

Tasman Flora, BS*, Mary Smallman, MS, Michelle Anne Kutzler, MBA, DVM, PhD

KEYWORDS

- APGAR • Lamb • Madigan squeeze • Time to stand • Time to suckle

KEY POINTS

- The use of resuscitation compression is a highly valuable method for improving abnormal behavior in newborns.
- In lambs with prolonged time to suckle and/or signs of neonatal maladjustment syndrome, resuscitation compression resulted in significantly improved behavioral scores and reduced time to stand, time to search, and time to suckle.
- Resuscitation compression has no side effects in healthy lambs.
- Resuscitation compression should be considered as a treatment for lambs with neonatal maladjustment syndrome-like symptoms or to stimulate nursing in lambs without a suckle reflex.

Video content accompanies this article at http://www.vetfood.theclinics.com.

INTRODUCTION

Neonatal maladjustment syndrome (NMS), or neonatal encephalopathy, is a central nervous system disorder characterized by lack of interest in the dam, reduced awareness in general, and inability to suckle, which can progress to more severe neurologic signs, including seizures.[1] Although NMS has been described in several species, NMS has been studied extensively in foals, where the prevalence is estimated at 1% to 2%.[2–4] Resuscitation compression (squeezing) has been used successfully in newborn foals and calves to reduce the behavioral symptoms of NMS.[5] The response to resuscitation compression is thought to be due to the release of neurohormones, which simulates compression like that occurring in the birthing process.[2] Weak newborn lambs demonstrate abnormal behaviors like those seen with NMS, and these lambs are at an increased risk for death within the first 48 hours after birth. In this report, the use of resuscitation compression in lambs was critically evaluated to

Department of Animal and Rangeland Sciences, Oregon State University, 112 Withycombe Hall, Corvallis, OR 97331, USA
* Corresponding author.
E-mail address: florata@oregonstate.edu

Vet Clin Food Anim 37 (2021) 175–181
https://doi.org/10.1016/j.cvfa.2020.10.006
0749-0720/21/© 2020 Elsevier Inc. All rights reserved.
vetfood.theclinics.com

determine if this technique would reduce the time to stand, time to search, and time to stand.

MATERIALS AND METHODS

Polypay lambs (n = 86) born at the Oregon State University Sheep Research Center in Corvallis, Oregon were included in this research. All procedures were approved by the Oregon State University Institutional Animal Care and Use Committee (Protocol #5152). Lambs were assessed within 5 minutes of birth using a modified APGAR scoring system[6] (**Table 1**). The time to stand, time to search, and time to suckle were recorded in minutes. At 40 minutes after birth, lambs were categorized into 3 groups based on total APGAR score, time to stand, and time to suckle. Group 1 lambs had an APGAR score of ≥3.6, a time to stand of less than 32.1 minutes, and a time to suckle of less than 40.7 minutes. Group 2 lambs had an APGAR score of ≥3.6 (like group 1) but had a time to stand of ≥32.1 minutes and a time to suckle of ≥40.7 minutes. Group 3 lambs had an APGAR score of less than 3.6 and/or symptoms characteristic of NMS.

A 21-point behavioral scoring system (21P-BSS; **Table 2**) was designed to assess all lambs at 45 minutes after birth and after lambs had suckled or been bottle fed. The 21P-BSS was performed on each lamb before treatment and within 60 minutes after treatment. There were 3 treatment groups: compression (n = 51), placebo (n = 17), and control (n = 18). Treatment was administered between 45 and 120 minutes of birth. Time to stand, time to search, and time to suckle were recorded again for lambs receiving the compression treatment.

The compression treatment was applied to lambs in group 1 (n = 20), group 2 (n = 28), and group 3 (n = 3) to evaluate differences in responses between normal lambs (group 1), susceptible lambs (group 2), and compromised lambs (group 3). The compression treatment was administered by tying a soft cotton rope (1/2-inch diameter and approximately 9 feet in length) around the chest of the lamb following the same procedure as described by Toth and colleagues[7] (**Fig. 1**). Approximately 1 lb of pressure was applied to the rope to tighten the loops and place the lamb into a sleepy, depressed state of movement (Video 1). The pressure was applied continuously for 5 minutes before the rope was removed, and the lambs were stimulated by rubbing their rump and sides (Video 2).

Table 1
The APGAR scoring system described by Flora and coworkers[7] was used to evaluate vitality of newborn lambs

Parameter	0 Points	1 Point	2 Points
Appearance (mucous membrane color)	Cyanotic	Pale	Pink
Pulse (beats/min)	<100	100–175	>175
Grimace (nasal stimulation)	No response	Moves head slightly	Sneezes/moves away/ shakes head
Attitude (rump stimulation)	No response	Moves with no attempt to stand	Attempts to stand
Respiration (oxygen saturation; Spo$_2$), %	<45	45–65	>65

The pulse and oxygen saturation were measured using a pulse oximeter (#CMS60D-VET, Contec Medical Systems Co, ltd, Qinhuangdao, China) attached to the lamb's dried ear or tail.

Table 2
A 21-point behavioral scoring system was developed to evaluate lambs before and after treatment

Parameter	Observation	Points Assigned
Standing	Not standing	1
	Standing but shaky	2
	Standing strongly	3
Seizure activity	Strong convulsions	1
	Mild convulsions	2
	No convulsions	3
Fear response	No movement away from humans	1
	Aware of humans/moves slightly away	2
	Avidly avoids humans	3
Attention to dam	Ignores dam, no attempt to be near her	1
	Aware of dam's presence but not staying close	2
	Attempts to stay close to dam, calls to her when she is far away	3
Interest in suckling	No interest in finding the teat	1
	Looks for teat when opportunistic timing	2
	Avidly searches for teat, attempting to suckle on dam	3
Attempt to stay warm	Lamb lays by itself	1
	Lamb attempts to lay close to others	2
	Lamb lays next to dam or siblings	3
Stargazing	Lamb stares off up into space/stares into corners	1
	Lamb stares/looks at odd items for several minutes	2
	Lamb does not stare up/into space/at odd objects	3

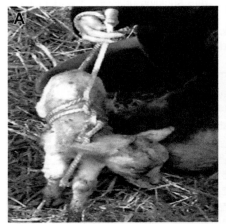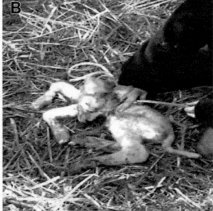

Fig. 1. (*A*) The compression treatment was administered by tying a soft cotton rope around the chest of the lamb following the same procedure as described by Toth and colleagues.[7] (*B*) Approximately 1 lb of pressure was applied to the rope to tighten the loops and place the lamb into a sleepy, depressed state of movement. The pressure was applied continuously for 5 minutes before the rope was removed, and the lamb's rump and side were stimulated.

The placebo treatment was applied to lambs in all 3 groups (group 1: n = 6; group 2: n = 10; and group 3: n = 1). The placebo treatment was administered by placing hands around the ribcage of the lamb (in the same region the rope would apply compression) and restraining the lamb continuously for 5 minutes. After the lambs were released, they were stimulated in the same manner as described for the compression treatment. The control treatment was also applied to lambs in all 3 groups (group 1: n = 10; group 2: n = 7; and group 3: n = 1) and involved administration of no treatment or human interaction with the lamb for 5 minutes.

Data were presented as mean $\pm$ standard deviation and analyzed using Microsoft Excel software (Redmond, Washington, USA). APGAR scores were compared with time to stand, time to search, and time to suckle using simple linear regression. The effects of treatment on time to stand, time to search, time to suckle, and behavioral score were compared within groups using a paired Student t test. Significance was defined as $P<.05$.

RESULTS

Before any treatment, time to stand, time to search, and time to suckle for all lambs was 24.2 ± 20.8, 26.5 ± 22.1, and 43.6 ± 19.8 minutes, respectively. There was no correlation ($R^2 < 0.2$) between APGAR score and the time to stand, time to search, and time to suckle for lambs with total APGAR scores ≥ 3.6 (groups 1 and 2; **Table 3**). The sample size for lambs with APGAR scores less than 3.6 was not large enough (n = 5) to perform the correlation.

During compression treatment, lambs maintained a sleeplike state for most of the treatment duration. Some lambs kicked and vocalized during compression treatment, and a few lambs defecated and urinated during the compression treatment. Somnolence and these other behaviors were not apparent in lambs receiving the placebo or control treatments. After compression treatment, there was a significant reduction in the time to stand, time to search, and time to suckle in both group 1 and group 2 lambs (**Table 4**). In addition, group 3 lambs that received the compression treatment had a significant reduction in the time to search and time to suckle, such that all group 3 lambs receiving the compression treatment were suckling unassisted within 21 minutes of treatment (see **Table 4**).

Compression treatment improved behavior scores in group 2 ($P = .047$) and group 3 lambs ($P = .013$), and there was a trend for compression treatment to improve

Table 3
Before treatment, there was no correlation between APGAR score and to time to stand (STAND), time to search (SEARCH), and time to suckle (SUCKLE) for lambs with total APGAR scores ≥ 3.6

	Group 1 (n = 36)			Group 2 (n = 45)		
	STAND	SEARCH	SUCKLE	STAND	SEARCH	SUCKLE
Appearance	$R^2 = 0.00$	$R^2 = 0.03$	$R^2 = 0.01$	$R^2 = 0.01$	$R^2 = 0.01$	$R^2 = 0.02$
Pulse	$R^2 = 0.02$	$R^2 = 0.02$	$R^2 = 0.18$	$R^2 = 0.00$	$R^2 = 0.00$	$R^2 = 0.01$
Grimace	$R^2 = 0.03$	$R^2 = 0.01$	$R^2 = 0.00$	$R^2 = 0.07$	$R^2 = 0.03$	$R^2 = 0.00$
Attitude	$R^2 = 0.02$	$R^2 = 0.00$	$R^2 = 0.01$	$R^2 = 0.01$	$R^2 = 0.00$	$R^2 = 0.00$
Respiration	$R^2 = 0.05$	$R^2 = 0.00$	$R^2 = 0.00$	$R^2 = 0.01$	$R^2 = 0.05$	$R^2 = 0.00$
Total	$R^2 = 0.03$	$R^2 = 0.00$	$R^2 = 0.02$	$R^2 = 0.02$	$R^2 = 0.00$	$R^2 = 0.00$

Group 1 lambs had a time to stand of less than 32.1 min and a time to suckle of less than 40.7 min, whereas group 2 lambs had a time to stand of ≥ 32.1 min and a time to suck of ≥ 40.7 min.

Table 4
Mean ± standard deviation (in minutes) for time to stand, time to search, or time to suckle measured in lambs before and after receiving compression treatment

	Group (n)	1 (20)	2 (28)	3 (3)
Time to stand	Before	15.5 ± 8.5	26.9 ± 11.3	88.3 ± 37.4
	After	4.00 ± 5.9	7.3 ± 9.6	8.3 ± 6.8
	P	.000[a]	.000[a]	.059
Time to search	Before	18.6 ± 8.74	25.8 ± 13.5	144.3 ± 20.8
	After	6.0 ± 6.3	10.2 ± 10.5	7.3 ± 5.0
	P	.000[a]	.000[a]	.003[a]
Time to suckle	Before	30.6 ± 6.8	47.9 ± 15.6	137.0 ± 38.0
	After	12.0 ± 10.5	15.4 ± 14.1	16.7 ± 3.7
	P	.000[a]	.000[a]	.022[a]

[a] Compression treatment significantly decreased time to stand, time to search, or time to suckle for lambs receiving compression treatment, with the exception of group 3 lambs in which there was a trend toward a reduction in time to stand.

behavior scores in group 1 lambs (P = .068) (**Table 5**). Placebo treatment did not affect behavior scores in group 1 or group 2 lambs, and no treatment did not affect behavior scores in group 2 lambs (see **Table 5**). However, behavior scores improved in group 1 lambs that received no treatment.

DISCUSSION

Application of physical stimulation to newborns has been shown to elicit a wide variety of behavioral responses.[8–13] Swaddling produces a tranquil state in most human infants.[11] Deep pressure techniques have been used to improve mood and adaptation to the environment in children with autism.[14] In addition, the use of a squeeze machine on both autistic and normal adults has a relaxing effect.[12] In rabbits, application of skin pressure was followed by "deactivated" EEG patterns, relaxed muscle tone, narrow lid aperture, and constriction of pupils.[8] Another study in rabbits found that positioning newborns on their abdomen with all limbs extended induced a state of "hypnosis."[15]

Table 5
Mean ± standard deviation for behavioral scores taken before and after each treatment for lambs in each group

Treatment	Compression			Placebo			Control		
Group (n)	1 (20)	2 (28)	3 (3)	1 (6)	2 (10)	3 (1)	1 (10)	2 (7)	3 (1)
Before	18.3	17.8	11.3	18.8	17.3	15.0	17.2	17.3	14.0
	± 2.1	± 2.6	± 1.2	± 1.1	± 2.87		± 2.6	± 1.9	
After	19.3	18.3	20.0	18.8	17.9	18.0	18.7	18.0	14.0
	± 1.8	± 2.6	± 0.8	± 1.2	± 2.3		± 1.8	± 2.3	
P	.068[b]	.047[a]	.013[a]	.500	.321	—	.003[b]	.285	—

[a] Compression treatment significantly improved behavior scores for lambs with either delayed time to stand or time to suckle (group 2) or low APGAR scores at birth (group 3).
[b] The behavior score in lambs with a normal APGAR score at birth and normal time to stand or time to suckle (group 1) improved significantly without treatment (control group), and there was a trend for improvement with compression treatment.

This report is the first to evaluate the use of resuscitation compression for the treatment of abnormal behavioral presentations in lambs. Group 1 lambs that received compression treatment showed no difference in behavioral scores, which indicates normal lambs neither benefit nor are harmed by this treatment. These results are similar to what was reported for normal foals and calves.[5,7] Lambs with prolonged time to stand or time to suckle and/or abnormal behavior (group 2 and group 3 lambs) showed a significant improvement in behavior after resuscitation compression. These results are similar to what was reported for foals and calves with NMS, in which all newborns stood immediately and approached their dam after the compression treatment.[2,5,7] This differed from what was seen in lambs. Of the 51 lambs squeezed, 8 (15.7%) stood immediately and another 13 (25.5%) stood within 1 minute of cessation of treatment. For all lambs receiving resuscitation compression, the time to stand, time to search, and time to suckle after cessation of treatment were 6.0 ± 8.3, 8.3 ± 8.9, and 14.3 ± 12.4 minutes.

Both foals and calves demonstrated depressed or dreamlike behavior during compression treatment,[5,7] like the lambs in the current study. It is of interest to note that it appeared that group 3 lambs kicked harder and more frequently during compression treatment when compared with lambs in group 1 and group 2. Although the sample size for group 3 lambs was small (n = 5), these results suggest that resuscitation compression is a valid method for improving abnormal behavior characteristic of NMS. Of the group 3 lambs that received compression treatment (n = 3), 2 lambs presented with no suckle reflex and 1 lamb had a minimal suckle reflex, whereas all lambs were unable to stand and showed disinterest in their dam. After compression treatment, lamb behavior improved markedly, and all lambs suckled from their dams within 21 minutes. The behavioral scores of these lambs improved from 11.3 ± 1.2 before treatment to 20.0 ± 0.8 after the treatment. The lamb behavior remained improved after treatment and did not regress.

SUMMARY

The use of resuscitation compression is a highly valuable method for improving abnormal behavior in newborns. In lambs with prolonged time to suckle and/or showing signs of NMS, resuscitation compression resulted in significantly improved behavioral scores and reduced time to stand, time to search, and time to suckle. The compression treatment also produced no side effects in healthy lambs. Resuscitation compression should be considered as a treatment for lambs with NMS-like symptoms or to stimulate nursing in lambs without a suckle reflex.

CLINICS CARE POINTS

- Neonatal resuscitation compression is a quick treatment that can be performed easily on the farm. However, care must be exercised while performing the procedure to avoid injuring the lamb.
- Neonatal resuscitation compression showed no negative effects when performed on normal lambs. However, when administered to lambs with abnormal behavior at birth, neonatal resuscitation compression markedly improves behavioral scores and vigor.
- It is important to note that neonatal resuscitation compression had no effect on the lamb acceptance by dams that had previously rejected them. Therefore, lambs experiencing dam rejection will still require additional care to ensure access to nourishment.

DISCLOSURE

This research was funded by the Oregon Sheep Commission (USA) and the College of Agricultural Sciences, Oregon State University, Continuing Researchers Support Program (USA).

SUPPLEMENTARY DATA

Supplementary data related to this article can be found online at https://doi.org/10.1016/j.cvfa.2020.10.006.

REFERENCES

1. Hess-Dudan F, Rossdale PD. Neonatal maladjustment syndrome and other neurological signs in the newborn foal: part 2. Equine Vet Educ 1996;8:79–83.
2. Aleman M, Weich KM, Madigan JE. Survey of veterinarians using a novel physical compression squeeze procedure in the management of neonatal maladjustment syndrome in foals. Animals 2017;7:69.
3. Rossdale PD, Leadon DP. Equine neonatal disease. J Reprod Fertil 1975;23:658–61.
4. Bernard WV, Reimer JM, Cudd T. Historical factors, clinicopathologic findings, clinical features, and outcome of equine neonates presenting with or developing signs of central nervous system disease. Proc Am Assoc Equine Pract 1995;41:222–4.
5. Stilwell G, Mellor DJ, Holdsworth SE. Potential benefit of a thoracic squeeze technique in two newborn calves delivered by caesarean section. N Z Vet J 2020;68:65–8.
6. Flora T, Smallman M, Kutzler M. Developing a modified Apgar scoring system for newborn lambs. Theriogenology 2020;157:321–6.
7. Toth B, Aleman M, Brosnan RJ, et al. Evaluation of squeeze-induced somnolence in neonatal foals. Am J Vet Res 2012;73:1881–9.
8. Kumazawa T. "Deactivation" of the rabbit's brain by pressure application to the skin. Electroencephalogr Clin Neurophysiol 1963;15:660–71.
9. Melzack R, Konrad KW, Dubrovsky B. Prolonged changes in central nervous system activity produced by somatic and reticular stimulation. Exp Neurol 1969;25:416–28.
10. Harlow HF, Zimmerman RR. Affectional response in the infant monkey. Science 1959;130:421–32.
11. Lipton EL, Steinschneider A, Richmond JB. Swaddling, a childcare practice: historical, cultural, and experimental observations. Pediatrics 1965;35:521–67.
12. Grandin T. Calming effects of deep touch pressure in patients with autistic disorder, college students and animals. J Child Adolesc Psychopharmacol 1992;2:63–72.
13. Giacoman SL. Hunger and motor restraint on arousal and visual attention in the infant. Child Dev 1971;42:605–14.
14. Bestbier L, Williams TI. The immediate effects of deep pressure on young people with autism and severe intellectual difficulties: demonstrating individual differences. Occup Ther Int 2017;7534972. https://doi.org/10.1155/2017/7534972.
15. Galashina AG, Kulikov MA, Bogdanov AV. Effects of "animal hypnosis" on a rhythmic defensive dominant. Neurosci Behav Physiol 2008;38:23–30.

Hematologic Conditions of Small Ruminants

Jennifer Johns, DVM, PhD[a],*, Meera Heller, DVM, PhD[b]

KEYWORDS

- Anemia • Goat • Hematology • Hemolysis • Parasitism • Regeneration • Ruminant
- Sheep

KEY POINTS

- Anemia is a clinically important syndrome in small ruminants and is divided into regenerative and nonregenerative anemia.
- Common causes of anemia in small ruminants include gastrointestinal and external parasitism resulting in chronic hemorrhage, and anemia of inflammatory or chronic disease.
- Iron deficiency can present as either mildly regenerative or nonregenerative anemia.
- Diagnostic testing is key to identifying the cause of anemia and selecting appropriate treatment and prevention strategies.

INTRODUCTION

Routine hematologic analysis in small ruminants is performed using a fresh whole blood sample placed in EDTA anticoagulant. Other anticoagulants can create dilution errors and/or interfere with morphologic analyses. Samples may be refrigerated within 1 hour of collection if immediate analysis is not possible. A maximum of 24 hours of refrigerated storage time before analysis is recommended. The mean corpuscular volume (MCV) and mean platelet volume may increase after 24 hours of storage and can increase hematocrit and packed cell volume (PCV).[1] Blood smears should be prepared immediately. The blood smear should be submitted with the sample if the sample is being submitted to an outside laboratory. Blood tubes should be shipped on cold packs but not allowed to freeze. Manual PCV determination via centrifugation of a microhematocrit tube should roughly match

Authors' note: This article covers only disorders of red blood cells and hemostasis in small ruminants. Although clinically important, disorders of white blood cells are not covered in this review.

[a] Department of Biomedical Sciences, Oregon State University Carlson College of Veterinary Medicine, 700 Southwest 30th Street, Corvallis, OR 97331, USA; [b] Department of Medicine and Epidemiology, University of California Davis School of Veterinary Medicine, One Garrod Drive, Davis, CA 95616, USA
* Corresponding author.
E-mail address: jennifer.johns@oregonstate.edu

Vet Clin Food Anim 37 (2021) 183–197
https://doi.org/10.1016/j.cvfa.2020.10.004
0749-0720/21/© 2020 Elsevier Inc. All rights reserved.

hematocrit values obtained from automated analysis. If PCV values are higher than hematocrit values, centrifugation may be insufficient. If recentrifuging the tube decreases the PCV value further, a centrifugation issue can be confirmed. Other causes of artifactual changes to PCV include red blood cell (RBC) shrinkage owing to excess EDTA (short sample volume in EDTA tube), causing falsely decreased hematocrit and PCV; patient hyperosmolarity (eg, marked hyperglycemia or hypernatremia) causing falsely increased hematocrit; and patient hypo-osmolarity (eg, marked hyponatremia) causing falsely decreased hematocrit. Gross changes in blood and plasma color may be noted with certain disease processes; for example, dark-colored whole blood may indicate methemoglobinemia, as can be seen in nitrate or nitrite poisoning, copper toxicity, and oak poisoning; pink-colored plasma can indicate intravascular hemolysis (or in vitro artifactual hemolysis); and bright yellow plasma can indicate hyperbilirubinemia (icterus or jaundice).

Normal values (reference intervals) for sheep and goats are shown in **Table 1**. In both species, polychromasia and reticulocyte counts in peripheral blood are minimal in health, but will increase in regenerative anemia. Both sheep and goats have relatively small RBCs and platelets compared with other domestic animal species. Automated hematology analyzers must have species-specific software to appropriately categorize blood cells in small ruminants and avoid mistaking RBCs for platelets. A manual blood smear review is necessary to confirm automated differential counting and to evaluate for the presence of abnormalities. Some goat breeds (eg, Angora) have substantial poikilocytosis normally (**Fig. 1**). Hemic parasites, polychromasia (see **Figs. 2** and **4**), nucleated RBCs (**Fig. 2**), and morphologic abnormalities (eg, neutrophil toxicity, left shift) can be detected on smear review.

POLYCYTHEMIA

Increased PCV or hematocrit indicative of polycythemia is most commonly relative polycythemia owing to dehydration and decreased plasma water. Absolute polycythemia is less common and is subdivided into appropriate and inappropriate responses. Appropriate polycythemia is due to increased erythropoietin levels

Table 1 RBC, platelet, and protein reference intervals for small ruminants		
Test	Ovine	Caprine
RBC count ($\times$ 10^6/µL)	9–15	8–18
Hemoglobin (g/dL)	9–15	8–12
Hematocrit (%)	27–45	22–38
MCV (fL)	28–40	16–25
MCH (pg)	8–12	5.2–8.0
Mean corpuscular hemoglobin concentration (g/dL)	31–34	30–36
Platelet count ($\times$ 10^3/µL)	2.5–7.5	3–6
Reticulocyte count (%)	0	0
Reticulocyte count absolute	Rare	Rare
Plasma protein (g/dL)	6.0–7.5	6.0–7.5

Reference intervals *courtesy of* Oregon State University Veterinary Diagnostic Laboratory. *Data obtained from* clinical healthy animals and analysis performed on a Siemens Bayer Advia 120. Blood smear review performed by trained medical technologists. Reference intervals constructed based on central 95% of data following removal of outlier data points.

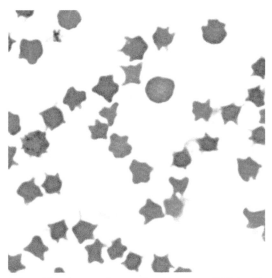

Fig. 1. Poikilocytosis in a blood smear from a healthy goat. Wright-Giemsa stain, original magnification ×100.

triggered by tissue hypoxia, for example, in animals living at high altitude, chronic cardiopulmonary disease. Inappropriate responses are those not in response to tissue hypoxia (eg, renal neoplasia causing increased erythropoietin secretion). Inappropriate polycythemia is rarely reported in small ruminants.

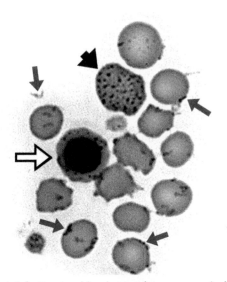

Fig. 2. *Mycoplasma ovis* infection in a blood smear from an anemic sheep. *Red (solid) arrows* indicate epicellular bacteria on surface of RBCs and as extracellular structures in the background. *Blue arrowheads* indicate polychromatophilic RBCs with basophilic stippling. *Black (open) arrow* indicates a nucleated RBC with basophilic stippling. Wright-Giemsa stain, original magnification ×100. (*Courtesy of* Dr. Melinda Camus, University of Georgia College of Veterinary Medicine, DVM, Athens, GA.)

ANEMIA

Causes of anemia are categorized based on the presence or absence of a regenerative response. Erythroid regeneration is indicated by the presence of polychromatophilic RBCs on a Wright-stained blood smear and/or by reticulocytes measured via automated analyzer or by manual new methylene blue staining. An increase in these immature RBCs that are larger with decreased hemoglobin concentration can cause an increase in the MCV (macrocytosis) and a decrease in the mean corpuscular hemoglobin and mean corpuscular hemoglobin concentration (hypochromasia). Increases in polychromatophils or reticulocytes, indicating a regenerative response, can be detected approximately 2 to 3 days after the onset of hemorrhage or hemolysis. For that reason, it is important to consider a "pre-regenerative" response as a differential for nonregenerative anemia.

Nucleated RBCs are often noted in blood smears from small ruminants with regenerative anemia. Increased nucleated RBCs (termed rubricytosis) is frequently associated with marked regeneration and/or marked anemia. Mechanisms for premature release of nucleated RBCs include release as part of the regenerative response and bone marrow hypoxic injury from severe anemia. Other insult or injury to bone marrow (eg, lead poisoning) or the spleen (eg, trauma) can also cause rubricytosis. In addition to polychromasia/reticulocytosis and rubricytosis, other common RBC abnormalities in regenerative anemia of small ruminants include basophilic stippling and Howell–Jolly bodies.

Regenerative Anemia

Regenerative anemia is classified into hemorrhagic and hemolytic based on the mechanism of RBC loss (**Table 2**). Physical examination findings can help to locate signs of external hemorrhage (eg, parasites, trauma) or hemolysis (eg, pigmenturia, icterus). A common cause of blood loss in small ruminants that may not be evident on physical examination is gastrointestinal loss owing to parasitism, abomasal ulceration, or hemorrhagic enteritis owing to *Clostridium perfringens* infection or enterotoxin.[2] Clinical signs of gastrointestinal blood loss include diarrhea and melena.

Table 2
Causes of hemorrhagic anemia in small ruminants

External Hemorrhage	Internal Hemorrhage with Variable Resorption of Blood	Hemostatic Disorders	
Ectoparasitism (eg, sucking lice, fleas, ticks)	Gastrointestinal or internal parasitism (eg, *Haemonchus* infection, coccidiosis)	Disorders of primary hemostasis (severe thrombocytopenia)	Disorders of secondary hemostasis (coagulopathies)
External trauma	Abomasal ulceration	Decreased platelet production	Sweet clover toxicosis
Hemostatic disorders	Hemorrhagic enteritis	Increased platelet consumption	Warfarin toxicosis
	Neoplastic and inflammatory lesions (eg, abscesses) causing internal hemorrhage	Increased platelet destruction	Interference with synthesis of vitamin K-dependent coagulation factors
	Abdominal hemorrhage (eg, abdominal trauma)		Consumptive coagulopathy

Hemostatic disorders can result from primary or secondary hemostasis problems. Severe thrombocytopenia (eg, <20,000 platelets/μL) is a primary hemostatic disorder that can result in spontaneous hemorrhage. Thrombocytopenia may occur alone or with pancytopenia (see causes of nonregenerative anemia elsewhere in this article). General causes of thrombocytopenia include decreased production owing to bone marrow disease or damage (eg, myelophthisis) or increased consumption. Consumptive coagulopathy (ie, disseminated intravascular coagulation) is an example of increased consumption that is often owing to viral vasculitis (eg, bluetongue infection of sheep). Increased platelet destruction (eg, immune-mediated thrombocytopenia) occurs in other species, but there is minimal evidence of this hemostatic disorder in small ruminants. Coagulopathies are a secondary hemostatic disorder that can occur from ingestion of moldy sweet clover hay or silage (known as "sweet clover toxicosis"). Coagulopathies can also occur from systemic accumulation of dicoumarol causing clinical warfarin toxicosis or by interference with hepatic synthesis of vitamin K–dependent coagulation factors leading to spontaneous hemorrhage.[3] Clinical signs of coagulopathies include epistaxis, melena, hematoma formation, and potentially fatal hemorrhage after trauma or surgery.

Hemolytic anemia from hemic parasitism

Anaplasma ovis is an obligate intracellular rickettsial pathogen infecting RBCs in domestic or wild sheep and goats.[4,5] Ixodid ticks vector *A ovis*, but mechanical transmission via fomite or biting flies can also occur. Subclinical or mildly clinical infection is most common, whereas severe clinical signs are uncommon but can include marked anemia and death.[6] High rates of endemic infection are described in regions with high levels of tick-borne transmission. Polymerase chain reaction (PCR) testing is sensitive and specific for diagnosis of active infection compared with blood smear evaluation; use of competitive enzyme-linked immunosorbent assay designed for *Anaplasma marginale* detection was validated for diagnosis of *A ovis* seropositivity.[5,7]

Mycoplasma ovis is a hemotrophic mycoplasma species that is globally distributed and often nonpathogenic in sheep and goats. However, multiple factors determine pathogenicity, including animal age and health and nutritional status, and severe hemolytic anemia is a potential outcome of infection.[8] Lambs suffer fatal infection more often than adult sheep[9]; goats develop lower levels of parasitemia than sheep.[10] Infection is transmitted via arthropod vector or iatrogenic means. Organisms can be seen on blood smears as small coccoid to rod shaped structures less than 1 μm in diameter adherent to RBCs and may be seen in the background as well (see **Fig. 2**). PCR is substantially more sensitive than blood smear evaluation for detection of the pathogen.[11]

Theileria spp. are tick-vectored protozoal parasites. In the erythrocytic piroplasm stage, this parasite causes variable hemolytic anemia in sheep and goats. Infection with *Theileria lestoquardi* is reported in Africa, south and east Asia, the Mediterranean and the Middle East.[12] Other *Theileria* species of small ruminants include *T luwenshuni* in sheep and *T uilenbergi* in goats in China.[13–15] *Theileria* organisms appear in blood smears as pleomorphic structures that are often round to piriform in shape. Maximum parasitism in an experimental study of sheep infected with *T lestoquardi* was 3% of RBCs.[16] PCR analysis of whole blood is likely more sensitive for detection of active infection than blood smear evaluation. Schizont stage organisms may be found in lymphocytes in lymphoid tissues, but are generally not seen in white blood cells in blood smears.

Hemolytic anemia from bacterial infectious organisms

In sheep, *Leptospira interrogans* (serovars Hardjo and Pomona) can cause a fatal intravascular hemolysis with resultant icterus, hemoglobinuria, and pigment nephropathy. The mortality rate in lambs is reported at 5%.[17–19] Goats are also susceptible to febrile illness from leptospirosis. In addition, subclinical *Leptospira* spp. infections in both sheep and goats are commonly associated with reproductive defects including abortion.[20]

Infection of sheep with *Clostridium novyi* type D (*Clostridium haemolyticum*) can result in febrile disease with severe hemolytic anemia and high morbidity.[21,22] *C novyi* type D is the agent of bacillary hemoglobinuria and produces phospholipase C that has potent hemolytic and necrotizing activity. As with other *C novyi* infections in sheep and cattle, endemic infection is associated with *Fasciola hepatica* (liver fluke) infection.

Hemolytic disease can also accompany *C perfringens* type A infection owing to the production of a hemolytic toxin, *C perfringens* alpha toxin. Enterotoxemia with high levels of *C perfringens* alpha toxin can cause severe hemolytic anemia in lambs ("yellow lamb disease") and adult sheep.[23] Rarely will other *C perfringens* genotypes produce high enough *C perfringens* alpha toxin to cause hemolytic disease.[2]

Hemolytic anemia from oxidant injury

Oxidant injury to RBCs can result in formation of Heinz bodies (aggregates of denatured hemoglobin that cause RBC membrane protrusion). Heinz bodies can be difficult to detect on routine Wright-stained blood smears (**Fig. 3**A). New methylene blue or other vital staining easily allows visualization of Heinz bodies (**Fig. 3**B). Heinz body hemolytic anemia is reported in lambs deficient in copper and selenium.[24] High susceptibility to copper intoxication in sheep can result in hemolytic anemia owing to oxidant damage and Heinz body formation.[25,26] Lambs are more susceptible than goats and adult sheep; British sheep breeds are more susceptible than Merino breeds.[27] Goats can also be affected and develop Heinz body hemolytic anemia, possibly with methemoglobinemia; hemolysis may not occur despite other signs of toxicity.[28,29] Additional stressors can precipitate a hemolytic crisis.[30] Sheep that are grazed on pastures low in molybdenum also can develop Heinz body hemolytic anemia owing to chronic copper toxicity.[27,31]

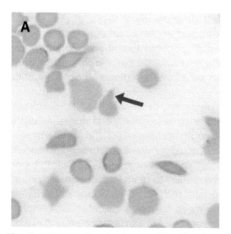
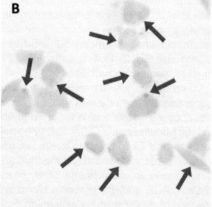

Fig. 3. Heinz bodies (*red arrows*) in blood smears from an anemic goat with Wright-Giemsa stain (*A*) and new methylene blue stain (*B*), original magnification ×100.

Sulfur compounds in brassicas (eg, cabbage, kale) are metabolized to oxidizing agents in ruminating animals, and high levels of *Brassica* spp. ingestion can result in Heinz body hemolytic anemia proportionate to the dietary intake. There are rare reports of natural and experimental toxicities in goats owing to kale ingestion; kids that were already anemic owing to hemonchosis were more susceptible naturally.[28] Sheep and goats are less susceptible to oxidant injury owing to ingestion of onions, garlic, and other *Allium* spp. than cattle, dogs, and cats, but can suffer from Heinz body hemolytic anemia with high levels of ingestion.[32] Ingestion of fresh oak acorns or leaves rich in tannic acid can result in accumulation of the metabolite pyrogallol that oxidizes hemoglobin to methemoglobin, causing hemolytic anemia. Edema and hemorrhagic enteritis are characteristic lesions on necropsy.[33] Clinical signs can appear 3 days after ingestion.[34] Sheep are more susceptible than goats; severe anemia was experimentally induced in goats fed oak tannins, but naturally occurring poisoning is rare in goats because they are relatively resistant.[33]

Hemolysis from miscellaneous causes

Postparturient hemoglobinuria in cattle owing to intravascular hemolysis is associated with marked hypophosphatemia, although concurrent copper and/or selenium deficiency may contribute to RBC fragility.[35] It is not known if this can occur in small ruminants.

Water toxicity can occur after ingestion of a large quantity of water that is rapidly absorbed and causes osmotic changes in the blood leading to rupture of RBCs. This finding is most commonly seen in small breed goats, especially around weaning, that are given water via a nipple bottle.[36]

Nonregenerative Anemia

Specific suppression of bone marrow erythropoiesis leads to nonregenerative anemia without other accompanying cytopenias. When bone marrow hematopoiesis is globally suppressed, pancytopenia including nonregenerative anemia can result. Nonregenerative anemia is normocytic (normal MCV) and normochromic (normal mean corpuscular hemoglobin concentration) unless specified elsewhere in this article.

Nonregenerative anemia without pancytopenia

Nonregenerative anemia without pancytopenia can result from pre-regenerative anemia owing to sudden (<48 hours) onset hemorrhage or hemolysis and can be severe. This condition differs from anemia with inflammatory or chronic disease, which is usually normocytic and normochromic but generally remains in a moderate range. Decreased iron availability for erythropoiesis results from inflammation-induced increases in inflammatory cytokines, hepcidin, and ferritin production.[37,38] The "chronic disease" term can be misleading because anemia can occur in less than 1 week after the onset of inflammation.[39]

Nonregenerative anemia without reticulocytosis or other evidence of regeneration can result from iron deficiency owing to nutritional deficiency or chronic blood loss and is well-described in confined lambs. Microscopically, microcytosis and hypochromasia may be evident.[40,41] The duration of hemorrhage and degree of blood reabsorption with gastrointestinal hemorrhage can determine the likelihood of iron deficiency anemia. Iron deficiency anemia owing to chronic gastrointestinal hemorrhage is often mildly regenerative owing to variable iron resorption. The location of hemorrhage (proximal vs distal gastrointestinal tract) may affect the likelihood of inadequate iron resorption resulting in deficiency. In contrast, nutritional iron deficiency and deficiency owing to external hemorrhage (eg, ectoparasitism) is generally nonregenerative.

Microcytosis and/or hypochromasia can occur with iron deficiency anemia, but microcytosis can be obscured by concurrent regeneration causing normal MCV or even macrocytosis (increased MCV). Increased poikilocytosis including RBC fragmentation can also be seen along with evidence of regeneration (**Fig. 4**). It is important to mention that hemolytic disorders do not cause iron deficiency, because the destroyed RBCs remain within the body, allowing for adequate recycling of heme iron.

Deficiency in adequate dietary copper can also lead to microcytic anemia in sheep. Goats may also be susceptible to deficiency when fed mineral supplements designed for sheep.[28] Excess dietary molybdenum, iron, or sulfur is a more common cause of copper deficiency than low copper levels in forage.[42] Cobalt (vitamin B_{12}) deficiency can also result in anemia in sheep under experimental conditions.[43]

Decreased erythropoietin production by diseased kidneys and resulting decreased erythropoiesis, decreased iron availability, and potentially shortened RBC half-life are mechanisms of anemia of renal failure.[44,45] Results from a complete blood count will show a progressive normocytic normochromic anemia in affected animals.

Lead poisoning of small ruminants can be associated with housing near junk piles or industrial sites or contact with lead-containing materials such as paint. Sheep grazing pastures near a zinc smelting facility developed microcytic hypochromic anemia.[46] Ruminants are more likely to develop acute lead poisoning with nervous system effects, but chronic lead poisoning can result in nonregenerative anemia, rubricytosis, and basophilic stippling of RBCs owing to interference with heme synthesis, along with neurologic and gastrointestinal signs.[47]

The effects of gossypol toxicity are multisystemic and vary by species and age. Immature ruminants are reportedly more susceptible than adult animals; lambs may suffer sudden death after exposure.[48] Potential hematologic effects of gossypol toxicity in ruminants include anemia and increased RBC fragility; complexing of iron by gossypol is one mechanism.

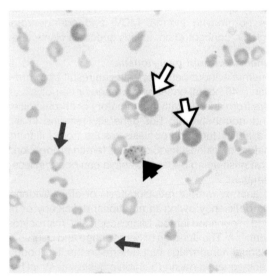

Fig. 4. Blood smear from a goat with iron deficiency anemia. *Red (solid) arrows* indicate hypochromic RBCs. *Black (open) arrows* indicate polychromatophilic RBCs. *Blue arrowhead* indicates polychromatophilic RBC with basophilic stippling. Wright-Giemsa stain, original magnification ×100.

Nonregenerative anemia with pancytopenia

Sheep are less susceptible than cattle to the toxicity of bracken fern (*Pteridium aquilinum*), but acute hemorrhagic disease, progressive retinal atrophy, and neoplasia of the proximal gastrointestinal tract and urinary bladder have been reported in sheep.[49] Hemorrhagic disease is due to bone marrow suppression resulting in pancytopenia (nonregenerative anemia, leukopenia, and thrombocytopenia). In cattle, monocytosis is proposed as a useful indicator of early toxicosis (bovine enzootic hematuria).[50]

Myelotoxicity causing pancytopenia has contributed to high mortality in a flock of sheep exposed to high levels of fungal toxins of *Stachybotrys chartarum*. Septicemia in affected sheep was likely due to severe leukopenia, whereas hemorrhagic anemia resulted from thrombocytopenia.[51] Myelophthisis, the effacement of normal hematopoietic tissue by infiltrating neoplasia or other cellular processes, is rarely reported in small ruminants. A single case of myelophthisis has been reported in a goat with systemic mastocytosis.[52] Primary myelofibrosis was reported in a series of Pygmy goat kids, with progressive pancytopenia resulting in death at 6 to 12 weeks.[53]

The tick-borne obligate intracellular bacterium *Anaplasma phagocytophilum* causes a febrile acute illness (granulocytic anaplasmosis; often called "tick-borne fever") that often includes nonregenerative anemia, leukopenia including neutropenia, and thrombocytopenia. Both sheep and goats can become infected (confirmed via whole blood PCR)[54] and can seroconvert,[55] but clinical illness is rarely reported in goats in comparison with sheep. One report describes confirmed granulocytic anaplasmosis with high mortality in a goat herd in the Northeastern Italian Alps.[56] In sheep, infection frequently leads to febrile illness, but mortality is rare unless other immune compromise is present. *A phagocytophilum* infection may predispose sheep to contracting other concurrent infections. *A phagocytophilum* infection of sheep can also be a persistent condition (ie, sheep may be a natural reservoir or carrier species).[57]

DIAGNOSIS

Signs of anemia include exercise intolerance, increased respiratory and heart rates, discolored mucous membranes, weakness, lethargy, and depressed mentation. Anemia can be clinically suspected based on pale mucous membrane color. The ocular mucous membranes and conjunctiva and third eyelid are especially sensitive and the FAMACHA system has used the color of these membranes as a reliable indicator of anemia.[58] As stated elsewhere in this article, hemolysis may also be clinically suspected based on jaundiced mucous membranes and intravascular hemolysis may result in visible pigmenturia. A complete blood count, including blood smear examination, is needed to classify the anemia as regenerative or nonregenerative. Blood smear examination can also be helpful in diagnosis of hemic parasites or oxidative damage (Heinz body hemolytic anemia).

Gastrointestinal and external parasitism is one of the most common causes of anemia in small ruminants. Careful examination of the hair coat for external parasites should always be performed on anemic patients to check for hematophagic parasites, including lice and ticks. Fecal examination can indicate presence of gastrointestinal parasites such as *Haemonchus contortus* or coccidia spp.; both are significant causes of anemia. A quantitative fecal analysis such as a fecal McMaster's count is advised to document the parasite burden and evaluate the success of treatment by means of a fecal egg count reduction test.[59] A fecal occult blood test can be useful to detect gastrointestinal hemorrhage; taking multiple samples can help improve the diagnostic value of this low-sensitivity test. Positive fecal occult blood tests can be associated with the gastrointestinal parasites mentioned elsewhere in this article, abomasal ulceration, or other less common causes of gastrointestinal hemorrhage.

It is useful to assess whether hemolysis is intravascular or extravascular. Intravascular hemolysis can be apparent grossly via pink to red urine and/or plasma color (discolored plasma can be seen in spun hematocrit tubes). Urinalysis is a more sensitive method for the detection of pigmenturia and can help to rule out a renal or postrenal cause of discolored urine. Diagnostics for extravascular hemolysis include blood smear evaluation, leptospirosis titers and testing for other infectious causes (eg, PCR for *M ovis*). In cases of intravascular hemolysis, copper should be considered, especially in sheep. It is important to note that goats with copper toxicity may present without any signs of hemolysis.[29]

THERAPEUTIC OPTIONS

Treatment for anemia should consider both the diagnosis and treatment of the root cause of the anemia, and treatment of the anemia itself. Blood transfusions are indicated when the hematocrit has decreased to less than 12%,[60] although patients with chronic anemia are able to tolerate lower hematocrit owing to physiologic compensation mechanisms. Whole blood transfusions are commonly given; however, if the animal is not hypoproteinemic or suffering from coagulopathy, transfusing with RBCs only is also appropriate. Clinical improvement in the patient is usually seen after transfusion, but this improvement may be short lived and animals with nonregenerative anemias or continued losses may require repeated transfusions. Transfused RBCs have a shortened half-life, although the exact lifespan is unknown in small ruminants. Studies using biotinylated or radiolabeled RBCs have shown a half-life of 20 days and 11 days, respectively, for transfused RBCs in horses.[61,62] Transfusion reactions are relatively rare in small ruminants,[63] but the risk of a transfusion reaction increases with subsequent transfusions because antibodies are produced by the host against the transfused cells. Blood typing for ruminants is generally not available. Blood for transfusion should be collected from a healthy donor of the same species, ideally screened for infectious diseases and with a normal hematocrit. Xenotransfusion has been reported in exotic or wildlife species using domestic ruminants as donors; however, this practice is not recommended if conspecific transfusion is possible.[64] Up to 20% of the donor's blood volume can be collected at one time (10–15 mL/kg of body weight), and donors should not be used for 3 weeks after a blood donation.[60] For further information regarding blood transfusions in ruminants, please see Vet Clinics of North America Food Animal Practice, Volume 30, July 2014. The following equations can be used to calculate the volume of donor blood needed for a transfusion:

Donor blood volume needed (L) = [(Desired PCV – Recipient PCV)/Donor PCV] × Recipient blood volume

Total blood volume (L) = Body weight (kg) × 0.08

Gastrointestinal parasitism is the most common cause of anemia in small ruminants. Treatment decisions regarding gastrointestinal parasites should consider physical examination findings, fecal analysis, farm history, and history of previous anthelminthic treatment. Anthelminthic resistance is a common problem. Fecal analysis can enumerate trichostrongyle and coccidia spp. burden to help direct treatment against worms versus coccidian parasites. Discussion of gastrointestinal parasite management has been covered extensively in 2 recent reviews.[65,66] External parasites, such as hematophagous lice, are often found concurrently in animals with gastrointestinal parasitism. These conditions can be treated with systemic ivermectin or less effectively with topical permethrin application.

The treatment of abomasal ulceration centers around 2 main goals: the maintenance of mucosal perfusion and increasing the pH of the abomasal compartment. Maintenance of perfusion can be achieved with intravenous fluid therapy and buffering of the abomasal compartment can be achieved by increasing long stem forage, decreasing concentrates in the ration, and by administration of histamine (H2) blockers or proton pump inhibitors. Information regarding performance of these pharmaceuticals in adult ruminants is sparse. However, injectable pantoprazole (PROTONIX IV, Pfizer, New York, NY) has been shown to be effective in camelids at 1 mg/kg intravenously once daily and 2 mg/kg subcutaneously once daily.[67] Intravenous famotidine is effective in cattle at 0.4 mg/kg every 8 hours, although tachyphylaxis occurs with multiple administrations.[68]

In cases of severe intravascular hemolysis, fluid therapy with a balanced polyionic fluid should be instituted to support the kidneys and avoid pigment nephropathy. Copper toxicity can be treated by providing copper chelators such as ammonium molybdate (50-500 mg/sheep once daily orally for 6 days), sodium thiosulfate (300-1000 mg once daily orally for 6 days) or D-penicillamine (52 mg/kg orally twice daily for 6 days).[27]

Specific discussion of treatment for infectious causes of hemolytic anemia (eg, leptospirosis, mycoplasmosis, anaplasmosis) is beyond the scope of this review; however, many causes can be treated with oxytetracycline (20 mg/kg subcutaneously every 48 hours). It is important to note that oxytetracycline can be nephrotoxic, and if given during an acute hemolytic crisis may exacerbate renal injury, especially if given without fluid support.

Iron deficiency can be treated by giving iron dextran parenterally; however, giving a blood transfusion will also supply iron as the transfused RBCs are broken down by the host and the iron is recycled. Veterinarians must exercise caution when administering iron dextran as repeat treatments can increase the risk of anaphylactic reaction. There is currently no iron dextran product labeled for use in ruminants. A dose of 20 mg/kg intramuscularly has been used in lambs.

For the treatment of coagulopathy owing to poisoning by sweet clover silage, or anticoagulant rodenticide, parenteral administration of synthetic vitamin K1 (phytonadione; recommended dosage in cattle is 1.0–1.5 mg/kg body weight given subcutaneous or intramuscular) is indicated, along with transfusion as needed to address anemia and coagulation factor deficiency.[69]

PREVENTION

Prevention of anemia in small ruminants largely entails effective gastrointestinal parasite control and providing adequate and appropriate nutrition. Parasite management has been discussed in 2 recent reviews.[65,66] The FAMACHA system can be a useful and practical method to monitor for anemia on a herd basis; its use is usually associated with hemonchosis control strategies.[58]

CLINICS CARE POINTS

- Differentials for regenerative anemia are hemorrhage and hemolysis; common causes include ectoparasitism, gastrointestinal parasitism, infectious agents and trauma.
- Differentials for non-regenerative anemia include nutritional and toxic causes, iron deficiency in very young animals, and renal failure.

- The FAMACHA system is a useful indicator of anemia in small ruminant herds/flocks.
- Hemoglobinuria can occur with intravascular hemolysis due to copper toxicity, leptospirosis and water toxicity.
- Effective control of gastrointestinal parasites is key to prevention of anemia in small ruminants.

DISCLOSURE

The authors declare that they have no relevant or material financial interests and received no funding in relation to this work.

REFERENCES

1. Pintér E, László K, Schüszler I, et al. The stability of quantitative blood count parameters using the ADVIA 2120i hematology analyzer. Pract Lab Med 2016;4: 16–21.
2. Giannitti F, Rioseco MM, García JP, et al. Diagnostic exercise: hemolysis and sudden death in lambs. Vet Pathol 2014;51(3):624–7.
3. Watson JL. Diseases of the hematopoietic and hemolymphatic Systems. In: Smith BP, Van Metre DC, Pusterla N, editors. Large animal internal medicine. 6th edition. St. Louis (MO): Elsevier; 2020. p. 1151–96.
4. Hornok S, Elek V, de la Fuente J, et al. First serological and molecular evidence on the endemicity of Anaplasma ovis and A. marginale in Hungary. Vet Microbiol 2007;122(3–4):316–22.
5. Mason KL, Gonzalez MV, Chung C, et al. Validation of an improved Anaplasma antibody competitive ELISA for detection of Anaplasma ovis antibody in domestic sheep. J Vet Diagn Invest 2017;29(5):763–6.
6. Allesandra T, Santo C. Tick-borne diseases in sheep and goats: clinical and diagnostic aspects. Small Rumin Res 2012;106(suppl):S6–11.
7. Shabana II, Alhadlag NM, Zaraket H. Diagnostic tools of caprine and ovine anaplasmosis: a direct comparative study. BMC Vet Res 2018;14(1):165.
8. Messick JB. Hemotrophic mycoplasmas (hemoplasmas): a review and new insights into pathogenic potential. Vet Clin Pathol 2004;33(1):2–13.
9. Allison RW, Meinkoth JH. Anemias caused by rickettsia, mycoplasma, and protozoa. In: Weiss DJ, Wardrop KJ, editors. Schalm's veterinary hematology. 6th edition. Ames (IA): Wiley-Blackwell; 2010. p. 199–210.
10. Jain NC. Hemolytic anemias associated with some infectious agents. [Chapter 10]. In: Jain NC, editor. Essentials of veterinary hematology. Malvern (PA): Lea & Febiger; 1993. p. 177-92.
11. Hampel JA, Spath SN, Bergin IL, et al. Prevalence and diagnosis of hemotrophic mycoplasma infection in research sheep and its effects on hematology variables and erythrocyte membrane fragility. Comp Med 2014;64(6):478–85.
12. Brown CGD, Ilhan T, Kirvar E, et al. Theileria lestoquardi and T. annulata in cattle, sheep, and goats: in vitro and in vivo studies. Ann N Y Acad Sci 1998;849:44–51.
13. Chen Z, Liu Q, Jiao FC, et al. Detection of piroplasms infection in sheep, dogs and hedgehogs in Central China. Infect Dis Poverty 2014;3:18.
14. Ge Y, Pan W, Yin H. Prevalence of Theileria infections in goats and sheep in southeastern China. Vet Parasitol 2012;186(3–4):466–9.
15. Yin H, Schnittger L, Luo J, et al. Ovine theileriosis in China: a new look at an old story. Parasitol Res 2007;101(Suppl 2):S191–5.

16. Yaghfoori S, Mohri M, Razmi G. Experimental Theileria lestoquardi infection in sheep: biochemical and hematological changes. Acta Trop 2017;173:55–61.

17. Schmitz JA, Coles BM, Shires GM. Fatal hemolytic disease in sheep attributed to Leptospira interrogans serotype hardjo infection. Cornell Vet 1981;71(2):175–82.

18. Hamond C, Silveira CS, Buroni F, et al. Leptospira interrogans serogroup Pomona serovar Kennewicki infection in two sheep flocks with acute leptospirosis in Uruguay. Transbound Emerg Dis 2019;66(3):1186–94.

19. Smith BP, Armstrong JM. Fatal hemolytic anemia attributed to leptospirosis in lambs. J Am Vet Med Assoc 1975;167(8):739–41.

20. Martins G, Lilenbaum W. Leptospirosis in sheep and goats under tropical conditions. Trop Anim Health Prod 2014;46(1):11–7.

21. Randhawa SS, Sharma DK, Randhawa CS, et al. An outbreak of bacillary haemoglobinuria in sheep in India. Trop Anim Health Prod 1995;27(1):31–6.

22. Songer JG. Clostridial diseases of small ruminants. Vet Res 1998;29(3–4): 219–32.

23. McDonnell AM, Holmes LA. Haemoglobinuria due to Clostridium perfringens type A mastitis in a ewe. Br Vet J 1990;146(4):380–1.

24. Suttle NF, Jones DG, Woolliams C, et al. Heinz body anaemia in lambs with deficiencies of copper or selenium. Br J Nutr 1987;58(3):539–48.

25. Maiorka PC, Massoco CO, de Almeida SD, et al. Copper toxicosis in sheep: a case report. Vet Hum Toxicol 1998;40(2):99–100.

26. Bostwick JL. Copper toxicosis in sheep. J Am Vet Med Assoc 1982;180(4):386–7.

27. Watson JL, George LW. Copper toxicosis. In: Smith BP, Van Metre DC, Pusterla N, editors. Large animal internal medicine. 6th edition. St. Louis (MO): Elsevier; 2020. p. 1174–5.

28. Smith MC, Sherman DM. Blood, lymph and immune systems. In: Smith MC, Sherman DM, editors. Goat medicine. 2nd edition. Ames (IA): Wiley-Blackwell; 2009. p. 275–317.

29. Cornish J, Angelos J, Puschner B, et al. Copper toxicosis in a dairy goat herd. J Am Vet Med Assoc 2007;231(4):586–9.

30. Arora RG, Andersson L, Bucht RS, et al. Chronic copper toxicosis in sheep. Nord Vet Med 1977;29(4–5):181–7.

31. Auza NJ, Olson WG, Murphy MJ, et al. Diagnosis and treatment of copper toxicosis in ruminants. J Am Vet Med Assoc 1999;214(11):1624–8.

32. Rae HA. Onion toxicosis in a herd of beef cows. Can Vet J 1999;40(1):55–7.

33. Smith MC, Sherman DM. Urinary system. In: Smith MC, Sherman DM, editors. Goat medicine. 2nd edition. Ames (IA): Wiley-Blackwell; 2009. p. 537–69.

34. Spier SJ, Smith BP, Seawright AA, et al. Oak toxicosis in cattle in northern California: clinical and pathologic findings. J Am Vet Med Assoc 1987;191(8):958–64.

35. Goff JP. Phosphorus deficiency. In: Current veterinary therapy: food animal practice. 5th edition. St. Louis (MO): Saunders Elsevier; 2009.

36. Middleton JR, Katz L, Angelos JA, et al. Hemolysis associated with water administration using a nipple bottle for human infants in juvenile pygmy goats. J Vet Intern Med 1997;11(6):382–4.

37. Douglas SW, Adamson JW. The anemia of chronic disorders: studies of marrow regulation and iron metabolism. Blood 1975;45(1):55–65.

38. Madu AJ, Ughasoro MD. Anaemia of chronic disease: an in-depth review. Med Princ Pract 2017;26(1):1–9.

39. Weiss DJ, Krehbiel JD. Studies of the pathogenesis of anemia of inflammation: erythrocyte survival. Am J Vet Res 1983;44(10):1830–1.

40. Bassett JM, Borrett RA, Hanson C, et al. Anaemia in housed newborn lambs. Vet Rec 1995;136(6):137–40.
41. Ullrey DE, Miller ER, Long CH, et al. Sheep hematology from birth to maturity. I. Erythrocyte population, size and hemoglobin concentration. J Anim Sci 1965; 24:135–40.
42. Minatel L, Carfagnini JC. Copper deficiency and immune response in ruminants. Nutr Res 2000;20(10):1519–29.
43. Mohammed R, Lamand M. Cardiovascular lesions in cobalt-vitamin B12 deficient sheep. Ann Rech Vet 1986;17(4):447–50.
44. Eschbach JW, Mladenovic J, Garcia JF, et al. The anemia of chronic renal failure in sheep. Response to erythropoietin-rich plasma in vivo. J Clin Invest 1984;74(2): 434–41.
45. Ruchala P, Nemeth E. The pathophysiology and pharmacology of hepcidin. Trends Pharmacol Sci 2014;35(3):155–61.
46. Shen X, Chi Y, Xiong K. The effect of heavy metal contamination on humans and animals in the vicinity of a zinc smelting facility. PLoS One 2019;14(10):e0207423.
47. Mount ME, Feldman BF. Practical toxicologic diagnosis. Mod Vet Pract 1984; 65(8):589–95.
48. Garland T. Overview of gossypol poisoning. In: Merck veterinary manual. 2015. Available at: https://www.merckvetmanual.com/toxicology/gossypol-poisoning/ overview-of-gossypol-poisoning. Accessed April 24, 2020.
49. Vetter J. A biological hazard of our age: Bracken fern [Pteridium aquilinum (L.) Kuhn] - a review. Acta Vet Hung 2009;57(1):183–96.
50. Perez-Alenza MD, Blanco J, Sardon D, et al. Clinico-pathological findings in cattle exposed to chronic bracken fern toxicity. N Z Vet J 2006;54(4):185–92.
51. Schneider DJ, Marasas WF, Dale Kuys JC, et al. A field outbreak of suspected stachybotryotoxicosis in sheep. J S Afr Vet Assoc 1979;50(2):73–81.
52. Khan KN, Sagartz JE, Koenig G, et al. Systemic mastocytosis in a goat. Vet Pathol 1995;32(6):719–21.
53. Cain GR, East N, Moore PF. Myelofibrosis in young pygmy goats. Comp Hematol Int 1994;4:167–72.
54. Yang J, Liu Z, Niu Q, et al. Anaplasma phagocytophilum in sheep and goats in central and southeastern China. Parasit Vectors 2016;9(1):1–7.
55. Gorman JK, Hoar BR, Nieto NC, et al. Evaluation of Anaplasma phagocytophilum infection in experimentally inoculated sheep and determination of Anaplasma spp seroprevalence in 8 free-ranging sheep flocks in California and Oregon. Am J Vet Res 2012;73(7):1029–34.
56. Paternolli S, Villotti S, Landi P, et al An outbreak of Anaplasma phagocytophilum in a goat herd in the Province of Trento (North-eastern Italian Alps): a case report. In: Proceedings of the 29th World Buiatrics Congress. Dublin, Ireland, July 3-8, 2016. p.220-221.
57. Stuen S. Anaplasma phagocytophilum - the most widespread tick-borne infection in animals in Europe. Vet Res Commun 2007;31(Suppl 1):79–84.
58. Kaplan RM, Burke JM, Terrill TH, et al. Validation of the FAMACHA© eye color chart for detecting clinical anemia in sheep and goats on farms in the southern United States. Vet Parasitol 2004;123(1–2):105–20.
59. Paras KL, George MM, Vidyashankar AN, et al. Comparison of fecal egg counting methods in four livestock species. Vet Parasitol 2018;257:21–7.
60. Balcomb C, Foster D. Update on the use of blood and blood products in ruminants. Vet Clin North Am Food Anim Pract 2014;30(2):455–474, vii.

61. Smith JE, Dever M, Smith J, et al. Post-transfusion survival of 50Cr-labeled erythrocytes in neonatal foals. J Vet Intern Med 1992;6(3):183–5.
62. Mudge MC, Walker NJ, Borjesson DL, et al. Post-transfusion survival of biotin-labeled allogeneic RBCs in adult horses. Vet Clin Pathol 2012;41(1):56–62.
63. Luethy D, Stefanovski D, Salber R, et al. Prediction of packed cell volume after whole blood transfusion in small ruminants and south American camelids: 80 cases (2006–2016). J Vet Intern Med 2017;31(6):1900–4.
64. Buck RK, Stegmann GF, Poore LA, et al. Xenotransfusion with packed bovine red blood cells to a wildebeest calf (Connochaetes taurinus). J S Afr Vet Assoc 2018; 89(0):a1669.
65. Keeton STN, Navarre CB. Coccidiosis in large and small ruminants. Vet Clin North Am Food Anim Pract 2018;34(1):201–8.
66. Zajac AM, Garza J. Biology, epidemiology, and control of gastrointestinal nematodes of small ruminants. Vet Clin North Am Food Anim Pract 2020;36(1):73–87.
67. Smith GW, Davis JL, Smith SM, et al. Efficacy and pharmacokinetics of pantoprazole in alpacas. J Vet Intern Med 2010;24(4):949–55.
68. Balcomb CC, Heller MC, Chigerwe M, et al. Pharmacokinetics and efficacy of intravenous famotidine in adult cattle. J Vet Intern Med 2018;32(3):1283–9.
69. Constable PD, Hinchcliff KW, Done SH, et al. Diseases of the hemolymphatic and immune systems. In: Constable PD, Hinchcliff KW, Done SH, Grünberg W, editors. Veterinary medicine: a textbook of the diseases of cattle, horses, sheep, pigs and goats. 11th edition. St. Louis (MO): Elsevier; 2017.

Update on Small Ruminant Lentiviruses

Cindy Wolf, DVM*

KEYWORDS

- Small ruminant lentivirus • Ovine progressive pneumonia virus
- Caprine arthritis encephalitis virus • Indurative mastitis

KEY POINTS

- Small ruminant lentiviruses (SRLVs) cause lifelong infections that manifest primarily subclinically.
- SRLVs target lungs, mammary glands, joints, and brain, causing production losses due to immunopathologic lesions that affect normal function.
- Control programs rely on sensitive ELISA tests used for surveillance accompanied by strict segregation of seronegative animals away from animals of unknown or test-positive status.
- Seronegative sheep and goats produce more milk and stay in the flock/herd longer.

INTRODUCTION

Small ruminant lentiviruses (SLRVs) have been recognized throughout the world for decades.

Originally these viruses were thought to be species specific. But SRLVs share phylogenetic proximity and natural cross-species infectivity, facilitating infections between sheep and goats and even into wild ruminants.[1] Maedi was first described as a sheep respiratory disease in South Africa in 1915.[2] Ovine progressive pneumonia virus (OPPV) was first reported in Montana in 1923. The affected sheep were also described as lungers because they lagged behind others in the group.[3] Maedi/visna virus (MVV) was reported in 1933 in sheep in Iceland introduced from an importation and dispersion of Karakul rams from Germany.[4]

Initially, the caprine arthritis encephalitis virus (CAEV) was first believed to be a hereditary disease in Europe due to the observational relationship of clinical disease in certain family lines. In the United States, CAEV was first described as a viral leukoencephalomyelitis in 1974; the virus was isolated from goats with chronic arthritis a few years later by researchers in the same laboratory.[5] A few major sheep-raising

College of Veterinary Medicine, University of Minnesota, Saint Paul, MN, USA
* PO Box 422, Rushford, MN 55971.
E-mail address: wolfx006@umn.edu

Vet Clin Food Anim 37 (2021) 199–208
https://doi.org/10.1016/j.cvfa.2020.12.003
0749-0720/21/© 2020 Elsevier Inc. All rights reserved.

countries in the world, including Iceland, New Zealand, and Australia, are free of SRLVs, but CAEV is more widespread throughout the world. For purposes of this article, these viruses are discussed as 1 virus except where differences are pointed out. Their close relationship is valuable in the development and use of diagnostic tests.

GENERAL CHARACTERISTICS AND EFFECTS ON PRODUCTION

SRLVs characteristically infect sheep or goat hosts for life, slowly cause the development of immunopathologic lesions in specific target tissues, adapt to persist in host populations due to their ability to mutate and evade the host's immune response, and are spread primarily horizontally via contact with infected herdmates.

SRLVs have been introduced into flocks and herds primarily through the introduction of infected live animals. Approximately 30% of infected animals develop disease; the rest have subclinical infections. These subclinical SRLVs' manifestations are easily missed unless producers are measuring data and analyzing ewe/doe and lamb/kid performance. Intensive management and detailed performance analysis often demonstrate the profit-robbing nature of SRLVs when infections are present.

Production data of breeding age ewes (n = 1446) indicated that the SLRV-negative ewes produced significantly more kilograms of lamb at weaning (3.84 kg) compared with their test-positive flock mates. Because more test-negative ewes lambed compared with their test-positive flockmates, this weight comparison increased to 4.95 kg when all ewes exposed were included in the analysis. Over the lifetime of a ewe, these differences become financially significant. The weight differences at weaning were reported to be due to test-positive ewes' decreased ability to successfully and profitably rear lambs. The nursery-reared lambs, regardless of their dams' test status, did not differ in growth rates and weaning weights, which were statistically different for lambs reared by ewes of positive versus negative SLRV infection status.[6] Producers with SLRV-affected ewes experience higher production costs due to need for lamb supplementation (ie, cost of purchased milk replacer and required labor).

In regard to MVV, milk production records were analyzed over a 10-year period in 3 flocks of Spanish Laxta dairy sheep, with medium to high seroprevalence; results indicated that MVV seropositive status reduced milk yield by 6.7%, which was an economically significant rate. Lost profit would have more than covered the costs of annual flock testing.[7]

Another retrospective study evaluated the effect of CAEV serologic status on milk production levels in 22 herds of dairy goats in Spain. Length of lactation, milk yield, and milk fat and lactose levels were significantly lower in seropositive goats versus seronegative and worsened as lactation number increased.[8]

VIRUS INTERACTION AND HOST REACTION

Unlike other mammalian lentiviruses, SRLVs do not cause an immunodeficiency. SRLVs result in an infection for life: their proviral DNA persists in monocytes and evades the host's immune system, thus permitting virus to disseminate to target tissues.[9]

Historically, concern focused on increased infection and subclinical disease susceptibility in certain breeds, specifically Border Leicester, Texel, and Finnsheep breeds,[10,11] but more recent research suggests these observations may be the effect of host genetics.[12]

Reduced lentivirus susceptibility has been documented in sheep with specific ovine transmembrane protein 154 (TMEM154) haplotypes. Although specific haplotypes were documented as protective, this finding was not an all-or-none phenomenon. Sheep possessing the ancestral form of TMEM154 gene were almost 3-times more likely to become infected in the same environment as age-matched pairs possessing the mutant forms. Haplotypes 2 and 3 were more predictive of OPPV infection.[12]

Another study of the same population of sheep showed that 39-month-old ewes with TMEM154 diplotypes 1,3 and 3,3 had an 8.5-times higher probability of nonmaternally acquired infection than ewes with TMEM154 1,1 diplotypes.[13] Neither of these studies determined the function of the TMEM154 protein, but findings suggest that sheep without TMEM154 function may have a selective advantage when exposed to OPPV. Heaton and colleagues[12] found that sheep with TMEM154 4,4 haplotypes (called knockouts) lived and reproduced normally. Lastly, a small percentage of sheep with haplotypes 1,1 were found to be infected with OPPV—consistent with the concept of conditional host genetic resistance. Contributing factors to overcoming host genetic resistance to OPPV include exposure to a high viral load, long duration of repeated viral doses, viral genetic adaptation to host defenses, and multiple routes of infection.[12]

SRLVs have been typed into A–E genotypes. To date, the SRLVs in the United States are A2 subtypes, which is based on *gag* and/or *pol* variation. Four subgroups of A2 have been identified in the United States. One of these subgroups has infected sheep with the TMEM154 4,4 diplotype.[14] Therefore, additional research will be helpful in guiding the development of genetically resistant flocks and genetic management of SRLVs interaction with available host genetics.

AWARENESS AND PREVALENCE

The Sheep 2011 study was conducted by the US Department of Agriculture National Animal Health Monitoring System (NAHMS) from sheep operations in 22 of the country's major sheep-producing States. These operations represented 70.1% of US farms with ewes and 85.5% of the ewe inventory. Half of all operations (53.5%) were familiar with OPPV. For the 53.5% of operations that were familiar with OPPV, 16.2% had a flock health management program directed to control or prevent OPPV. Of the total, 18.7% reported never being infected with OPP, 5.4% indicated their flock currently was infected with OPP, and 3.3% indicated their flock was previously infected but now was OPP negative. Approximately three-fourths of operations (72.7%) did not know their current OPP status.[15] These statistics are based on producers' views but not corroborated by serologic data.

OPPV antibody ELISA testing was performed on sera collected from 1415 sheep from 54 flocks in Wyoming during the NAHMS Sheep 2011 study. The seropositivity rates of OPPV in this regional sample were 18% in the sheep and 47.5% in the flocks. These flocks ranged in size and grazing types.[16]

CLINICAL SIGNS AND LESIONS

SRLVs target 4 specific organ sites, which include the lungs (primarily OPPV), mammary glands (both OPPV and CAEV), joints (largely CAEV), and the central nervous system (CNS) (both OPPV and CAEV). SLRVs do not infect lymphocytes, unlike other immunodeficiency-causing lentiviruses; instead, characteristic lymphoproliferative lesions slowly develop in target tissues. Viral replication occurs in the monocytes as they leave the blood or bone marrow and mature to macrophages and localize in the target tissues. Infection causes a humoral and cell mediated response but neither confers immunity. Instead, the disease is immunopathologic in nature because the host immune system reacts to viral antigens, especially surface glycoproteins.

CAEV-infected adult goats present most commonly with a chronic arthritis, which progresses over time, is unresponsive to treatment except for palliative care, and ultimately produces an animal welfare situation indicating euthanasia. The carpi are the primary joints involved but others affected can include tarsal, femorotibial, femoropatellar (stifle), metatarsal and metacarpal, and coxofemoral joints in addition to the atlanto-occipital and carpal bursae. Any number of joints can be affected at the same time. Examinations should include comparison to joints of unaffected herdmates. With time, the affected joint capsule and adjacent soft tissue become progressively mineralized, bony exostoses form, and joint(s) collapse with eventual ankylosis. The decreased range of motion and constant pain from the changes, discussed previously, result in persistent weight loss. Diagnostic testing should include arthrocentesis in conjunction with serum ELISA, herd history, and radiographic findings.

SRLV-infected adult does and ewes can both develop bilateral indurative mastitis. Around the time of parturition, the udder appears normal unless palpated. Both halves feel diffusely firm without pitting edema. Even with stimulation to assist with milk letdown, scant quantities of milk are present bilaterally. Often the flock owner does not realize there is an insufficient quantity of milk produced until an affected ewe's lambs are noted to be starving or have died. In dairy sheep and goats, this condition is detected earlier due to the more frequent and intimate nature of human-small ruminant udder interaction at milking. Affected animals usually are culled. Affected mammary glands have characteristic lymphoproliferative lesions on histopathologic examination, evident as increased smooth muscle and fibrous connective tissue; lymphoid follicle proliferation adjacent to ductules; lymphocytic, mononuclear, and plasma cell infiltrates in the mammary parenchyma; and a net loss of milk-secreting alveoli. These histologic changes are similar to those observed in SRLV-induced interstitial pneumonia. A diagnosis is based on the combination of herd history, serum or milk ELISA, milk polymerase chain reaction (PCR), and potentially biopsy of mammary tissue.

The clinical presentation of SRLVs interstitial pneumonia is that of a progressive dyspnea. Affected animals often are thought to need treatment with broad-spectrum antimicrobial agents for a presumed bacterial pneumonia, which, if present, is a sequela of a primary SRLV infection. Initially, treated animals may improve slightly only to relapse from their primary SRLV lung disease. Affected animals lose body condition as they become increasingly dyspneic. Fine-needle aspirate on a sedated small ruminant can produce sufficient lung sample for histologic examination. Characteristic histopathologic changes resemble those found in the mammary gland (ie, lymphoid nodule proliferation; increased smooth muscle and fibrous connective tissue; alveolar wall thickening; and peribronchial and perivascular accumulations of mononuclear cells). At necropsy, gross findings are diffusely firm, enlarged, gray-colored lungs that may show rib impressions and enlarged mediastinal lymph nodes.

The neurologic form of CAEV affects kids between 1 month and 6 months of age, with some cases occurring in older goats. In contrast, visna affects mature sheep. Like the other clinical syndromes, the disease in both species is progressive and ultimately results in the need for humane euthanasia. The condition in kids starts as a rear limb paresis that develops into paralysis affecting all 4 limbs. Initially, the kid is bright and alert and has a normal appetite. In sheep, there are 2 forms. The brain form presents as a slight head tilt and circling toward the affected side due to lesions in the lateral ventricles. Some animals may have hindlimb ataxia and are hypermetric. Progression occurs over a couple of months necessitating euthanasia. When visna affects the spinal cord, the classic sign is knuckling of 1 of the rear limb fetlocks even while the limb stays weight bearing.[17] These presentations of CAEV kid leukoencephalomyelitis and visna CNS disease notably are seen more commonly in populations with high seropositive rates.

TRANSMISSION

Historically the lactogenic route of transmission was considered the primary means of spread for both OPPV and CAEV. But over the past decade, research has proved that nonmaternal transmission is truly the primary mode of OPP viral spread.[13] Major factors in transmission include the length of time that uninfected sheep experience exposure while mixed with infected groups, animal density, and housing type.[13] Confinement housing, which is correlated with high stocking rates, strongly influences transmission compared with pasture-based flock transmission rates.[18]

There are concerns about more minor routes of transmission in eradication programs. For instance, semen has been implicated yet the rate of transmission via semen has not been well quantified. SRLVs are known to be present in ovine male genital tracts when a concurrent orchitis, epididymitis, or posthitis is present,[19,20] whereas seropositive bucks have been identified as a risk factor influencing herd seroprevalence. The breeding behavior of bucks and in estrus does results in a shared airspace where aerosolization of nasal secretions, saliva, urine, and semen occurs. Transmission may be influenced more by such normal behavior than infected semen alone. Intrauterine transmission with the OPPV is reported to occur infrequently (5%) but has not been reported with CAEV.[21,22] Standard International Embryo Transfer Society protocols can make embryos of unknown status safe to transfer.

Fomite transmission of CAEV and OPPV occurs through use of contaminated milking equipment and poor milking practices (ie, milking mixed infection status groups together, use of common preparatory equipment across groups and exposure to spilled milk and contaminated cloths and hands). Many goat dairies practice artificial rearing of neonatal kids. Even with prompt removal of newborn kids, a small percentage of kids can be seropositive when first tested. Possible explanations include in utero transmission, transmission during the kidding process either via vaginal contact, unobserved accidental colostral ingestion, or exposure to the dam's oral and respiratory contaminated secretions during normal immediate postpartum licking of the kid.[23] Lastly, could a seropositive test result actually indicate persistence of maternal antibody, dependent on the efficacy of the heat treatment of colostrum and pasteurization of milk? The role of shared fomites used during routine management, such as common needles, tattoo pliers, and hot iron disbudders, is difficult to confirm. Disinfection of equipment and employment of single-use needles or needleless vaccine injectors are effective control practices to reduce risk of transmission.[24] Greenwood and colleagues[25] suggested that certain behaviors also may contribute to spread of infection in goats. These include self-teat sucking, biting, and eye licking as documented in hot weather environments; nasal and oral contact with anal and vaginal areas; milk leaking; drinking of urine; and anal intercourse among bucks.

CONTROL

In general, effective SRLV control programs rely on an understanding of how SRLVs are spread and the use of testing regimens that rely on highly sensitive, specific, and frequent tests. Control protocols need to be written and reviewed quarterly. Seropositive animals need to be removed from the tested group as soon as test results are available.

Challenges inherent with effective control programs include:
the variable time between infection and seroconversion
the virus transmission possible from a retained animal that has fluctuating test
    results

the occassional false-positive test results due to unknown reasons. Because of these testing challenges, control programs can become expensive, stretch patience, and strain commitment on thepart of the flock or herd owner.

TESTING

Key points in a control and ultimately eradication program are as follows[26,27]:

- There is not a perfect 1-time test. Most control programs are based on using sensitive serum-based ELISA tests that are performed repeatedly on the population that the flock/herd owner is working toward making seronegative and virus-free. This approach can test (1) weaned, potential replacement lambs to enable producers to keep their own genetics (and may be less expensive in the long run than purchasing seronegative animals); (2) yearlings that have not yet cohabited with mature ewes; and/or (3) ewes and rams of unknown status.
- Seropositive animals must be removed from the tested group as soon as test results become available. From a practical standpoint, they need to be moved to a well-fenced area and have a special, highly visible tag or paint brand placed such that they can easily be identified if an accidental mixing of groups occurs.
- Negative lambs can be raised by positive ewes. A majority of new infections occur postweaning via adult-to-adult contact after young replacement sheep join the infected or uncharacterized adult flock. Therefore, producers can salvage their genetics as they rebuild to a seronegative flock.
- Highly sensitive ELISAs can detect new infections but also present challenges of yielding false-positive results for no apparent reason. Also, ELISAs cannot immediately detect new infections.
- Seronegative animals must be kept entirely separate from seropositive sheep/ goats and away from animals of unknown status. Weaned healthy lambs/kids as young as 6 months can be tested. Animals scheduled to be tested should not be vaccinated in the preceding 2 weeks to 3 weeks ahead of their blood draw because this practice may result in transient false-positive results.
- Repeated testing at 2-month to 3-month intervals is crucial for early detection and subsequent removal of newly infected animals.
- This high-frequency testing is continued until 2 to 3 consecutive, whole-group negative tests have occurred. Usually, when starting with weaned lambs that are an average of 6 months of age, a total of 3 to 4 tests is required to achieve 2 consecutive whole-group negative tests.
- Purchasing negative replacements may bring in other health problems worse than OPPV. At least OPPV travels with the sheep, in and out—it does not persist around the farm after the sheep leave.
- Control programs require producer commitment to the financial, time, and management costs. Ideally a budget is prepared
  - For the cost of repeated testing
  - For facilities needed for appropriate separation of seropositive and seronegative groups
- To cull animals that are showing clinical signs of SRLV, which often serve as an aerosol source of virus and should be removed promptly from the operation.[28]
- To ELISA test incoming animals on arrival and 60 days later, prior to release from quarantine. These include newly purchased animals as well as those returning from shows in contact with other sheep/goats.

A phenomenon exists where an individual ewe can repeatedly test negative but serves as a source of virus. This is suspected to occur in the situation when a flock culls the seropositive sheep after each test and on the next whole-flock test all are seronegative, but then a few seropositive sheep are detected on the next consecutive test. Eradication is challenged by the necessity to diagnose 1 or more clinically normal yet persistently infected animal(s), and a very small number of those escape most current detection methods. Worldwide, SRLV control program and laboratory managers have suspected the occurrence of this phenomenon. An accelerated testing approach has been tried that uses an improved real-time (RT)-PCR in conjunction with ELISA testing at 60-day to 90-day intervals to address this situation.[29] One protocol that has been applied to contend with this challenge is described by Brinkhof and colleagues in 2010.[30] Short interval testing every 3 months using a highly sensitive ELISA and PCR which was used to detect proviral SRLV sequences that had been integrated into the host genome. The disadvantage of this approach is cost. Otherwise, this technique returned the study flock to SRLV negative status after 3 rounds of testing at 2-month to 3-month intervals. The leader-gag RT-PCR found some infected animals before they were antibody positive. The leader-gag sequence was chosen due to being highly conserved, which is valuable with SRLV due to likelihood of mutation. It also could be applied to resolve inconclusive results, such as sheep that unexpectedly are antibody positive in a previously seronegative flock as well as confirming infection status where an individual animal's test results fluctuate. Currently, there is not yet a universally recommended protocol to resolve confounding results.

CONTROL IN GOATS VIA PASTEURIZED REARING SYSTEM

- Remove newborn kids immediately from dams and herdmates at birth to prevent kids from being licked or touched by any doe's secretions.[23] Parturition may be induced in dams with known breeding dates that have reached greater than or equal to day 145 of pregnancy by intramuscular injection of 2 mL to 3 mL of prostaglandin (dinoprost tromethamine injection, 10–15 mg). Kidding should be expected an average of 32 hours later, with a range of 30 hours to 36 hours. By inducing parturition, kidding may be anticipated and attended to permit immediate removal of newborn kids from their dam.
- Wash off amniotic fluid and placenta from newborn kids followed by drying them to prevent chilling; place in an isolated nursery that is separated by 2 m from other goat pens or housing.
- Feed heat treated colostrum (heat and hold at 56°C for 1 hour) for first 24 hours of life.
- Raise on pasteurized milk (heat to 73.9°C for 15 seconds).
- Perform serologic testing of all kids reared via this strict artificial rearing method every 6 months with prompt removal of seropositive kids until 2 consecutive whole-group negative tests. This seronegative group needs separate housing throughout the goats' lifetime. This housing should not be adjacent to seropositive or unknown status goats. Airborne virus has been documented from air breathed out of seropositive cull sheep.

Even though the OPP virus has been found in saliva, respiratory secretions, colostrum and milk, urine, and feces, control programs are effective that focus on minimizing or even preventing nonmaternal contact transmission from infected adult animals. Because the role that contact with infected sheep plays now is understood, lambs no longer need to be snatched at birth and artificially reared. This alleviates the need to attend lambing around the clock since ewes are much less responsive to induction of parturition compared with goats. The role of nonmaternal transmission needs to be evaluated in goats, which is especially relevant as the numbers of meat goats continue to rise in the United States.

Also of critical significance is the mathematical model of transmission devised by Illius and colleagues,[18] which estimates the transmission rates were 1000-times faster in housed ewes compared with pastured ewes. Prevalence is expected to double each year in housed ewes even when the initial incidence starts at a low level.[18]

Depopulation and restocking with virus-free animals are no longer required to make a farm SRLV-free.

SUMMARY

SRLV surveillance and control programs require significant time and financial commitment on the part of small ruminant producers, their veterinary health advisors, and SRLVs program managers.

Interested producers are motivated for the following reasons:
- They own small purebred flocks.
- They have access to facilities for running 2 flocks (a seronegative population and seropositive population).
- They have experienced first-hand with the decreased levels of production and resultant costs associated with a high seropositive rate.
- They have an increased demand and receive a better sale price for their seronegative breeding stock.

It is reported that flocks and herds that are highly productive (ie, lamb and kid in confinement multiple times per year) experience the negative effects of SRLV infection more profoundly than herds with less productive animals. Producers report that test positive ewes have a shorter productive life due to development of dyspnea or lower production levels in flocks and herds that monitor individual performance levels. A higher culling rate of female sheep and goats in their prime of life costs the producer by increasing replacement costs. Progress toward maintaining flock/herd genetics while growing the seronegative group size in a flock/herd is possible by following the rigorous protocols described. Ultimately, most producers phase out the seropositive group.[31]

CLINICS CARE POINTS

- SRLVs cause a lifelong infection, which can be either subclinical or clinical.
- SRLVs target lungs, mammary glands, joints, and the central nervous system and cause characteristic clinical signs and lesions.
- SRLVs can be controlled through rigorous serum ELISA and PCR testing programs and management grouping based on test results.

DISCLOSURE

The author has nothing to disclose.

REFERENCES

1. Caroline L, Minardi CJC, Jean-Francois M. SRLVs: a genetic continuum of lentiviral species in sheep and goats with cumulative evidence of cross species transmission. Curr HIV Res 2010;8:94–100.
2. Smith MC, Sherman DM. Goat medicine. 2nd edition. Ames (IA): Wiley-Blackwell; 2009. p. 96–106, 192-196.
3. Marsh H. Progressive pneumonia in sheep. J Am Vet Med Assoc 1923;62: 458–72.
4. Gislason G. Experiments and further studies on a few diseases: maedi. In: Report for a special committee of the Icelandic ministry of agriculture on import of domestic animals and karakul diseases. Icelandic Ministry, Reykjavik, Iceland; 1947. p. 238-46.
5. Crawford TB, Adams DS, Cheevers WP, et al. Chronic arthritis in goats caused by a retrovirus. Science 1980;207:997–9.
6. Keen JE, Hungerford LL, Littledike ET, et al. Effect of ewe ovine lentivirus infection on ewe and lamb productivity. Prev Vet Med 1997;30:155–69.
7. Juste RA, Villoria M, Leginagoikoa I, et al. Milk productions losses in Laxta dairy sheep associated with small ruminant lentivirus infection. Prev Vet Med 2020;176: 104886.
8. Martínez-Navalón B, Cristòfol P, Ernesto AG, et al. Quantitative estimation of the impact of caprine arthritis encephalitis virus infection on milk production in dairy goats. Vet J 2013;197:311–7.
9. Larruskain Amaia, Jugo Begoña. Retroviral infections in sheep and goats: small ruminant lentiviruses and host interaction. Viruses 2013;5(8):2043–61.
10. Cutlip RC, Lehmkuhl HD, Brogden KA, et al. Breed susceptibility to ovine progressive pneumonia (maedi/visna) virus. Vet Microbiol 1986;12:283–8.
11. Houwers DJ, Visscher AH, Defize PR. Importance of ewe/lamb relationship and breed in the epidemiology of maedi-visna virus infections. Res Vet Sci 1989; 46:5–8.
12. Heaton MP, Clawson ML, Chitko-Mckown CG, et al. Reduced lentivirus susceptibility in sheep with TMEM154 mutations. PLoS Genet 2012;8(1):e1002467.
13. Leymaster KA, Chitko-McKown CG, Heaton MP. Incidence of infection in 39-month-old ewes with TMEM154 diplotypes "1 1," "1 3," and "3 3" after natural exposure to ovine progressive pneumonia virus. J Anim Sci 2015;93(1):41–5.
14. Clawson ML, Reid R, Gennie S, et al. Genetic subgroup of small ruminant lentiviruses that infects sheep homozygous for TMEM154 frameshift deletion mutation A4Δ53. Vet Res 2015;46:22.
15. National animal health monitoring system. Sheep 2011. Part 1: reference of sheep management practices in the United States, 2011. Fort Collins (CO): USDA APHIS Veterinary Services Centers for Epidemiology and Animal Health; 2012. Available at: www.aphis.usda.gov/animal_health/nahms/sheep/downloads/sheep11/Sheep11_dr_Part1pdf.
16. Gerstner S, Jeffrey JA, John VD, et al. Prevalence of and risk factors associated with ovine progressive pneumonia in Wyoming sheep flocks. J Am Vet Med Assoc 2015;247:932–7.
17. Scott PR. Sheep medicine. 2nd edition. Boca Raton (FL): CRC Press; 2015. p. 216–8.
18. Illius AW, Lievaart-Peterson K, McNeilly TN, et al. Epidemiology and control of maedi-visna virus: curing the flock. PLoS One 2020;15(9):e0238781.

19. de la Concha Bermejillo A, Magnus-Corral S, Brodie SJ, et al. Venereal shedding of ovine lentivirus in infected rams. Am J Vet Res 1996;57:684–8.
20. Peterson K, Brinkhof J, Houwers DJ, et al. Presence of pro-lentiviral DNA in male sexual organs and ejaculates of small ruminants. Theriogenology 2008;69: 433–42.
21. Cross RF, Smith CK, Moorhead PD. Vertical transmission of progressive pneumonia of sheep. Am J Vet Res 1975;36:465–8.
22. Cutlip RC, Lehmkuhl HD, Jackson TA. Intrauterine transmission of ovine progressive pneumonia virus. Am J Vet Res 1981;42:1795–7.
23. Rowe JD, East NE. Risk factors for transmission and methods for control of caprine arthritis-encephalitis infection. Vet Clin North Am Food Anim Pract 1997;13:35–53.
24. Herrmann-Hoesing LM. Diagnostic assays used to control small ruminant lentiviruses. J Vet Diagn Invest 2010;22(6):843–55.
25. Greenwood PL, North RN, Kirkland PD. Prevalence, spread and control of caprine arthritis-encephalitis virus in dairy goat herds in New South Wales. Aust Vet J 1995;72:341–5.
26. Available at: https://www.bah.state.mn.us/media/OPP-Final-Guidelines-2020.pdf.
27. Kalogianni AI, Bossis I, Ekateriniadou L, et al. Etiology, epizootiology and control of maedi-visna in dairy sheep: a review. Animals (Basel) 2020;10:616.
28. Villoria M, Leginagoikoa I, Lujan L, et al. Detection of Small Ruminant Lentiviruses in environmental samples of air and water. Small Rumin Res 2013;110:155–60.
29. Brinkhof JMA, van Maanen C, Wigger R, et al. Specific detection of small ruminant lentiviral nucleic acid sequences located in the proviral long terminal repeat and leader-gag regions using real-time polymerase chain reaction. J Virol Methods 2008;147:338–44.
30. Brinkhof JMA, Moll L, van Maanen C, et al. Use of serology and polymerase chain reaction for the rapid eradication of small ruminant lentivirus infections from a sheep flock: a case report. Res Vet Sci 2010;88:41–3.
31. Pérez M, Muñoz JA, Biescas E, et al. Successful Visna/maedi control in a highly infected ovine dairy flock using serologic segregation and management strategies. Prev Vet Med 2013;112:423–7.

Secure Sheep and Wool Supply Plan for Continuity of Business

Danelle A. Bickett-Weddle, DVM, MPH, PhD[a],*,
Renée D. Dewell, DVM, MS[b], Charles E. McIntosh, BS[c]

KEYWORDS

- Foot and mouth disease • Veterinarians • Preparedness • Biosecurity
- Secure sheep and wool supply plan

KEY POINTS

- The Secure Sheep and Wool Supply (SSWS) Plan for Continuity of Business (COB) facilitates sheep industry preparedness for, and response to, a foot and mouth disease (FMD) outbreak in the United States.
- Clinical signs of FMD in sheep are often inapparent or very subtle.
- US Department of Agriculture strategies to control FMD include stopping movement of susceptible animals and their products, rapid identification of infected animals, strategic depopulation with proper disposal, and vaccination.
- Movement into, within, or out of FMD Control Area(s) will occur by permit only and will be based on the risk posed by that movement and the premises' ability to meet permit requirements.
- The SSWS Plan includes guidance for producers and packers (when requesting) and officials (when evaluating requests) for animal and/or animal product movement permits, once animal movement resumes.

INTRODUCTION

The Secure Sheep and Wool Supply (SSWS) Plan for Continuity of Business (COB) was created as a collaborative effort between the US sheep industry and state, federal, and academic partners and is available at www.securesheepwool.org. It facilitates sheep industry preparedness for, and response to, a foot and mouth disease (FMD) outbreak in the United States. FMD is a highly contagious foreign animal

[a] Center for Food Security and Public Health, Iowa State University, 2176 VMPM, Ames, IA 50014, USA; [b] Center for Food Security and Public Health, Iowa State University, 2124 VMPM, Ames, IA 50014, USA; [c] Center for Food Security and Public Health, Iowa State University, 2160 VMPM, Ames, IA 50014, USA
* Corresponding author.
E-mail address: DBWEDDLE@IASTATE.EDU

Vet Clin Food Anim 37 (2021) 209–219
https://doi.org/10.1016/j.cvfa.2020.11.002
0749-0720/21/© 2020 Elsevier Inc. All rights reserved.
vetfood.theclinics.com

disease that affects sheep and other cloven-hooved animals, such as swine, cattle, goats, and deer. The United States eradicated FMD in 1929, yet it remains endemic in two-thirds of the countries of the world.[1] FMD is not a public health or food safety concern, but its impact on animal health, welfare, and production affects food and animal product availability and trade from countries with this animal disease. If introduced into the United States, FMD will have a devastating impact on animal health; the agriculture industry; and the livelihood of producers, veterinarians, transporters, packers, and processors, other allied industries, and food security for the American consumer.

FMD is caused by a picornavirus that can be spread animal-to-animal through direct contact and via bodily secretions and excretions (breath, saliva, urine, manure, milk, semen). Fomites like vehicles, equipment, footwear, and clothing that become contaminated can also spread FMD indirectly among animals and between premises. Aerosol spread has also been implicated in outbreaks.[2] Sheep are primarily infected through direct contact with FMD-infected animals.[3] Clinical signs in sheep are often inapparent or very subtle. Transmission between sheep may also occur before clinical signs are noted.[3,4] The movement of infected but undetected sheep presents a major risk for spreading the virus during an FMD outbreak.[5] The ease of virus spread necessitates strict control measures if a country aims to contain and eradicate FMD.

If FMD were diagnosed in the United States, the US Department of Agriculture (USDA) strategies to control this contagious animal disease include stopping movement of susceptible animals and their products, rapid identification of infected animals, strategic depopulation with proper disposal, and vaccination.[6] Regulatory officials (local, state, tribal, and federal officials, as appropriate) have the authority and responsibility to establish regulatory Control Areas around FMD-infected premises (those diagnosed with positive animals). They also can regulate animal, animal product (wool, semen, embryos), and other movements that pose a risk for virus spread within, into, and out of these Control Areas.[7] Sheep producers and wool processors will be affected by the movement restrictions even if their animals are not infected or wool is not contaminated with the FMD virus. The SSWS Plan for COB also provides opportunities for producers with animals that have no evidence of infection to maintain business continuity during an FMD outbreak.

BACKGROUND

On the first diagnosis of FMD in the United States, the USDA Animal and Plant Health Inspection Service (APHIS) will be the lead federal agency in charge of managing the outbreak response. The USDA APHIS will work together with the State Animal Health Officials (SAHO) who have infected premises within their state and are authorized to issue premises quarantines. The USDA has a series of guidance documents that address controlling, containing, and eradicating FMD, the most comprehensive being the Foot-and-Mouth Disease Response Plan: The Red Book, available at: www.aphis.usda.gov/animal_health/emergency_management/downloads/fmd_responseplan.pdf.

The USDA APHIS also provides Ready Reference Guides, which are brief summaries about many relevant critical activities for an FMD response, that are available at: www.aphis.usda.gov/aphis/ourfocus/animalhealth/emergency-management/ct_fadprep_readyreferenceguides.

One critical activity involves movement controls to contain FMD. The USDA recommends a 72-hour national movement standstill of susceptible species and animal products (wool, semen, and embryos) once FMD is diagnosed. Pending the outbreak investigation, the movement standstill may be extended. It may take several days or weeks for the livestock industry and state and federal officials to understand the extent of the outbreak and have confidence that animals with no evidence of infection can move without spreading FMD.[7]

Once the national movement standstill lifts, movement restrictions may remain for the regulatory Control Areas(s) to limit risk of disease spread by animals, animal products, vehicles, and other equipment. Movement into, within, or out of Control Area(s) will be by permit only and based on the risk posed by that movement and the premises' ability to meet permit requirements. Regulatory Officials managing the incident will determine the movement permitting requirements.[7]

CONTINUITY OF BUSINESS PLANS

Prolonged movement restrictions will negatively impact the livestock industry and animal welfare. Livestock operations affected by movement restrictions, but with animals not infected with FMD, will need to restart movement as soon as possible to support business continuity in a way that is consistent with mitigating the risk of spreading FMD.[7] A delicate balance must be struck between controlling an FMD outbreak while not economically destroying the affected industries. Pre-planning is critical to minimize the impact. Providing opportunities for premises that meet permitting criteria and have no evidence of FMD infection to move their animals or animal products to market or the next phase of production also benefits American consumers and livestock-related industries. The USDA has developed *FAD PReP/NAHEMS Continuity of Business (COB) Guidelines,* which are available at: www.aphis.usda.gov/animal_health/emergency_management/downloads/nahems_guidelines/cob_nahems.pdf.

The USDA also funded several of the Secure Food Supply Plans for Continuity of Business, beginning in 2007 with the egg industry due to the global consequences that highly pathogenic avian influenza (HPAI) was causing. The Secure Egg Supply Plan evolved over a decade, and several HPAI outbreaks in the United States, resulting in the Secure Poultry Supply Plan, which encompasses eggs, turkeys, and broiler chickens. This business continuity plan was applied by the poultry industry and state and federal agencies during the 2014 to 2015, 2016, and 2017 HPAI outbreaks and the 2018 to 2020 virulent Newcastle Disease outbreak.

COB Plans have been created for several livestock sectors, including milk, pork, beef, sheep, and wool. Sheep operations that follow the SSWS Plan guidance will be better prepared to request a movement permit once movement restarts.[7]

SECURE SHEEP AND WOOL SUPPLY PLAN FOR CONTINUITY OF BUSINESS

In 2019, the American Sheep Industry (ASI) Association provided funding to the Center for Food Security and Public Health (CFSPH) at Iowa State University, College of Veterinary Medicine, to create the SSWS Plan for COB. The process to create the resources involved the formation and engagement of a very collaborative and diverse group of stakeholders. Individuals involved in the daily management of sheep on pasture, range, public lands, in feedlots, and at packing plants, as well as wool processors reviewed documents and offered insight, perspective, and alternatives. Likewise, stakeholders involved in the regulatory aspects at the state and federal levels provided review and expertise. Educators in extension and academia across the United States provided input.

Building on all the resources created through the other Secure Food Supply Plans and aligning with the guidance in the USDA response documents, the SSWS Plan for COB and 27 other supporting documents ranging in length from 1 to 44 pages were created and posted on the Web site at www.securesheepwool.org. The guidance and language are consistent wherever possible with the other Secure Food Supply Plans and supporting documents. Unique aspects of the sheep and wool industries were included where applicable. FMD infects multiple species; producers and Regulatory Officials need consistency in messaging for effective preparedness and response. Lessons learned through stakeholder discussions then contributed to the improvement of the Secure Milk, Beef, and Pork Supply Plans and resources.

DISCUSSION

The SSWS Plan includes guidance for producers and packers (when requesting) and officials (when evaluating requests) for animal and/or animal product movement permits, once animal movement resumes. Regulatory Officials also may implement additional requirements depending on the scope of the outbreak. All interstate movements also must meet existing movement/state entry requirements in addition to outbreak-specific conditions. Implementing the guidance outlined in the SSWS Plan before an outbreak may decrease the risk of disease exposure and spread. It also facilitates the eventual issuing of movement permits for sheep premises with no evidence of infection, and for allied industries.[7] **Table 1** provides a summary of movement permit guidance.

TRACEABILITY

One of the first steps in requesting a movement permit during an FMD outbreak is to provide Regulatory Officials with traceability information, that is, "who" wants to move "how much of what item" to "where." The USDA will need traceability information throughout the outbreak to inform the epidemiology of the outbreak. Trading partners

Table 1
Summary of movement permit guidance[a] for sheep, semen, and embryos located within a control area during an FMD response

Permitting Guidance for Movement of Sheep, Semen, Embryos	Condition Met?
1. Traceability information is available (PIN, GPS Coordinates, and information on type and number of animals/quantity of wool/semen/embryos moved)	Yes
2. Biosecurity measures listed in the Biosecurity Checklist are in place and acceptable to Responsible Regulatory Officials	Yes
3. Trace back/forward information is acceptable; premises is not designated as Infected, Suspect, or Contact	Yes
4. Destination premises and state are willing to accept the sheep/semen/embryos	Yes
5. No evidence of infection based on disease monitoring (surveillance)	Yes
Permit guidance to move sheep/semen/embryos if all above responses are "Yes"	Consider Issuing MOVEMENT PERMIT

Abbreviations: FMD, foot and mouth disease; GPS, global positioning system; PIN, premises identification number.
[a] For information on issuing permits for wool movement out of a Control Area, as well as FMD virus survivability in wool, inactivation recommendations, and traceability refer to the *SSWS Wool Handling during an FMD Outbreak* document available at: https://securesheepwool.org/Assets/SSWS_Wool-Handling-During-FMD-Outbreak.pdf.
From Secure Sheep and Wool Supply. Secure Sheep and Wool Supply (SSWS) Plan for Continuity of Business. Available at https://securesheepwool.org/Assets/Secure-Sheep-and-Wool-Supply-Plan-for-Continuity-of-Business.pdf; with permission.

expect the United States to provide accurate traceability information during the outbreak to document where disease is and is not. To progress toward disease freedom, provision of traceability information to the World Organization for Animal Health (OIE) to describe the control, containment, and eradication procedures will be necessary. Accurate and complete record keeping is a critical part of traceability to manage an FMD outbreak and move toward disease freedom.

With respect to a movement permit request, the "who" is the physical location of the animals on the premises. During an FMD outbreak, a premises identification number (PIN or PremID) will be required for all livestock operations that want to move items into, within, or out of a Control Area. A PIN is a 7-digit alphanumeric number that can be requested from the office of the relevant SAHO. Veterinary clinics with haul-in facilities also should request a PIN. The USDA provides information about how to obtain a PIN on their Web site at: https://www.aphis.usda.gov/aphis/ourfocus/animalhealth/traceability/state-pin/state-pin. The PIN is uniquely linked to the geospatial location reflecting the actual location of the animals on the premises. This includes a valid 911 address and a set of matching coordinates (latitude and longitude).

The "how much of what item" is the quantity of animals (number of head) or animal product (ie, semen, embryos, bales of wool) that needs to move. Although some risk is assumed when moving animals or animal products during an FMD outbreak, potential movements are carefully evaluated before permits are issued. Movement permit decisions will be determined based on the estimated risk of the requested movement, which is partially affected by the type of item (live animals pose a greater risk than wool that has been stored using an appropriate time and temperature protocol designated by the OIE to inactive FMD virus). "Where" the item is moving is an important component of the risk assessment. Does the item stay within the Control Area? Or, is it being transported to another state? A PIN is required for both the premises of origin and the destination premises. The business transaction and communication between the supplier (sheep producer/rancher) and the buyer (next phase of production) must occur before requesting a movement permit. The buyer at the destination site must be willing to accept the item from a Control Area. The buyer may require additional assurances, such as evidence of enhanced biosecurity or diagnostic test results, before agreeing to accept the movement. Those aspects are covered next.

Producers may already have a national PIN assigned if they have received official sheep tags in the past (sometimes referred to as scrapie tags) as part of the National Scrapie Eradication Program. A PIN also is required to obtain a 15-digit "840" tag or implant used to identify sheep.[7]

Producers, packers, markets, and veterinarians with haul-in clinic facilities are encouraged to validate their PIN with SAHOs to ensure their data accurately represents the location of the animals and not a mailbox at a residence or business affiliated with the animal premises. Validated PINs speed up communication and response during an outbreak.[7]

WOOL TRACEABILITY

Movement of wool and wool products will likely be restricted during an FMD outbreak because wool can harbor virus. Traceability of wool bales/bags from infected farms or commingled wool from multiple flocks will be needed in an FMD outbreak. Every bale/bag within a shipment should be uniquely identified so that it can be traced back to the individual flock(s) of origin.

Establishing a bale/bag identification system before an outbreak is recommended because it is possible that FMD-infected sheep could be shorn and their wool stored before the sheep are diagnosed. Once the bale/bag is uniquely identified, the wool should remain in the original bale/bag, without additional sorting and re-baling. For additional details, see the Secure Sheep and Wool Supply Plan: Wool Handling During a Foot and Mouth Disease (FMD) Outbreak available at: https://securesheepwool.org/Assets/SSWS_WoolHandling-During-FMD-Outbreak.pdf.[8]

ENHANCED BIOSECURITY

Existing biosecurity plans may offer protection against endemic diseases, but stringent biosecurity measures are essential to protect the flock from FMD virus exposure. The SSWS Plan provides enhanced biosecurity recommendations based on the known disease exposure routes for FMD. Operations with susceptible species raised outdoors (on pasture, in dry lots, and on private and public rangelands) may have more difficulty preventing FMD exposure depending on their proximity to infected premises and the presence of wildlife in the area. Veterinarians are a critical resource in educating sheep owners/managers/shepherds and helping them develop written, operation-specific enhanced biosecurity plans against FMD exposure.

The written plan should address all the items listed in the *Self-Assessment Checklist for Enhanced Biosecurity for FMD Prevention for Sheep Feedlots* or *Sheep on Rangeland/Pasture*. These checklists describe the steps needed to decrease the risk of FMD virus exposure from multiple routes (eg, personnel, vehicles, semen, manure, carcasses). The 2 Biosecurity Checklists, the 2 corresponding *Information Manuals for Enhanced Biosecurity for FMD Prevention* (assists in writing a biosecurity plan), and a single enhanced biosecurity plan template are available on the SSWS Web site at: https://securesheepwool.org/producers/biosecurity/. Producers are encouraged to implement as many items as is practical before an FMD outbreak occurs to help protect the flock from virus exposure. Owners/managers/shepherds should be capable of implementing the remaining biosecurity measures in an acceptable manner if an FMD outbreak occurs, as this is a component of the permit guidance.[9]

Producers who graze sheep on public lands face unique challenges and are encouraged to review the *Considerations for Enhanced Biosecurity for Livestock Grazing on Public Land Allotments* document at: https://securesheepwool.org/Assets/SSWS_Enhanced-Biosecurity-Considerations-Public-Lands.pdf.

SURVEILLANCE

Producers who wish to move their sheep or their products into, within, or out of a Control Area will need to demonstrate a lack of evidence of infection with FMD based on surveillance. FMD causes mild, often subclinical disease in sheep and the disease may go undetected for a relatively long time.[10] Sheep are often referred to as the "silent spreaders" because subtle signs of FMD may be easily overlooked or attributed to other diseases. This greatly impedes early identification of disease. It also prevents relying solely on observational surveillance because of the high probability of false negatives. Due to the difficulty in clinical recognition of FMD in sheep, they are thought to have significantly contributed to further spread of the disease to other susceptible flocks and herds during past FMD outbreaks.[3]

The typically subtle or subclinical signs reported for FMD-infected sheep is starkly contrasted to FMD infection in naïve cattle and swine that commonly show obvious clinical signs with vesicles on the mouth and feet resulting in anorexia, severe lameness, and a reluctance to move. The Secure Food Supply Plans for cattle and swine (beef, milk, pork) include guidance for conducting active observational surveillance (AOS) as an initial screening test to demonstrate a lack of evidence of infection.

AOS is a systematic method for routinely monitoring livestock for potential signs of early FMD infection during an outbreak. AOS does not replace diagnostic testing or periodic inspections of animals on farm by Regulatory Officials; it is meant to supplement other surveillance methods. The use of AOS in sheep is not reliable as a primary surveillance technique because FMD-infected sheep do not typically manifest overt clinical signs of FMD. The SSWS Plan document, *Factors to Consider Regarding Surveillance, Biosecurity and Movement Permitting of Sheep in a Foot and Mouth Disease Outbreak,* available at www.securesheepwool.org, describes the challenges across a variety of surveillance options. Highlights are presented in this section.

Veterinarians should educate producers about the signs of FMD infection in their animals because, if identified, they indicate a potentially serious situation. Producers should be educated and reminded about the importance of reporting suspicious clinical signs to their veterinarian or the state and federal animal health officials in a timely manner. As a refresher, some potential signs of FMD in sheep include the following[3,11–13]:

- Lameness, which may have a sudden onset and affect multiple flock members
- Anorexia
- Panting
- Increased perinatal lamb mortality
- Increased frequency of stillbirths and abortions
- Obtundation, particularly among lambs

During physical examination of FMD-infected sheep, the following may be noted[3,11–13]:

- Pyrexia (>40°C)
- Oral vesicles/lesions (**Fig. 1**)
- Interdigital vesicles/lesions
- Coronary band vesicles/lesions
- Teat lesions

Veterinarians involved with sheep and other livestock susceptible to FMD are encouraged to maintain their status as a USDA Category II Accredited Veterinarian, as they may be a necessary component of disease monitoring and sample collection or overseeing the collection of diagnostic samples during an outbreak. Collecting samples from animals with clinical signs is done by Foreign Animal Disease Diagnosticians who are state or USDA-employed veterinarians who have had additional training in disease recognition, sample collection, and biosecurity to contain disease.

DIAGNOSTIC TESTS FOR FOOT AND MOUTH DISEASE INFECTION IN SHEEP

The United States has excellent validated diagnostic techniques to identify FMD virus infection in animals with clinical signs. Diagnostic tests used to identify FMD include virus isolation (VI), virus neutralization (VN), FMD viral infection-associated antigen, enzyme-linked immunosorbent assay, electron microscopy, and complement fixation. Additionally, polymerase chain reaction (PCR) tests are frequently used to diagnose FMD.[14] The National Animal Health Laboratory Network (NAHLN) laboratories are approved by APHIS to test sheep for FMD virus using the National Veterinary Services Laboratories (NVSL)-NAHLN PCR protocol.[13] In contrast to available FMD diagnostic tests for animals, as of September 2020, there are no approved tests for detection of FMD virus in wool.[13]

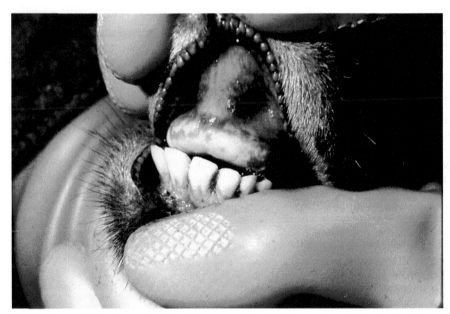

Fig. 1. Ulceration in the oral cavity of a sheep with FMD. (*Courtesy of* Charles Louis Davis and Samuel Wesley Thompson DVM Foundation, Gurnee, IL. Available at: https://noahsarkive.cldavis.org/cgi-bin/show_image_info_detail.cgi?image=F16056 Accessed on September 29, 2020.)

For business continuity in the SSWS Plan, a lack of evidence of infection needs to be demonstrated in animals with no identified clinical signs consistent with FMD infection. Oral swab samples, compared with plasma samples, have been reported to be superior for detecting FMD virus infection in sheep.[15] (Note: Plasma is not an approved sample type for sheep in the United States as of September 2020.) There is no practical sampling protocol for laboratory testing available as of September 2020 for a flock of adult sheep that provides a high degree of confidence that a flock is not infected with FMD. Additional research on sampling and diagnostic testing protocols that do not rely on individual animal sampling (such as pooled oral fluid sampling) is needed for managing an FMD outbreak and for eventual eradication.[16] A large percentage of the flock would need to be tested to provide confidence that the flock is truly negative, because, in some cases, only a minority of the sheep in a flock may be infected.

If the flock could potentially be exposed to FMD virus, then testing within 2 or 3 days of movement would be necessary to establish with a high degree of confidence that the flock was FMD-free. Perhaps testing for FMD antibodies after 3 weeks of isolation and enhanced biosecurity for a closed flock would provide Regulatory Officials with confidence that the flock is truly negative. However, as of September 2020, the NAHLN laboratories are not approved to test for antibody to FMD virus. Diagnostic tests to be performed and sampling protocols may evolve throughout an FMD outbreak based on new knowledge and technology.

WOOL AND FOOT AND MOUTH DISEASE VIRUS

Wool handlers and processors rely on sheep producers for their product, making them integral to business continuity. In the event of an FMD outbreak, it is possible that infected sheep could be shorn and their wool stored before the sheep are diagnosed.[17] Reported survival times of FMD virus (FMDV) on wool is approximately 2 months at 4°C (39.2°F) (with significantly decreased survival at 18°C [64°F]).[2] FMDV can be inactivated in acid conditions (below 6.0 pH) or alkaline conditions (above 9.0 pH).[2]

Wool from an infected flock, and perhaps all wool from a Control Area, will be considered by Regulatory Officials to be contaminated with FMDV. It must be assumed that, in some cases, wool from infected yet undetected flocks will enter the supply chain.

MOVEMENT AND DECONTAMINATION OF WOOL DURING A FOOT AND MOUTH DISEASE OUTBREAK

It is critical that any wool harvested during, or just before, a US FMD outbreak is handled in a biosecure manner that does not contribute to disease spread. FMDV can be carried on clothing, footwear, equipment, and personal items, making it imperative that wool handlers, shearers, processors, and others who have contact with raw wool follow proper biosecurity protocols to avoid transmitting the FMDV to susceptible animals. Wool and wool-handling equipment can also serve as a fomite to spread FMDV unless proper procedures are followed.

The OIE describes procedures to inactivate FMDV in wool and hair. Details are described in the OIE Terrestrial Animal Health Code, Foot and Mouth Disease, Article 8.8.32: *Procedures for the inactivation of FMDV in wool and hair* available at: https://www.oie.int/index.php?id=169&L=0&htmfile=chapitre_fmd.htm. Wool to be transported to a decontamination site must be sealed in an airtight container with biosecurity steps taken to prevent spread of infection by the truck or driver. Wool that cannot be treated to standards established by the OIE should be disposed of on the premises. Wool disposal options will be guided by regulatory officials managing the outbreak. Some examples are described in the guidance document: Secure Sheep and Wool Supply Plan: Wool Handling During a Foot and Mouth Disease Outbreak available at: https://securesheepwool.org/Assets/SSWS_Wool-Handling-During-FMD-Outbreak.pdf.

PREPARING WOOL FOR STORAGE TO INACTIVATE FOOT AND MOUTH DISEASE VIRUS

Proper handling of wool is necessary to ensure the FMDV is eliminated and the wool does not become recontaminated during handling. The equipment used to harvest and bale wool also must be treated as potentially contaminated. Cleaning and disinfecting equipment are important to minimize contamination, especially if the equipment is to be used on other premises. USDA guidance on disinfectants labeled for FMDV is available at: https://www.aphis.usda.gov/animal_health/emergency_management/downloads/fmdvirus-disinfectants.pdf.

SUMMARY

Veterinarians have a tremendous opportunity to positively impact producers by helping them prepare for an FMD outbreak and maintain some semblance of COB during an outbreak. Staying abreast of the latest information about FMD can begin by reviewing the resources listed in this article and visiting www.fmdinfo.org. This reliable resource was created and is maintained by the FMD Cross-Species Team representing US sheep, pork, beef, and dairy industries. Maintaining awareness about FMD preparedness and response efforts can be done by visiting the USDA Emergency Management FMD Web site at: https://www.aphis.usda.gov/aphis/ourfocus/animalhealth/emergency-management/em-fmd/ct_fmd.

Sheep operations will be subject to movement controls during an FMD outbreak and should be prepared to manage animal and product movement disruptions. The voluntary SSWS Plan for COB was developed to help producers, and their veterinarians, prepare for and respond to an FMD outbreak. The SSWS Plan is science-based and risk-based, funded by the ASI Association, and developed collaboratively with industry, government officials, and veterinarians at Iowa State University. The SSWS Plan provides producers and veterinarians with the tools they need to contingency plan, and write enhanced, operation-specific biosecurity plans, as well as to learn about surveillance opportunities and challenges. For more information, visit www.securesheepwool.org.

ACKNOWLEDGMENTS

The authors express sincere gratitude to Dr. Jim Roth at the Center for Food Security and Public Health (CFSPH) for providing expertise and intellectual input; the American Sheep Industry Association for providing funding for the creation of the Secure Sheep and Wool Supply Plan and associated documents; the advisory group for reviewing, editing, and improving the guidance documents; and the graphic designers and instructional technologist at the CFSPH for creating aesthetically pleasing resources and a user-friendly Web site.

DISCLOSURE

D.A. Bickett-Weddle: The author works for the Center for Food Security and Public Health (CFSPH) at Iowa State University, which received funding from the American Sheep Industry (ASI) Association to develop the Secure Sheep and Wool Supply (SSWS) Plan for Continuity of Business (COB), supporting documents, and Web site. The CFSPH also received funding from USDA APHIS for the maintenance of the Secure Beef and Milk Supply Plans, supporting documents, and Web site. R.D. Dewell: The author works for the CFSPH at Iowa State University, which received funding from the ASI Association to develop the SSWS Plan for COB, supporting documents, and Web site. The CFSPH also received funding from USDA APHIS for the maintenance of the Secure Beef and Milk Supply Plans, supporting documents, and Website. C.E. McIntosh: The author works for the CFSPH at Iowa State University, which received funding from the ASI Association to develop the SSWS Plan for COB, supporting documents, and Web site. The CFSPH also received funding from USDA APHIS for the maintenance of the Secure Beef and Milk Supply Plans, supporting documents, and Web site.

REFERENCES

1. Leon EA. Foot-and-mouth disease in pigs: current epidemiological situation and control methods. Transbound Emerg Dis 2012;59:1–14.
2. Spickler AR. Foot and mouth disease. 2015. Available at: http://www.cfsph.iastate.edu/DiseaseInfo/factsheets.php. Accessed September 18, 2020.
3. Kitching R, Hughes G. Clinical variation in foot and mouth disease: sheep and goats. Rev Sci Tech 2002;21:505–12.
4. Hughes G, Mioulet V, Kitching R, et al. Foot-and-mouth disease virus infection of sheep: implications for diagnosis and control. Vet Rec 2002;150:724–7.

5. Barnett P, Cox S. The role of small ruminants in the epidemiology and transmission of foot-and-mouth disease. Vet J 1999;1999:6–13.
6. USDA APHIS. FAD PReP, FMD response plan. 2014. Available at: https://www.aphis.usda.gov/animal_health/emergency_management/downloads/fmd_responseplan.pdf. Accessed September 18, 2020.
7. Secure sheep and wool supply plan for continuity of business. 2020. Available at: https://securesheepwool.org/Assets/Secure-Sheep-and-Wool-Supply-Plan-for-Continuity-of-Business.pdf. Accessed September 18, 2020.
8. Wool handling during a foot and mouth (FMD) disease outbreak. In: Secure Sheep and Wool Supply Plan. 2019. Available at: https://securesheepwool.org/Assets/SSWS_Wool-Handling-During-FMD-Outbreak.pdf. Accessed September 18, 2020.
9. Information manual for enhanced biosecurity for FMD prevention: sheep on pasture/rangeland. 2020. In: Secure Sheep and Wool Supply. Available at: https://securesheepwool.org/Assets/SSWS_Info-Manual-Enhanced-Biosecurity-FMD-Pasture-Rangeland.pdf. Accessed September 18, 2020.
10. Goris NE, Eblé PL, de Jong MCM, et al. Quantification of foot-and-mouth disease virus transmission rates using published data. ALTEX 2008;26:52–4.
11. Muthukrishnan M, Balasubramanian NS, Alwar SV. Experimental infection of foot and mouth disease in indian sheep and goats. Front Vet Sci 2020;7:356. Available at: https://www.frontiersin.org/articles/10.3389/fvets.2020.00356/full. Accessed September 24, 2020.
12. Rout M, Subramaniam S, Sanyal A, et al. Foot and mouth disease in sheep, goats, semi-domesticated and wild animals. Indian Farming 2012;61:24–9.
13. Factors to consider regarding surveillance, biosecurity and movement permitting of sheep in a foot and mouth disease outbreak. In: Secure Sheep and Wool Supply Plan. 2019. Available at: https://securesheepwool.org/Assets/SSWS_Factors-to-Consider-Movement-Permit-FMD.pdf. Accessed September 24, 2020.
14. Neumann EJ, Ramirez A, Schwartz KJ. Swine disease manual, 4th edition. 2009. Available at: https://vetmed.iastate.edu/vdpam/about/production-animal-medicine/swine/swine-disease-manual. Accessed September 24, 2020.
15. Eblé P, Orsel K, van Hemert-Kluitenberg F, et al. Transmission characteristics and optimal diagnostic samples to detect an FMDV infection in vaccinated and non-vaccinated sheep. Vet Microbiol 2015;177:69–77.
16. Poonsuk K, Giménez-Lirola L, Zimmerman JJ. A review of foot-and-mouth disease virus (FMDV) testing in livestock with an emphasis on the use of alternative diagnostic specimens. Anim Health Res Rev 2018;19:110–2.
17. McColl K, Westbury H, Kitching RP, et al. The persistence of foot-and-mouth disease virus on wool. Aust Vet J 1995;72:286–92.

Reindeer Veterinary Care for Small Ruminant Practitioners

N. Isaac Bott, DVM

KEYWORDS

• Antlers • Artificial insemination • Caribou • Cervid *Rangifer* • Theriogenology

KEY POINTS

- Nutritional needs of reindeer greatly differ between summer and winter—as intermediate feeders, they alternate between consuming lush nutritive vegetation and carbohydrate-rich lichens, respectively.
- Pharmacologic considerations and anatomic features of reindeer largely resemble those applied to sheep and goats.
- Reindeer bulls during the breeding season are exceptionally sensitive to anesthetics, and practitioners should avoid procedures whenever possible until the rut has ended.
- Antler development and growth occur independently from gonadal activity in reindeer.
- Reindeer steers continue to grow normal-sized antlers but frequently encounter abnormalities, such as antleromas, incomplete velvet removal, and failure to shed or cast.
- The average standing estrus time reported in reindeer ranges between 1 hour and 3 hours, one of the shortest durations described in ruminant species.
- The unique and variable gestational lengths in *Rangifer* species are theorized as synchronized adaptations for optimal predation safety and plant phenology.
- Transrectal ultrasonography is a modality frequently utilized for fetal viability but limited until 20 weeks of gestation.
- Reindeer cannot be housed adjacent to goats and sheep due to contracting potentially fatal diseases, such as malignant catarrhal fever.

 Video content accompanies this article at http://www.vetfood.theclinics.com.

INTRODUCTION

Reindeer (*Rangifer tarandus tarandus*) and caribou (*Rangifer tarandus granti*) are members of the same species, which is further subdivided into 2 main groups, with 7 extant subspecies, all with a circumboreal and circumarctic distribution.[1,2] Although caribou

Mountain West Animal Hospital Inc, 410 South 450 West, Springville, UT 84663, USA
E-mail address: isaac@docbott.com

Vet Clin Food Anim 37 (2021) 221–236
https://doi.org/10.1016/j.cvfa.2020.10.008
0749-0720/21/© 2020 Elsevier Inc. All rights reserved.

appeared in North America by crossing the Bering land bridge centuries ago, reindeer first arrived in Alaska in 1892. They were imported by boat from Siberia to establish them as a foundation for red meat production.[3]

Reindeer have been domesticated for centuries. They provide an economic mainstay for many native populations. In northern latitudes, they are kept primarily for meat production. Studies have shown that meat from reindeer is more tender compared with beef aged for the same period.[4,5] In the lower 48 states, they are used primarily for seasonal exhibition and for zoologic displays. An organization of reindeer owners, called the Reindeer Owners and Breeders Association, is an active group of reindeer farmers in North America who meet regularly and share information regarding reindeer ownership, government regulations, and overall reindeer health.

Because reindeer are managed extensively, environmental factors have a significant impact on fecundity. Current evidence suggests that management of these factors—of which reproduction, nutrition, herd health, and herd composition seem to be the most important—will enable the productivity of reindeer herds to be markedly improved. A recent move toward a more intense production of reindeer, using traditional agricultural methods, requires intensified management and a thorough understanding of reindeer management.

A review of both female and male reproductive management is presented as a guide for practicing veterinarians to understand and apply in clinical practice the peculiarities of this species. This article also discusses restraint, examination, anesthesia, and common problems that a small ruminant practitioner likely encounters when treating this species.

RESTRAINT

Most reindeer in the lower 48 states are accustomed to handling and are comfortable with a halter and lead rope. Restraint devices are a simple crush design and are lined with soft material (ie, foam, carpet, or vinyl) to provide comfort and minimize trauma to antlers in velvet[6] (**Fig. 1**). These devices typically do not have a head catch. Physical restraint of the head is attained by cautious grasping of the antlers or halter (**Fig. 2**). With this type of restraint, venipuncture can be accomplished from the jugular, cephalic, or lateral saphenous veins with relative ease. Hoof trims, vaccinations, and physical examinations can be performed easily while an animal is in the crush. A systematic approach to the physical examination always should be followed (**Box 1**).

NUTRITION

Pluralities of deer species are classified as browsers, meaning that they are highly selective of food and travel tremendous distances in search of a specific diet. Only approximately a quarter of all deer species are true grazers.[7] Reindeer are unique in that they do not fall into either category but are classified as intermediate feeders, meaning they switch naturally between browsing and grazing, which usually depends on the seasonal availability of their preferred food.[8] For example, during summer, their diet consists of green vegetation with high nutritive value. Alternatively, in the winter, their diet is dominated by lichens. Lichens are rich in digestible carbohydrates but low in protein and essential minerals. Timothy grass (*Phleum pratense*) is used commonly to make hay and silage. Slender wheat grass (*Elymus trachycaulus*) is highly palatable and also often is used for supplemental feeding of reindeer in North America.[9] The digestive system of reindeer is poor at accommodating large quantities of fibrous forage. Pelleted or mixed dry feeds are fed primarily as part of a total mixed ration.

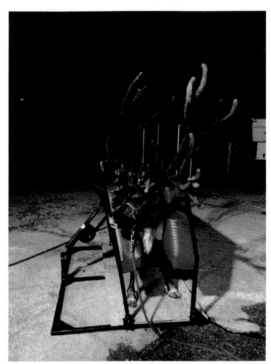

Fig. 1. An example of a functional reindeer squeeze or crush properly restraining an adult male reindeer.

Cereal grains, primarily barley and oats, are the main ingredient in most reindeer mixed feeds. Occasionally corn is used in some rations.[10] These rations vary greatly regarding crude protein and carbohydrate fractions as well as mineral content. A pelleted ration developed in Oregon is included for reference (**Fig. 3**).

ANESTHESIA

Often anesthesia is required in the field where animals cannot be intubated and maintained on an inhalant anesthetic. Wherever possible, the animals should be placed in sternal recumbency, the head elevated, and the oral cavity pointing toward the ground to minimize complications that also occur in other ruminant species.

Pharmacologic agents and doses used in reindeer are similar to those in other small ruminant species. Specific drug doses for reindeer and caribou have been published.[11] Commonly used α_2-adrenoceptor agents include xylazine and dexmedetomidine. Reversal agents, such as atipamezole, commonly are used.

Cyclohexamines, such as ketamine and tiletamine, also are used in conjunction with α_2-adrenoceptor agents. Ketamine is preferred by practitioners, because tiletamine is associated with extended recovery times due to its longer elimination half-life. A preparation of butorphanol-azaperone-medetomidine is available commercially in the United States through ZooPharm (ZooPharm, https://www.zoopharm.com, Laramie, WY) and commonly is used with reindeer.[11]

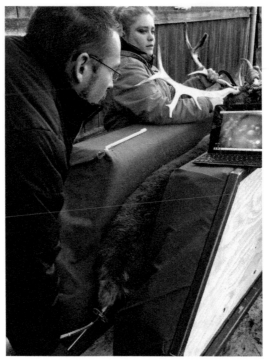

Fig. 2. Proper antler and body restraint demonstrated.

Rutting male reindeer and caribou have an unacceptably high mortality rate under anesthesia. Avoiding anesthesia wherever possible in male reindeer is the best practice during the breeding season.[2]

ANTLERS

Antlers are the fastest growing tissue and the only example of the regeneration of an entire organ in mammalian species.[12] Reindeer and caribou are unique among cervids because both sexes bear antlers. This suggests that antler development is largely

---

Box 1
Systematic approach to the physical examination in reindeer

- Examine antlers.
  - As a safety precaution, first take note of the size and position of antlers, including all points and tips.
  - Growing antlers are palpably warmer than mature antlers.
  - Inspect antler base and skin around pedicles.
- Examine eyes, ears, nose, mouth, and teeth.
- Auscult heart, lungs, and abdomen.
- Examine tail, rectum, vulva, or scrotum and take rectal temperature.
- Visually inspect legs and hooves.

RIV	Name	(PR) Product
		PU51, SANTA REINDEER PLT
	Ext.Reference	5097714
	GR BARLEY	14.171
	GR CORN FINE	4.500
	GR GRAIN SCRNINGS.	13.000
	SUNCRD ALFALFA ML	10.000
	WHEAT MIDDLINGS	50.000
	DEHULLED SOYMEAL........	1.179
	SUPER-BIND BG	0.500
	CAL CARB FINE325BK	1.700
	MONO-DICALPHOS VIB	0.200
	FAT,YELO GR MIXER	0.600
	MOLASSES AT COND	4.000
	SELENIUM PX{.06%}	0.050
	TM PMX	0.050
	VIT PMX	0.050
		100.000
	DRY MATTER	87.492 %
	PROTEIN	14.000 %
	FAT EE	2.656 %
	FIBER MAX	9.816 %
	ADF	12.679 %
	CALCIUM	1.038 %
	PHOSPHORUS	0.768 %
	MAGNESIUM	0.306 %
	POTASSIUM	1.147 %
	COBALT TT	0.750 PPM
	COPPER TT	24.014 PPM
	IODINE TT	0.860 PPM
	MN TT	121.487 PPM
	SE AD	0.301 PPM
	ZINC TT	124.118 PPM
	VIT A AD	7.500 KIU/LB
	VIT D3 AD	2.500 KIU/LB
	VIT E AD	20.000 IU/LB

Fig. 3. A list of ingredients in a reindeer pellet commonly used in Oregon, Utah, and Washington State. Product values (PR) are given as percentage.

independent of gonadal activity.[13] The presence of antlers is used as a taxonomic feature for the genus *Rangifer*.[2]

Antlers are a good indicator of overall health of the animal. Heavy parasite loads have been shown to cause antler asymmetry. Chronic lameness and limb amputation also have been shown to affect the antler contralateral to the affected limb, resulting in asymmetric growth.[12]

Female antler growth is driven largely by estrogen.[14] Female antler cycles have been experimentally controlled by estradiol implantation. Removal of estradiol implants after 4 months cause antler shedding.[15] Cows shed their antlers between the months of February and April.[15]

In bulls, the sequential activation of the reproductive system, and antler growth, starts with an almost simultaneous elevation of luteinizing hormone and with follicle-stimulating hormone in April.[16] Male antler growth occurs at the rapid rate of 3 cm to 5 cm of new growth per day. Antlers begin to develop in late winter and continue growing through the end of July. A spike in testosterone initiates velvet rubbing and shedding.[2,12,16] Male reindeer cast their antlers typically during the first week of December.[17]

Antler development and casting in castrates has some interesting characteristics not found in other species. Unlike many other deer species, reindeer steers continue to grow massive antlers after castration (**Fig. 4**). Steers occasionally experience incomplete velvet removal and delayed antler shedding. Subcutaneous implants containing estradiol benzoate (10 mg) and progesterone (100 mg) (Synovex-C, Zoetis, Parsippany, NJ) commonly are placed at the base of the ear of castrates during October. Two pellets are inserted in each animal.[2] After administration, steers then rub velvet and cast their antlers similarly to intact male reindeer. Subsequent antler cycles then continue without interruption.[2]

Veterinarians frequently are sought to treat antler injuries. Reindeer steers sporadically develop large, multinodular, hyperplastic fibropapillomatous growths that resemble perruques in other castrated deer species (**Fig. 5**). The etiology of these lesions is unclear, but they may be associated with papilloma virus infection.[18] Such lesions are treated with surgical excision and usually are curative.[17] These velvet accumulations often occur in the lower portion of the antler, near the shovel and proximal portions of brow tines. Adequate cauterization and hemostasis are required because of the highly vascular nature of this tissue.

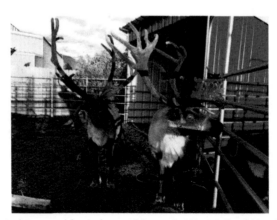

Fig. 4. Two castrated 8-year-old reindeer at Mountain West Animal Hospital.

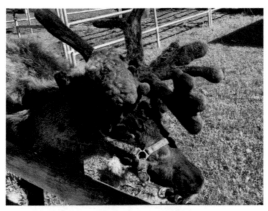

Fig. 5. An antleroma in a 9-year-old castrated male reindeer.

MALE REPRODUCTIVE MANAGEMENT

Male reindeer have the largest antler to body size ratio among deer species.[19] As with other cervids, the male's body, antler size, and fighting ability determine access to receptive female reindeer.[20,21] The first sign of the pending rut is the cleaning of velvet from the antlers. Antler cleaning is triggered by rising levels of testosterone in late August. Complete removal of velvet occurs rapidly, often within a 12-hour period. Intense aggressive displays follow with territorial marking and sparring like other deer species. Rut behavior also includes a self-marking display of hunching and urinating on the hind limbs, termed trampling-urination (Video 1).[2] This is accompanied by distinctive vocalizations referred to as grunting or barking. Bulls are territorial and exhibit a scraping behavior that involves aggressively rubbing the nose on the ground, leaving scent from the nasal, preorbital, and forehead glands (Video 2). The rut generally lasts through late November (**Fig. 6**).

Voluntary food intake dramatically decreases at the onset of the rut. Male reindeer often display anorexia at the height of rut. Studies suggest that it is common for male reindeer to lose up to 23% of lean mass.[22] This body mass reduction occurred in all male reindeer over 2 years of age, regardless of social hierarchy.[2] Cautionary management is required for all male reindeer during the rut. Even the most docile bulls become extremely aggressive and cannot be trusted until the rut has ended (**Fig. 7**).

Many reindeer farmers elect to remove hard antlers after velvet is shed and sensation is lost. A reciprocating saw blade is used to remove antlers approximately 2 cm to 3 cm above the antler pedicle (Video 3). Although this lessens the ability of male reindeer to use antlers as a weapon, they often still resort to pawing and using their broad hooves in a threatening manner. Extreme caution always must be used by the veterinarian when working on intact bulls in rut.

Anesthetic unpredictability is reported in nearly all species of rutting males, but reindeer are particularly susceptible to the effects of cylohexamines (ketamine) and α_2-agonists (xylazine).[11] Deaths have been reported from a single 15-mg dose of xylazine.[2] Due to this high mortality, general anesthesia should be avoided in male reindeer during the breeding season.[2,11]

Historically, medroxyprogesterone acetate (Depo-Provera, Pharmacia and Upjohn Company, Kalamazoo, MI) has been used to calm male reindeer and reduce aggression during rut. Although it is not approved for use in reindeer, it often is administered

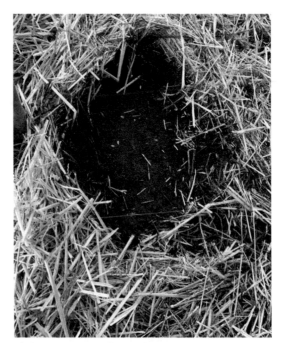

Fig. 6. A scrape made by a rutting male reindeer.

in a set of 2 injections (200–400 mg, intramuscularly [IM]) administered in August and October.[2] No specific studies have evaluated the long-term impact of this drug on spermatogenesis, fertility, semen quality, or subsequent breeding ability.

FEMALE REPRODUCTION MANAGEMENT

Reindeer are highly seasonal breeders. The breeding season coincides with the decreasing photoperiod in the fall. They are seasonally polyestrus, with an estrous cycle length of approximately 24 days ±3.4 days in North American reindeer.[23]

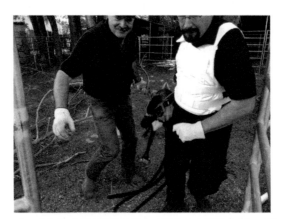

Fig. 7. A bulletproof vest is worn by the author when working with rutting male reindeer.

Considerable variation has been reported in primiparous Norwegian reindeer, with an average estrous cycle length of 19.4 days ±5.7 days.[24] Seasonal ovarian activity is initiated in late August. As in other ruminant species, a small transient rise in plasma progesterone, lasting 4 days to 9 days, precedes the first fertile estrous cycle. The detailed endocrine profiles of the estrous cycle in reindeer generally are in accordance with those found in sheep. Current research suggests that some female reindeer may experience 2 or more short cycles prior to the onset of full-length cycles.[2,15]

A peculiarity in reindeer is the relatively short length of standing estrus compared with that of other ruminants. Studies conducted at the University of Alaska revealed an average standing estrus time of 1 hour (range 1 hour to 3 hours).[23,24] Female reindeer continue to cycle well into spring (as late as April), having 6 cycles to 8 cycles through the winter. The transition into anestrus has been reported to occur with abrupt cessation of luteal activity or the formation of a persistent corpus luteum, which can persist into the next breeding season.[2]

As reported in other small ruminant species, the introduction of a bull prior to the initiation of estrous cycles significantly hastens the onset of ovarian activity by 2 weeks. This subsequently results in synchronicity of calving the following spring.[23]

Estrus synchronization, superovulation, and artificial insemination (AI) in reindeer requires special attention. Growing interest in the truncation of the breeding season and AI have largely focused on synchronizing estrus.[25] Among captive reindeer in Alaska, 2 injections of prostaglandin $F_{2\alpha}$ (15 mg, IM) (Lutalyse, Pharmacia and Upjohn Company, Kalamazoo, MI) administered 10 days apart resulted in luteolysis, and a single 15-mg injection at 6 weeks after conception terminated pregnancies.[2] Cloprostenol (0.25 mg, IM) also has been shown to induce luteolysis in reindeer calves and abortion in adult female reindeer.[26,27]

Attempts at AI in reindeer have been met with mixed results.[28,29] Most published reports provide little to no information on either the methods employed or the results obtained. As with AI in other species, it is a labor-intensive process. It requires the ability to collect and store semen as well as the ability to synchronize or recognize estrus in the female reindeer for appropriately timed insemination.[30] Frozen semen AI successes have been reported in only a handful of cases.[31,32] The use of an ovine controlled internal drug release (CIDR) device has been described in both 7-day and 14-day protocols, with timed AI occurring 44 hours to 60 hours after CIDR removal.[32,33] In 1 study, an injection of cloprostenol (250 μg, IM) administered at CIDR removal and a gonadotropin-releasing hormone injection (100 μg, IM) administered at the time of AI (44 hours post-CIDR removal) resulted in a 66% pregnancy rate.[32]

A challenge frequently encountered in reindeer transcervical AI is within the reindeer cervix. It anatomically resembles that of the ewe, thus hindering the ability to readily pass the inseminating tube successfully into the uterus.[28] Superovulation has been attempted with follicle-stimulating hormone and resulted in a poor embryo recovery rate of 20%.[34]

PREGNANCY DETECTION

Studies have been published on both Norwegian and Alaskan reindeer detailing the endocrinology of pregnancy. Progesterone concentrations show significant variability during pregnancy (range 2.4–14.28 ng/mL), both within and between individual animals. Progesterone levels reliably increase immediately after conception to mean levels of 5.89 ng/mL ± 0.09 ng/mL, where it remains until parturition.[2,23,35,36] This remains consistent with other species that are dependent on luteal progesterone production throughout pregnancy. Studies show that the reindeer placenta does produce some progesterone; however, this contribution is not clearly evident in the progesterone profile.[37] As with other species, cyclic progesterone levels in nonpregnant female reindeer can overlap those found in pregnant female reindeer and thus make peripheral progesterone an unreliable method of pregnancy detection.[2]

Pregnancy-Specific Protein B

Pregnancy-specific protein B (PSPB) has been used to detect pregnancy successfully in populations of wild and domestic caribou and reindeer. PSPB appears in maternal plasma at 4.4 weeks (range 4 weeks to 5 weeks) after mating.[38,39] Blood samples should be collected 6 weeks after breeding. Due to exhibition demand during the holidays, reindeer owners in the United States typically postpone PSPB testing until late December.

Transrectal Ultrasonography

Given that reindeer are habituated to handling and restraint, transrectal ultrasonography has become a useful modality for pregnancy detection. Advantages of ultrasonography are the application in the field and its ability to produce immediate results. It also allows for fetal measurements and assessment.[40]

It is used routinely between 35 days and 60 days of gestation, although earlier detection is achievable.[41] Once week 20 of gestation is reached, it becomes increasingly difficult to detect the fetus because the gravid uterus is displaced ventrally and becomes unreachable for the ultrasound transducer (Video 4).

Antler Retention

Retention of antlers in pregnant reindeer cows long has been a technique of wildlife biologists to assess pregnancy status in wild caribou.[42] In reindeer, it is not always a reliable predictor of pregnancy. Antler retention into mid-April can be used to infer pregnancy, although the contrary is not true. A portion of pregnant female reindeer often cast their antlers prior to calving.[2,43,44]

Gestation Length and Parturition

Reindeer have short and highly synchronized mating and calving seasons. Reported gestation length is highly variable. Published gestations range from 198 days to 240 days.[2,45] It also has been hypothesized that part of this variability is due to the limited reliability of breeding observations and, therefore, inaccurate estimates of conception date. Nevertheless, an estimated 90% of female reindeer are bred in a 10-day to 21-day interval and calve in an equally synchronized manner.[46] Several studies have documented a negative correlation between gestation length and conception date.[47] Although the underlying mechanisms responsible for this gestational plasticity and enhanced calving synchrony are not understood fully, it is assumed that the primary advantage of synchronized parturition is that fewer neonates are lost to predation.[48] Another hypothesis is that synchronicity of parturition is correlated with optimal plant phenology.[45]

Twinning is unusual in domestic reindeer and caribou, with a plurality of twins not surviving birth.[49,50] Dystocias are uncommon in reindeer but do occasionally occur. As with other cervids and small ruminants, manual correction of the malpresentation can be accomplished easily by a skilled veterinarian (Video 5). Malpresentations in reindeer are the same as those described in sheep and goats. Successful caesarian sections have been performed in a field setting using a lumbar approach like that commonly used in sheep and goats. Muscular layers of the reindeer abdomen are much thinner than other cervids, and closure is difficult without a surgical assistant aiding in apposition of the lateral abdomen.

REINDEER HEALTH
Respiratory Disease

Sick reindeer often separate themselves from the herd. Posturing with a hanging head and extended neck often indicates illness. Feed intake decreases and often the hair coat has a dull and unkempt appearance.[51]

Reindeer can adapt well to extreme climate variations. In summer, the normal respiratory rate of a reindeer at rest is 20 breaths per minute to 50 breaths per minute. During extremely cold winter months, this resting respiratory rate decreases to 8 breaths per minute to 16 breaths per minute. Stress, such as capture or restraint, may increase the respiratory rate to 100 breaths per minute to 180 breaths per minute.[52,53] As with other cervids and small ruminants, coughing occurs in the context of a variety of respiratory diseases and is reported to be observed best in the morning.[54]

Parainfluenza virus type 3 (PIV3) is a viral disease that infects cattle and is known to infect reindeer also. A study of semidomesticated reindeer in Sweden revealed that PIV3 antibodies were present in 54% of animals.[55] Other pathogens, such as *Pasteurella*, can combine and induce a syndrome referred to as bovine respiratory disease complex in cattle.[54] Often, an intranasal infectious bovine rhinotracheitis virus–PIV3 cattle vaccine is administered prior to beginning the travel associated with the holiday display season.

Chronic Wasting Disease

The first chronic wasting disease (CWD) case identified in free ranging cervids outside of North America occurred in a wild Eurasian tundra reindeer (*Rangifer tarandus tarandus*) in Norway in 2016. This is the first known natural case documented in reindeer.[56] The first case of CWD in North American reindeer was found in a captive reindeer herd in northern Illinois in 2018. Emerging knowledge that CWD occurs in reindeer will dramatically change the selling and interstate exhibition of reindeer in the intercontinental United States. There currently is no evidence that suggests CWD can cause clinical disease in humans. Further studies are needed with respect to interspecies CWD transmission, including its zoonotic potential.[57,58]

Malignant Catarrhal Fever

Reindeer are susceptible to malignant catarrhal fever (ovine herpesvirus 2) with a clinical presentation, including generalized neurologic signs, oculonasal discharge, and sudden death. It is of paramount importance to not house reindeer near sheep and goats.[59–61]

Parasites

Captive reindeer seem to be particularly predisposed to acquiring parasitic infections. Northern facilities are especially prone to warble fly (*Hypoderma tarandi*) infestations. Ivermectin (Ivomec, Merial, Duluth, GA) is labeled for the treatment and control of warbles *(Oedemagena tarandi)* in reindeer (200 μg/kg, subcutaneously). Myiasis frequently occurs after antler velvet has been damaged. Other external parasites of concern are tick species (*Amblyomma, Dermacentor*, and *Ixodes* spp) and their associated pathogens. *Babesia* and *Anaplasmosis* cause a high rate of morbidity and mortality. Internal parasites of importance are the meningeal worm (*Dictyocaulus viviparus*) and

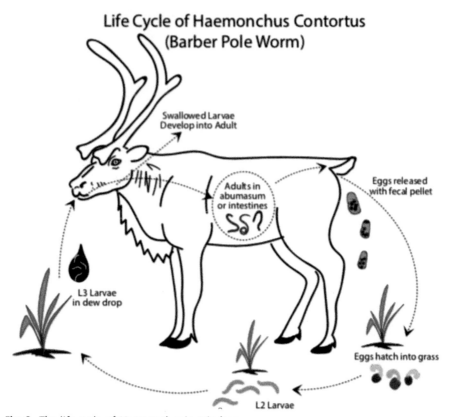

Fig. 8. The life cycle of *Haemonchus* in reindeer.

nematodes of which the barber pole worm (*Nematodirus* sp) seem to be of significant pathogenicity in reindeer (**Fig. 8**).[54]

CLINICS CARE POINTS

- Numerous environmental factors have a significant impact on success of reindeer fecundity and overall reproduction within the continental United States.
- Reindeer bulls in rut are exceptionally aggressive. Even the most docile of bulls cannot be trusted until the rut has ended.
- Reindeer bulls during the breeding season are exceptionally sensitive to anesthetics, and practitioners should postpone, where possible, all procedures until the rut has ended.
- Antler removal after velvet shedding often is performed in rutting bulls as a safety precaution for owners and practitioners.
- Reindeer steers continue to grow normal-sized antlers but frequently encounter abnormalities, such as antleromas, incomplete velvet removal, and failure to shed or cast.
- The average standing estrus time reported in reindeer ranges between 1 hour and 3 hours, one of the shortest durations described in ruminant species.
- A negative correlation exists between gestation length and conception date. The earlier in the breeding season a cow conceives, the longer her gestation length.

- Peripheral progesterone concentration is an unreliable pregnancy detection method in reindeer due to frequent overlap of cyclic progesterone levels also observed in nonpregnant female reindeer. PSPB can be used after week 6 of gestation to confirm pregnancy.
- Transrectal ultrasonography is a modality frequently utilized to confirm pregnancy and assess fetal viability but is limited beyond 20 weeks of gestation.

DISCLOSURE

The author has nothing to disclose.

SUPPLEMENTARY DATA

Supplementary data related to this article can be found online at https://doi.org/10.1016/j.cvfa.2020.10.008.

REFERENCES

1. Leader-Williams N. Reindeer on South Georgia: the ecology of an introduced population. Cambridge (United Kingdom): Cambridge University Press; 1988. p. 319.
2. Blake JE, Rowell JE, Shipka MP. Reindeer reproductive management. In: Youngquist RS, Threlfall WR, editors. Large animal theriogenology. St. Louis (MO): Saunders Elsevier; 2007. p. 970–4.
3. Finstad G. Reindeer in Alaska: Under new management. Agroborealis 2007; 38:22–8.
4. Wiklund E, Farouk M, Finstad G. Venison: meat from red deer (Cervus elaphus) and reindeer (Rangifer tarandus tarandus). Anim Front 2014;4(4):55–61.
5. Rincker PJ, Bechtel PJ, Finstad G, et al. Similarities and differences in composition and selected sensory attributes of reindeer, caribou and beef. J Muscle Foods 2006;17:65–78.
6. Finstad GL, Renecker LA. Design for a portable reindeer crush. Fairbanks (AK): University of Alaska Fairbanks, Agricultural and Forestry Experiment Station, School of Agriculture and Land Resources Management; 2001.
7. Brown RD, Mississippi State University. International symposium on the biology of deer. In: The biology of deer. New York: Springer-Verlag; 1992.
8. Hofmann R. Evolutionary steps of ecophysiological adaptation and diversification of ruminants: a comparative view of their digestive system. Oecologia 1989;78(4): 443–57.
9. Finstad GL, Kielland K. Landscape Variation in the diet and productivity of reindeer in Alaska based on stable isotope analyses. Arct Antarct Alp Res 2011; 43(4):543–54.
10. Ahman B, Finstad GL, Josefsen TD. Feeding and associated health problems. In: Tryland M, Kutz SJ, editors. Reindeer and caribou health and disease. Boca Raton (FL): Taylor and Francis Group; 2019. p. 135–56.
11. Lian M, Evans AL, Beckam KB, et al. Restraint and immobilization. In: Tryland M, Kutz SJ, editors. Reindeer and caribou health and disease. Boca Raton (FL): Taylor and Francis Group; 2019. p. 465–92.
12. Markusson E, Folstad I. Reindeer antlers: Visual indicators of individual quality? Oecologia 1997;110:510–7.

13. Lincoln GA, Tyler NJC. Antler growth in male and female reindeer calves occurs in the absence of the gonads. In: Brown RD, editor. The biology of deer. New York: Springer; 1992. p. 493–8.

14. Lincoln GA, Tyler NJC. Role of gonadal hormones in the regulation of the seasonal antler cycle in female reindeer, Rangifer tarandus. J Reprod Fertil 1994; 101:129–38.

15. Lincoln GA, Tyler NJC. Role of oestradiol in the regulation of the seasonal antler cycle in female reindeer, Rangifer tarandus. J Reprod Fertil 1999;115:167–74.

16. Bubenik GA, Schams D, White RJ, et al. Seasonal levels of reproductive hormones and their relationship to the antler cycle of male and female reindeer (Rangifer tarandus). Comp Biochem Physiol B 1997;116(2):269–77.

17. Fletcher J, Foster A, Goddard P, et al. Managing antler problems in deer. In Pract 2016;38(10):513–9.

18. Foster AP, Barlow AM, Nasir L, et al. Fibromatous lesions of antler velvet and haired skin in reindeer (Rangifer tarandus). Vet Rec 2013;172(17):452.

19. Holand Ø. Rangifer males' mating strategy. Reprod Domest Anim 2019;54(Suppl S3):57–62.

20. Body G, Weladji RB, Holand Ø, et al. Highly competitive reindeer males control female behavior during the rut. PLoS One 2014;9(4):e95618.

21. Strong JS, Weladji RB, Holand Ø, et al. Personality and fitness consequences of flight initiation distance and mating behavior in subdominant male reindeer (Rangifer tarandus). Ethology 2017;123(6–7):484–92.

22. Tyler NJ, Blix AS. Survival strategies in arctic ungulates. Rangifer 1990;3:211–30.

23. Shipka MP, Rowell JE, Sousa MC. Steroid hormones of the estrous cycle and pregnancy and gestation length in farmed Alaskan reindeer. J Anim Sci 2007; 85:944–51.

24. Ropstad E. Reproduction in female reindeer. Anim Reprod Sci 2000;60:561–70.

25. Hirth AM. Estrous synchronization in reindeer. Master's thesis. Germany: University of Bayreuth; 2004. p. 52.

26. Ropstad E, Lenvik D. The use of Cloprostenol and prostaglandin $F_{2\alpha}$ to induce luteolysis in reindeer calves (Rangifer tarandus). Rangifer 1991;11(1):13–6.

27. Ropstad E, Kindahl H, Nilsen TA, et al. The effect of cloprostenol in non-pregnant and pregnant Norwegian semi-domestic reindeer (Rangifer tarandus tarandus). Anim Reprod Sci 1996;43(4):205–19.

28. Dott HM, Utsi MN. Artificial insemination of reindeer. J Zool 1973;170:505–8.

29. Bott N. Reproductive management of reindeer (Rangifer tarandus). In: Am Assoc of Bovine Practitioners. Louisville (KY): Proceedings of the Annual AABP Conference. 2018. p. 188–91.

30. Mysterud A, Bonenfant C, Loe LE, et al. The timing of male reproductive effort relative to female ovulation in a capital breeder. J Anim Ecol 2008;77:469–77.

31. Shipka MP, Rowell JE, Bychawski S. Artificial insemination in reindeer using frozen-thawed semen. Dairy Sci 2010;93:124.

32. Bott I, Merkley R, Robinson T, et al. Preliminary results of estrus synchronization and timed artificial insemination in domesticated reindeer (Rangifer tarandus). Clin Ther 2011;3:326.

33. Fadden AN, Bott NI, Kutzler MA. Breeding management in a reindeer (Rangifer tarandus) with a history of reproductive failure. Clin Ther 2014;6:359.

34. Lindeberg H, Aalto J, Vahtiala S, et al. Recovery and cryopreservation of in vitro produced reindeer embryos after oestrous synchronization and superovulatory treatment. Rangifer Rep 1999;4:76.

35. Krog J, Wika M, Savalov P. The development of the foetus of the Norwegian reindeer. In: Reimers E, Gaare E, Skjenneberg S, editors. Second International reindeer/caribou symposium. Røros (Norway): Direktoratet for vilt og ferskvannsfisk; 1980. p. 306–10.

36. Ropstad E, Veiberg V, Sakkinen H, et al. Endocrinology of pregnancy and early pregnancy detection by reproductive hormones in reindeer (Rangifer tarandus tarandus). Theriogenology 2005;63:1775–88.

37. Blom AK, Sjaastad V, Jacobsen E. Plasma levels of progesterone and oestradiol-17b in reindeer (Rangifer tarandus tarandus) during pregnancy. Acta Vet Scand 1983;24:287–94.

38. Ropstad E, Forsberg M, Sire JE, et al. Plasma concentrations of progesterone, oestradiol, LH and 15-ketodihydro- PGF2a in Norwegian semi-domestic reindeer (Rangifer tarandus tarandus) during their first reproductive season. J Reprod Fertil 1995;105:307–14.

39. Rowell JE, Russell DE, White RG, et al. Appearance of PSPB following mating and its disappearance after induced abortion in caribou and reindeer. Rangifer Rep 1999;4:77.

40. Vahtiala S, Säkkinen H, Dahl E, et al. Ultrasonography in early pregnancy diagnosis and measurements of fetal size in reindeer (Rangifer tarandus tarandus). Theriogenology 2004;61(4):785–95.

41. Ropstad E, Johansen O, King C, et al. Comparison of plasma progesterone, transrectal ultrasound and pregnancy specific proteins (PSPB) used for pregnancy diagnosis in reindeer. Acta Vet Scand 1999;40(2):151–62.

42. Adams LG. Reproductive performance of female Alaskan caribou. J Wildl Manag 1988;62:1184–95.

43. McEwan EH, Whitehead PE. Reproduction in female reindeer and caribou. Can J Zool 1972;50:43–6.

44. Cronin MA, Hasklell SP, Ballard WB. The frequency of antlerless female reindeer and caribou in Alaska. Rangifer 2003;23(2):67–70.

45. Post E, Boving PS, Pedersen C, et al. Synchrony between caribou calving and plant phenology in depredated and non-depredated populations. Can J Zool 2003;81:1709–14.

46. Shipka MP, Rowell JE. Gestation length in Alaskan reindeer. J Anim Sci 2006; 84:58–9.

47. Bergerud AT. The reproductive season of Newfoundland Caribou. Can J Zool 1975;53:1213–21.

48. Flydal K, Reimers E. Relationship between calving time and physical condition in three wild reindeer (Rangifer tarandus) populations in southern Norway. Wildl Biol 2002;8:145–52.

49. Godkin GF. Fertility and twinning in Canadian reindeer. Rangifer Spec 1986;1: 145–50.

50. Cuyler C, Ostergaard JB. Fertility in two west Greenland caribou Rangifer tarandus grornlandicus populations during 1996/97: Potential for rapid growth. Wildl Biol 2005;11:221–7.

51. Laaksonen S, Nieminen M. Poron terveyden mittarit. [The health indicators of reindeer]. Poromies 2005;2:42–5.

52. Blix AS, Walløe L, Folkow LP. Regulation of brain temperature in winter-acclimatized reindeer under heat stress. J Exp Biol 2011;214(22):3850–6.

53. Nikolaevskii LD. General Outline of the anatomy and physiology of reindeer. In: Zhigunov PS, editor. Reindeer husbandry. Jerusalem: Israel Program for Scientific Translations; 1961. p. 5–56.

54. Laaksonen S. Assessment and treatment of reindeer diseases. In: Tryland M, Kutz SJ, editors. Reindeer and caribou health and disease. Boca Raton (FL): Taylor and Francis Group; 2019. p. 383–444.

55. Zarnke RL. Serologic survey for selected microbial pathogens in Alaskan wildlife. J Wildl Dis 1983;19(4):324–9.

56. Benestad SL, Mitchell G, Simmons M, et al. First case of chronic wasting disease in Europe in a Norwegian free-ranging reindeer. Vet Res 2016;47(1):88.

57. Osterholm MT, Anderson CJ, Zabel MD, et al. Chronic wasting disease in cervids: implications for prion transmission to humans and other animal species. mBio 2019;10(4):e01091-19.

58. Hornlimann B, Riesner D, Kretzschamar H. Prions in humans and animals. New York: De Gruyter Berlin; 2006. p. 683.

59. Vikøren T, Li H, Lillehaug A, et al. Malignant catarrhal fever in free-ranging cervids associated with OvHV-2 and CpHV-2 DNA. J Wildl Dis 2006;42(4):797–807.

60. Das Neves CG, Ihlebæk HM, Skjerve E, et al. Gammaherpesvirus infection in semidomesticated reindeer (Rangifer tarandus tarandus): a cross-sectional, serologic study in northern Norway. J Wildl Dis 2013;49(2):261–9.

61. Bartlett SL, Abou-Madi N, Messick JB, et al. Diagnosis and treatment of Babesia odocoilei in captive reindeer (Rangifer tarandus tarandus) and recognition of three novel host species. J Zoo Wildl Med 2009;40(1):152–9.

Moving?

Make sure your subscription moves with you!

To notify us of your new address, find your **Clinics Account Number** (located on your mailing label above your name), and contact customer service at:

Email: journalscustomerservice-usa@elsevier.com

800-654-2452 (subscribers in the U.S. & Canada)
314-447-8871 (subscribers outside of the U.S. & Canada)

Fax number: 314-447-8029

Elsevier Health Sciences Division
Subscription Customer Service
3251 Riverport Lane
Maryland Heights, MO 63043